BIBLE ANSWERS FOR ALMOST ALL YOUR QUESTIONS

ELMER TOWNS

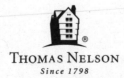

THOMAS NELSON
Since 1798

NASHVILLE   DALLAS   MEXICO CITY   RIO DE JANEIRO

Published in Nashville, Tennessee, by Thomas Nelson. Thomas Nelson is a registered trademark of Thomas Nelson, Inc.

All scripture quotations, unless otherwise indicated, are taken from the New King James Version. © 1982 by Thomas Nelson, Inc. Used by permission. All rights reserved.

Verses marked CEV are taken from the Contemporary English Version. © 1995 American Bible Society. Used by permission.

Verses marked NASB are from the *New American Standard Bible®*, © The Lockman Foundation 1960, 1962, 1963, 1968, 1971, 1972, 1973, 1975, 1977, 1995. Used by permission. (www.Lockman.org)

Verses marked KJV are from the King James Version of the Bible.

Library of Congress Cataloging-in-Publication Data
Towns, Elmer L.
    Bible answers for almost all your questions / Elmer Towns.
        p. cm.
    Includes index.
    ISBN 978-0-7852-6324-1 (pbk.)
        1. Christian life--Biblical teaching. I. Title.
BS680.C47T69 2003
230--dc21   2003000254

Printed in the United States of America
13 14 15 16 17 RRD 38 37 36 35 34 33

TO HAROLD WILLMINGTON
Dean, Liberty Bible Institute

To Harold Willmington, whom I met in October 1958 before either of us wrote a book, or held a Bible conference, or were considered "Bible scholars." Our lives have been pilgrimages of learning the Bible together and teaching others what we have learned.

Because of our journey together in the Bible, and because of Harold's love for the Word of God, I dedicate this book to him with much gratitude and respect.

Sincerely yours in Christ,
Elmer L. Towns

CONTENTS

INTRODUCTION

Have you ever been asked a question, and you didn't know the answer? How did you feel? Did it bug you? Did it discourage you? Did it motivate you to go find an answer? If you can't find answers, this book is for you. I haven't answered every question asked about the Bible, but you'll find a lot of them here.

Maybe you weren't asked a question, but something caught your eye when reading the Bible, or you heard something in a sermon that puzzled you. You've got a question. Good chance you'll find an answer in these pages.

I haven't answered every question you have, nor have I answered every question about the Bible that's ever been asked. There are multiple thousands of questions; I could have filled this book with questions just from Genesis or just from the gospel of Matthew. So where did these questions come from?

Because I'm a teacher, I love questions. Answering questions is the mortar that holds the bricks of knowledge together. Without questions, a teacher couldn't build the lives that his or her students live. Without questions, teachers couldn't construct the sanctuaries in which our students worship.

I've been teaching college and seminary students for forty-five years and ministering in churches for over fifty years. The questions in this book came from those I've answered or are like the ones I've answered.

There's no question too dumb ("Did Adam have a navel?"), no question too trite ("Where did Cain get his wife?"), no question too controversial ("Should a Christian have a tatoo?"), and no question too political. Notice I answer questions about abortion, homosexuality, social drinking, and body piercing. I've tried to be straightforward in my answers. Sometimes I've given the answers to both sides of the question. When I give two or more answers to a question, sometimes I tell you which answer

I prefer. Sometimes I don't know which answer is correct, so I give equal time to two or more answers.

Most of the answers are the kind I give at the front door of a church after I've preached a sermon. At the front door of a church, people don't want deep theological answers to their questions. What do they want? They want straight, direct answers—without a lot of reasons. However, some of the answers in this book are involved, like those I would give to a puzzled student after a class.

The following principles have helped me answer these questions: (1) when the Bible is clear, I tell you exactly what the Bible says; (2) when the Bible gives only part of an answer, I use terms like "apparently" and "perhaps," suggesting my answers are not dogmatic; (3) when the Bible is silent, I don't make rules and can't be dogmatic; (4) I answer these questions out of a good conscience before God, answering according to my moral sense of right and wrong; (5) a vast number of Christians have already answered many of these questions, so many times I say, "Evangelical scholars teach . . ." or "Most conservative Christians believe . . . "; (6) when it comes to what the vast numbers of Christians believe about a question, I follow the rule of "the priesthood of believers," that is, what the majority of Christians believe is probably true. Each person has direct access to God, but there is probably a consensus of truth when they agree. The old slogan will help us here: *If it's new, it's not true; and if it's true, it's not new.* (7) these answers are my opinions, formed after years of questioning other believers and studying the Bible for myself. No one else is responsible for them, just me. If they help you—fine! If you want to make these answers your answers—fine! However, don't believe them because I say so; believe them when they have been demonstrated to you.

May you enjoy reading these answers as much as I did writing them. May God help you through my answers to find your way to the Word of God. After all, the Bible is the court of last appeal. As Jesus said, "Your word is truth" (John 17:17).

Written from my home at the foot of the Blue Ridge Mountains of Virginia,

—Elmer L. Towns

QUESTIONS
ABOUT
GENERAL MATTERS

Where is the ark of the covenant today?

Ever since the motion picture *Raiders of the Lost Ark*, there has been great speculation that the ark of the covenant still exists. But what does history say?

First, there is a Jewish tradition that Jeremiah took it out of the Holy of Holies—because Jeremiah was from the Levitical priestly line—and had the ark buried in one of the Judean hills, perhaps in a cave in the wilderness.

Second, the Samaritan Plesheba (the Samaritans' sacred book) says that the ark of the covenant was buried on Mount Nebo.

Third, some say the ark was lost or buried in Egypt. We know that Jeremiah traveled to Egypt after Jerusalem was destroyed, and he probably died in Egypt. A strong tradition tells us that he carried the ark of the covenant to Egypt.

Fourth, some believe the ark could be in the "Valley of the Kings." When the Israelites built a temple on the Island of Taphanhes (Jeremiah 2:16; 43:1–7) in the Nile Delta, they reestablished temple sacrifices—and perhaps the ark of the covenant—in that temple. Later, the Egyptians destroyed the temple and took all the treasures that were contained in the temple into their treasury houses. If the ark was in that temple, from there it could have gone on to be buried in one of the burial treasure houses in the "Valley of the Kings," where the tombs are located in the Nile River Valley. This gives some credibility to Indiana Jones's search for the ark of the covenant in that area.

Fifth, there are at least seven known man-made tunnels under the Temple Mount in Jerusalem that would have existed under Solomon's temple in Jerusalem. Some believe that when the Babylonians destroyed Jerusalem and the temple, the ark of the covenant was taken into one of these caverns and sealed behind a rock wall and is still there today. A rumor has it that Rabbi Yehuda Getz, Chief Rabbi of the Western Wall, claimed to have gone into one of the caves and, holding a small mirror in a crack of the wall, saw the ark of the covenant. Thus many believe it still exists under the Temple Mount.

Sixth, some believe that the original ark of the covenant is within a church in Axum, Ethiopia. When the queen of Sheba (Ethiopia) came to visit Solomon (1 Kings 10:1–10), tradition tells us she was shown the ark of the covenant. She withheld sexual favors from Solomon until he gave her the ark of the covenant, then had a replica made and placed in the temple. Some proof of this theory is that the ark is called the ark of the Lord when the original ark was in Solomon's temple. But after Solomon, the ark is always called just "the ark," or the "ark of the covenant." It is not called the "ark of the Lord" after Solomon's time. When the Queen of Sheba returned home, she conceived a child, and the lineage to the throne in Ethiopia always carried the motto, "The root of the tribe of David" and each succeeding king traced his heritage back to Solomon. When Haile Selassi died in 1974, he was the last king in the line of Solomon.

Seventh (this suggestion is offered tongue in cheek because of Indiana Jones), some think the ark of the covenant is located at a warehouse in Washington, D.C.

Eighth, during the Tribulation, heaven is opened and the ark of the covenant is revealed (Rev. 11:19). Some feel this ark in heaven is the same ark that was used by Israel. Others believe the ark in heaven is the pattern from which the first ark was constructed on earth.

Who were the twelve disciples according to the Bible?

The original twelve were chosen in succession at a very early period of the Savior's public life. They were chosen as follows: First came *Andrew* and his brother *Simon (Peter)*; *James* and *John*, the sons of Zebedee (Matt. 4:18–22; 10:2–3; Mark 1:16–20; Luke 6:14; John 1:35–42); then *Philip* and *Nathanael* (also named *Bartholomew*) (John 1:43–51). Subsequently, there came *Matthew*, also known as *Levi* (Matt. 9:9; Mark 2:14; Luke 5:27–28); *Thomas, James* (the son of Alphaeus), *Simon the Canaanite* (also called *Zelotes*), *Lebbaeus (Thaddaeus)* (also called *Judas*, John 14:22), and *Judas Iscariot* (Matt. 10:1–4; Mark 3:19; Luke 6:13–16; Acts 1:13). In Luke 6:13 Jesus called these disciples "apostles."

After Judas's betrayal and death, two men possessing the necessary qualifications of apostleship were put forward. The Bible says the requirement of an apostle was that he had to be an eyewitness of the events of the life of Jesus, he had to see Him after His resurrection, and he had to testify to mankind concerning Him (Matt. 10:2–42; Acts 1:21–22; 1 Cor. 9:1). One nominated to be an apostle was Joseph (called Barsabas and Justus) and the other was Matthias. Lots were cast to choose which one would replace Judas, and the lot fell upon Matthias, who was consequently elected (Acts 1:23–26).

However, the title "apostle" was not limited to the Twelve, for Barnabas (Acts 14:14) and James (the Lord's brother, Gal. 1:19; 1 Cor. 15:7) were also called apostles.

Paul was divinely chosen and called to preach the gospel to the Gentiles (Acts 9:1–31; 22:5–21; 26:1–20). He had not traveled with Jesus on earth, but he possessed the apostolic qualifications of having seen Jesus after His resurrection. On the way to Damascus, Jesus appeared to him and spoke to him, changing his hostility into passionate devotion. Paul was able to say, "Am I not an apostle? am I not free? have I not seen Jesus Christ our Lord?" (1 Cor. 9:1 KJV). Perhaps the early church should not have elected Matthias to replace Judas, but should have waited for the apostle Paul.

How did the apostles die?

The Bible does not tell us a great deal about the individual lives of the apostles. However, we do find an account how the apostle *James* (the son of Zebedee) died. King Herod Agrippa I killed him with a sword (Acts 12:2).

The last Scripture account of *Andrew* is found in Acts 1:13 when he was with ten other disciples in the Upper Room, prior to Pentecost. According to tradition it was in Achaia, Greece, in the town of Patra that Andrew died a martyr. The governor Aepeas's wife was healed and converted to the Christian faith, and shortly after that the governor's brother became a Christian. Aepeas was enraged and arrested Andrew. He condemned him to die on the cross. Andrew, feeling unworthy to be crucified on the same-shaped cross as his Lord, begged that his be different. So he was crucified on a cross shaped like the letter *X,* which is called Saint Andrew's cross.

Tradition also has it that *Peter* was crucified. He requested to be hung upside-down because he felt unworthy to die as his Lord had died. John 21:18, 19 alludes to the fact that Peter would die a martyr's death when our Lord prophesied that one day Peter's freedom would cease.

A fifth-century church historian relates that *Matthew* was martyred in Ethiopia where he had gone as a missionary.

Thomas (Didymus) is last mentioned in the Upper Room with the disciples (Acts 1:13), after which tradition says he labored in Parthia, Persia, and India and suffered martyrdom near Madras, at Mount St. Thomas. He was killed with a spear.

James (the son of Alphaeus), known as *James the Less,* preached in Palestine and Egypt, where early church history says he died as a martyr and his body was sawed in pieces.

Lebbeaus or *Thaddaeus,* also known as *Judas,* is believed to have died for Christ after preaching in Persia and Assyria. He was killed with arrows at Ararat.

Simon the Zealot was a "right-wing" member of a political party called the Zealots. Tradition says he was crucified.

Tradition also tells us that, following the last Passover supper, *Philip* went as a missionary to Phrygia and was martyred and buried at Hierapolis. It is said he died by hanging. While he was hanging, he requested that his body be wrapped not in linen, but in papyrus, for he was not worthy that even his dead body be treated as the body of Jesus was treated.

The last Scriptural account we have of *Nathanael (Bartholomew)* is found in John 21:2 when he was present at the lake breakfast prepared by the Savior on the Galilean shore. Tradition has it that he preached in India and Armenia and was flayed alive with knives.

Judas Iscariot, of course, betrayed Christ and subsequently committed suicide (Matt. 27:3–10).

John was banished to the Isle of Patmos during the reign of Nero (or perhaps Domitian). While at Patmos he received the vision of Revelation. He was later liberated and died a natural death while pastoring at Ephesus.

Are automobiles mentioned in the Bible?

Some Bible students have interpreted as a possible reference to the modern-day automobile: "The chariots rage in the streets, they jostle one another in the broad roads; they seem like torches, they run like lightning" (Nah. 2:4). However, the verse properly indicates the ease and access that invading armies and their armaments had to a city during a predicted siege. The attackers took the city by surprise, and the defenders could not restrain them.

What do *B.C.* and *A.D.* mean?

The proper meaning for the abbreviation *B.C.* is "Before Christ." The abbreviation *A.D.* represents the period of time after the birth of Christ known as the beginning of the Christian Era. *A.D.* is actually an abbreviation for the Latin words *Anno Domini,* which mean "in the year of our Lord."

In A.D. 532 a monk by the name of Dionysius Exiguus introduced the present custom of regarding time by counting the years from the birth of Christ. Thus, the period of time during Christ's earthly ministry would have been known as A.D.

What does the Bible teach about capital punishment?

God originally allowed the use of capital punishment when He instructed the families after the Flood, "Surely for your lifeblood I will demand a reckoning; from the hand of every beast I will require it, and from the hand of man. From the hand of every man's brother I will require the life of man" (Gen. 9:5). Capital punishment was reinforced under the Law: "He who strikes a man so that he dies shall surely be put to death" (Ex. 21:12). "He who kidnaps a man and sells him, or if he is found in his hand, shall surely be put to death" (Ex. 21:16). Numbers 35:16–18 tells us, "the murderer shall surely be put to death" (KJV).

Some people are against capital punishment, quoting the commandment, "Thou shalt not kill." They have taught that this particular command means there should be no capital punishment. This is not what the sixth commandment means. In the Hebrew language it reads, "Thou shalt not murder."

God's Word clearly teaches capital punishment should be the judgment on those who commit deliberate, willful murder. In Romans 13:1–7, God clearly commands us to be subject to the civil and governmental authority. This passage refers to armed officers who bear "the sword" (v. 4). This is a weapon used to put people to death when the need arises. This indicates we should use force to protect ourselves against aggressors, and against murderers who take innocent lives. The death penalty should be applied for crimes such as cold-blooded murder.

Jesus Himself suggests His support of capital punishment (Luke 13:1–5). He used this to indicate that His listeners, though not guilty of criminal offenses against the law, would perish if they did not repent of their sins against God.

Why should a Christian celebrate Christmas, when we don't know the actual date or time Jesus was born?

The answer is not to find the actual date of His birth, but to worship Christ and celebrate properly the entrance of the Son of God into humanity. Christians should recognize the date that society has agreed upon when Christ was born, and use that "birthday" to spread the gospel.

Technically, Jesus probably was born close to December 25, although we don't know the actual date. Jesus was baptized when He was thirty years old near the time of his birthday (Luke 3:23). According to the chronology of John 1:29–2:12, He immediately ministered for approximately two weeks. Then Jesus spent forty days being tempted (Mark 1:12–13). Jesus then went on His first Galilean preaching tour (Mark 1:14–45), approximately two months. Next Jesus went to Jerusalem for the Passover Feast (John 2:13–25). There are approximately three to four months between December 25 and Passover, a strong suggestion that Jesus was born on or near December 25.

What does the Bible teach about the religious meaning of circumcision?

God instituted the rite of circumcision for Abraham and his descendents through Isaac as the token of the Abrahamic covenant (Gen. 17:1–10, 21). All Jewish males eight days old were required to be circumcised, although Abraham was eighty-nine years old when he was circumcised. Any non-Jews who wished to become members of the commonwealth of Israel were required to submit to the rite of circumcision, whatever their ages might be (Gen. 34:14–17, 22).

The term *circumcision* is often used in reference to people of the Jewish community just as the term *uncircumcision* is used for Gentile people (Gal. 2:7–8; Col. 3:11). Circumcision, in the New Testament, also signifies the putting away of all carnal lusts of the flesh (Col. 2:11).

The apostle Paul addressed the issue of circumcision in Romans 2–4 and in several of the other letters he wrote in the New Testament. Paul concluded that circumcision was not necessary for someone to be saved, but faith was necessary in order to be saved and go to heaven. "Since there is one God who will justify the circumcised by faith and the uncircumcised through faith" (Rom. 3:30). "Circumcision is nothing and uncircumcision is nothing, but keeping the commandments of God is what matters" (1 Cor. 7:19).

There is no need for a Gentile convert to be circumcised: "Indeed I, Paul, say to you that if you become circumcised, Christ will profit you nothing" (Gal. 5:2). On the other hand, there is no obligation incumbent upon a Jewish convert to remain uncircumcised. "For in Christ Jesus neither circumcision nor uncircumcision avails anything, but faith working through love" (Gal. 5:6).

To accept the rite of circumcision as a condition of salvation is to abandon the liberty for which Christ liberated us and to bind oneself to the slavery of legalism. Depending on circumcision, or any other work, means renouncing justification by grace through faith (in Christ) and puts one under the law.

Why do some believe dogs or cats will *not* go to heaven?

While animals that are pets respond to us, show us affection, and give us great companionship, the Bible teaches that they do not have a mortal soul in the same sense that a person does. Animals are not made in the image of God; there is nothing in the Bible about them being redeemed from sin. They have no knowledge of sin and cannot experience conversion. Therefore, they have no life after death.

The Bible seems to indicate that in the Millennium there will be lions that will eat straw like an ox, and many other animals on the earth will become tame. But this is life on *earth* during the thousand-year Millennium, not a description of our life in heaven. When Jesus returns, there seems to be an indication that the armies of heaven will be riding horses; however, there is no indication that these will be the same identical animals that lived on the earth. Even then, some Bible commentators believe the horses will not be animals, but angels. There does not seem to be any Scriptural teaching that animals are raised from the dead to live with God.

Why do some believe their dogs and cats *will* be in heaven?

Many Christians are attached to their pets and have convinced themselves that their animal pets will be with them in heaven. They argue that animals have souls and that Acts 3:21 speaks about the "restoration of all things" (the King James Version says "restitution of all things"), so this could include pets. When Jesus returns, He will be riding a horse (Rev. 19:11). So if horses are in heaven, they say, why not dogs and cats? Finally, they look to the passage that says the wolf shall dwell peacefully with the lamb, and the calf and the young lion shall lie together (Isa. 11:6).

What is the difference between the eastern gate and the gate beautiful?

The eastern gate (one of twelve gates into Jerusalem) led from outside the city of Jerusalem through the city wall into the temple area, that is, the Temple Mount. Once through the eastern gate, a traveler immediately faced a second gate: the beautiful gate into the temple (Acts 3:2). There are several Scriptures that mention the eastern gate. A specific passage that mentions the eastern gate is Ezekiel 44:1–2.

The eastern gate is on the east side of the city of Jerusalem facing the Mount of Olives. The Turkish governor of Jerusalem closed the gate in A.D. 1530 with the intent of postponing the Day of Judgment and the end of the world. Many Christians believe that when Jesus comes again (the second coming of Christ), the gate will be opened and He will once again enter the Holy City by this gate. Notice the prophecy that this gate would be closed: "Then He brought me back to the outer gate of the sanctuary which faces toward the east, but it was shut. And the LORD said to me, 'This gate shall be shut; it shall not be opened, and no man shall enter by it, because the LORD God of Israel has entered by it; therefore it shall be shut'" (Ezek. 44:1–2).

What does the Bible teach about men's hair length?

The following passage addresses the issue: "Does not even nature itself teach you that if a man has long hair, it is a dishonor to him?" (1 Cor. 11:14). This is a difficult passage, especially in a culture where long hair on men is controversial. The passage cannot mean that nature naturally grows short hair on men and long hair on women, since biologically this is not the case. Several factors must be considered. First, the context: Paul is talking about differentiating between the sexes. "Ha[ve] long hair" means to wear long hair like a woman. It cannot be said that Paul has in mind a specific kind of haircut. Paul is simply saying that it is shameful for a man to wear his hair in an effeminate way. Men should have shorter hair than women; conversely, women should have longer hair than men (1 Cor. 11:5–12).

Another factor regarding length of men's hair has to do with culture. Worldwide cultures emerge with the same sense of propriety regarding long hair on men. The vast majorities of cultures regard effeminacy of hair and dress as distasteful to a man.

It should be noted that Scripture does not dictate "spirituality" by the length of one's hair. The real issue here is submission to divine authority. Therefore, every aspect of the believer's life should reflect his obedience and submission to the Lord Jesus Christ and His divinely established authority. It should also be noted that the only exception in Scripture to the rule that prohibits men from wearing long hair was in the case of the Nazarite vow found in Numbers 6:5 and Judges 13:5.

What are the keys to the kingdom? (Matthew 16:19)

"And I will give you the keys of the kingdom of heaven, and whatever you bind on earth will be bound in heaven, and whatever you loose on earth will be loosed in heaven" (Matt. 16:19). There has been much confusion associated with "Peter's keys." Some have misunderstood the passage to mean that Christ had granted Peter exclusive right to open or close heaven to individuals. When the Lord promised Peter and the other apostles "the keys of the kingdom," it meant that through the preaching of the gospel they would open the kingdom of heaven to all believers and shut it against unbelievers. Peter used the "keys" at Pentecost (Acts 2:14), at Samaria (Acts 8:14), and at the house of Cornelius the Gentile (Acts 10).

The expressions "shall be bound in heaven" and "shall be loosed in heaven" are examples in Greek (the original language of the New Testament) of the future perfect passive construction and should therefore be translated "shall have been bound already" and "shall have been loosed already." In other words, Peter's pronouncement of "binding" or "loosing" is dependent upon what people will do with the gospel rather than upon earth's giving direction to heaven.

What are graven images (second commandment)?

The first commandment forbids the worship of any false god, seen or unseen. The second commandment forbids the worship of an image of any sort, whether the figure of a false deity or one symbolic of Jehovah. The presence of the invisible God was to be marked by no symbol of Himself, but by His words.

The actual Hebrew word for *graven image* means "carved image." The Hebrew means something hacked or chiseled into some "likeness." These idols were normally of wood (though the word could cover stone carvings as well), usually with some precious metal covering. The condemnation of images clearly means images that were idols.

The children of God—Israel—were monotheistic, in that they worshiped one God. The Israelites lived, however, in the midst of a polytheistic world. God would not share their worship with any other god. The commandment, therefore, would be "You must not make for yourself an idol."

What is the meaning of Halloween?

Halloween came into being during the first century as a day of remembrance for those who suffered martyrdom for their belief in and faithfulness to Jesus Christ. So large a number died as martyrs that a day was appointed to honor them and was called *All Saints Day*. The evening preceding this day was *All Hallows Eve*, which later, in the fourth century, became known as *Halloween* (or *Holy Evening*).

During the Middle Ages the custom of causing mischief and begging for the poor arose, along with the idea that demons roamed that night because they were powerless to do so on All Saints Day. While some Christians have an aversion to celebrating Halloween, the semiholiday does remind the general public of the reality of Satan.

Although Halloween had a very legitimate beginning, unfortunately, through the centuries it has deteriorated into an event with very negative, even sinister, overtones. Halloween generally connotes something dark and evil. God forbids us to be involved with evil spirits and those things pertaining to the netherworld (Deut. 18:10–12).

What does the Bible teach about Mary, the mother of Jesus?

The doctrine of Maryology states that Mary's soul was never touched by original sin, that it was full of grace from the instant of its creation in the womb of her mother, Anne. The doctrine further teaches that God the eternal Father made her "Queen of Heaven."

All who are God's children appreciate the great contribution of Mary. However, the doctrinal teaching of Maryology cannot be found in the Bible. God's Word does not teach that Mary was immaculately conceived. Further, it nowhere teaches that the eternal Father made Mary the Queen of Heaven. She was an ordinary woman, and though she was greatly used of God as the human mother of the Lord Jesus Christ, Mary was a sinner and needed a Savior like everyone else. She prayed to "God my Savior" (Luke 1:47).

We know from God's Word that Mary was a virgin and thus was pure. She was undoubtedly a very virtuous woman and devoted to God. She was perhaps the greatest woman ever born (Luke 1:28, 30). Her immediate submission to the news brought by the angel and her praises to God show her to be a believer in God and His promises. From reading her prayer in Luke 1:46–55, it is obvious that Mary was familiar with God's Word, knew the Scriptures well, and was close to God. It is wonderful that God chose her as the mother who would give birth to Jesus. However, the Bible does not say that she remained a virgin all her life.

There is serious harm done when people put Mary above Jesus. Mary was a wonderful woman and chosen of God for motherhood to the Baby Jesus. But many have attempted to say that Mary was sinless, and that even she herself can help redeem sinful man. The Bible nowhere tells us this. We must be careful to believe what God's Word says about Jesus: "Nor is there salvation in any other, for there is no other name under heaven given among men by which we must be saved" (Acts 4:12). We should respect Mary and Joseph; however, none should be put above Jesus and none should be put equal to Jesus (Phil. 2:10–11).

What is the love of money?

Riches are neither good nor bad. It is the attitude toward money that is good or bad. From a study of 1 Timothy 6:9–10, we learn that money can cause lust that produces temptations, snares, and other hurtful lusts. It is not money that does this; it is the *love* of money. "But those who desire to be rich fall into temptation and a snare, and into many foolish and harmful lusts which drown men in destruction and perdition. For the love of money is a root of all kinds of evil, for which some have strayed from the faith in their greediness, and pierced themselves through with many sorrows" (1 Tim. 6:9–10).

First Timothy 6:6–8 instructs individuals to be content with what they possess: "Now godliness with contentment is great gain. For we brought nothing into this world, and it is certain we can carry nothing out. And having food and clothing, with these we shall be content."

How should a Christian observe the Sabbath?

This question in our contemporary society is usually a reference to our observances on Sunday, not the Sabbath. The word *Sabbath* means rest, and is a reference to the seventh day of the week, that is, Saturday. In the Old Testament the Jews observed the Sabbath very rigorously; they did not build fires to cook their meals, did not prepare food, did not walk long distances, and set aside the day strictly for rest. The Ten Commandments teach, "Remember the sabbath day, to keep it holy" (Ex. 20:8 KJV). This says that we are to keep the day holy. Since holy means "set apart," we are to set the day apart for the Lord—we are to worship Him.

But when Jesus came, "He said unto them [the Pharisees], 'The sabbath was made for man, and not man for the sabbath'" (Mark 2:27 KJV). Jesus broke the scribes' and Pharisees' tradition of the Sabbath. He healed on the Sabbath day (John 5:1–17), and He allowed His disciples to eat from the fields on the Sabbath day (Mark 2:23). Yet, at the same time, Jesus went into the synagogue for worship and study on the Sabbath day.

We should not regard Sunday as the Jewish Sabbath, but should realize that the Lord's Day should be observed in a way that glorifies the Lord. We should not do things on Sunday that we do during the week. Certainly, a Christian shouldn't do anything that would be a reproach to unsaved people or would lead other Christians away from church and worship of the Lord.

A Christian should set out to enjoy Sunday by attending church and spending time singing, listening to sermons, learning, and worshiping God. Sunday should also be a time of serving the Lord, for example, visiting the sick, performing Christian service, and witnessing, or for private Bible reading, rest, meditation, and Christian fellowship with other people. It is not wrong to be happy on Sunday or to have quiet recreation that goes with rest. But recreation should probably be incidental, not a major part of the day. Most types of recreation such as hunting, fishing, playing golf, and attending athletic events do not seem the proper use of Sunday; however, they are not strictly prohibited.

Are we sure that the day on which we worship is the same as the original Sunday of the New Testament church?

We are not sure that Sunday is actually Sunday; actually the day we celebrate as Sunday could actually have been Tuesday in New Testament times. Chronologists tell us the calendar has lost count of actual days. The answer is to use the Sunday that society recognizes as the Lord's Day for worship.

What is the third heaven?

Paul mentions a third heaven in his second epistle to the Corinthians: "I know a man in Christ who fourteen years ago—whether in the body I do not know, or whether out of the body I do not know, God knows—such a one was caught up to the third heaven" (2 Cor. 12:2). Although this man is not mentioned by name, it is clear that Paul is speaking of himself, because of the context (vv. 6–10). With reference to the location of the third heaven, commentaries suggest that a threefold division was employed among the Jews: the air (nubiferum), the sky (astriferm), and heaven (angeliferum). The first heaven is atmospheric, the second is comprised of the stellar universe, and the third is the unique dwelling place of God. During the experience described by Paul, he was caught up into the localized presence of God, that is, the third heaven.

What is the basis of God's judgment of those who have never heard the gospel?

Many wrongly believe that those who have never heard of Jesus Christ in this life will have an opportunity to be saved after death. First, God has spoken to them through nature, but they have rejected the voice of God that spoke to them. "Because what may be known of God is manifest in them, for God has shown it to them. For since the creation of the world His invisible attributes are clearly seen, being understood by the things that are made, even His eternal power and Godhead, so that they are without excuse" (Rom.

1:19–20). Notice the Bible says that they are without excuse, so God cannot overlook their sin and let them into heaven after they die.

Second, every man who judges another for not living up to the Law realizes that he himself has broken the Law. "Therefore you are inexcusable, O man, whoever you are who judge, for in whatever you judge another you condemn yourself; for you who judge practice the same things" (Rom. 2:1). Therefore, the unsaved know they are sinners before God.

Finally, every person has an inner conscience and is reflective of the laws of God. When one goes against his conscience, he violates the moral law of God. "Who show the work of the law written in their hearts, their conscience also bearing witness, and between themselves their thoughts accusing or else excusing them in the day when God will judge the secrets of men by Jesus Christ, according to my gospel" (Rom. 2:15–16).

What does the Bible teach about being a vegetarian? Is it wrong to eat meat?

In Genesis 3:18b, after the fall of man, God instructed Adam, "And you shall eat the herb of the field." At that time man was condemned to exhausting manual labor to make a living. This was because of God's curse upon the ground (Gen. 3:17–18). Adam was to work before the Fall, but after the Fall it would be "in the sweat of your face you shall eat bread till you return to the ground" (Gen. 3:19).

Permission to eat animals appears later in Genesis 9:3: "Every moving thing that lives shall be food for you. I have given you all things, even as the green herbs."

In the New Testament, the apostle Paul instructs Timothy about the issue of abstaining from meat: ". . . forbidding to marry, and commanding to abstain from foods which God created to be received with thanksgiving by those who believe and know the truth. For every creature of God is good, and nothing is to be refused if it is received with thanksgiving; for it is sanctified by the word of God and prayer" (1 Tim. 4:3–5).

The vision Peter had concerning all manner of animals also gives support for the allowance of man to eat meat: "And a voice came to him, 'Rise, Peter; kill and eat.' But Peter said, 'Not so, Lord! For I have never eaten anything common or unclean.' And a voice spoke to him again the second time, 'What God has cleansed you must not call common'" (Acts 10:13–15).

Though God's point was that Peter was not to consider Gentiles "unclean," He also made it clear that eating the "unclean" meats was permitted.

The dietary laws (Lev. 11:41–44; 20:25; Deut. 14:3–20) for the Jews were very strictly adhered to by even the apostles. But on the cross of Calvary, God broke down the middle wall of partition (Eph. 2:14–18) between the Jews and Gentiles. The dietary laws were put aside along with the temple law. Therefore, we can partake of meat without any prohibitions. However, we are admonished by the apostle Paul regarding offending a brother, "Therefore, if food makes my brother stumble, I will never again eat meat, lest I make my brother stumble" (1 Cor. 8:13).

What does the Bible teach about wine?

The Bible implies that there are two kinds of wine. First, wine is described as a poison that will result in misery. This is called "mixed wine" (Prov. 23:29–30), "strong drink" (Isa. 28:7 KJV), "venomous poison" (Prov. 23:32; Deut. 32:33), "wine of astonishment" (Ps. 60:3 KJV), "mixture" (Ps. 75:8 KJV), "the cup of trembling" (Isa. 51:17), and "the wine cup of fury" (Jer. 25:15). Drinkers of this type of wine are described as being "sick" and "inflamed with wine" (Hos. 7:5).

Second, wine is described as a good drink, and the consequences of its use are desirable. It is called "the best of the wine" (Num. 18:12 KJV) and "new wine" (Neh. 10:37, 39). Wine is mentioned as part of the blessing of prosperity in the land (Gen. 27:28; Deut. 11:14), as something that "cheereth God and man" (Judg. 9:13 KJV), and finally, as a drink that "makes glad the heart of man" (Ps. 104:15).

We should reject intoxicating wine because it brings violence and misery (Prov. 23:29). Second, we should reject intoxicating wine because it turns a man away from God (Is. 28:7). In the third place we reject wine because it destroys life (Prov. 23:32; Deut. 32:33; Hos. 7:5). The fourth reason for rejecting wine is that its use leads to condemnation (Isa. 5:22; 1 Cor. 8:10). And finally, we reject wine because it leads to eternal ruin (Isa. 51:17, 22; Jer. 25:15; Rev. 14:19).

On the other hand the Bible teaches the benefits of wine. It was used as an offering to God (Num. 18:12; Neh. 10:37; Lev. 2:11). A second good result of wine is that it quenches thirst. This applies the necessary refreshment to life (Gen. 27:28, 37; Deut. 7:13; Deut. 11:14; Prov. 3:10). And finally, wine was a symbol of spiritual blessing and/or a symbol of the Holy Spirit (Judg. 9:13; Prov. 9:2; Song 5:1; Eph. 5:18).

Leaven was forbidden with all sacrifices (Ex. 23:18, 34:25). Remember, leaven or yeast was a sign of sin, and could not be present in one's home on Passover. Since leaven was used to make wine intoxicating, we can only assume that intoxicating wine would never be used in offering to God. Therefore, God's children should abstain from intoxicating wine.

Why should a Christian not drink alcoholic beverages?

The most serious drug problem in America is not marijuana, LSD, or some other drug. Alcohol has caused more physical, mental, and psychological damage to more people of all ages than all of the hallucinogenic drugs combined.

Most Americans feel liquor is acceptable in some forms, but I disagree. The following reasons tell us why drunkenness is wrong.

1. God rejects drunkenness because it degrades human dignity. The Bible teaches, "And do not be drunk with wine, in which is dissipation; but be filled with the Spirit" (Eph. 5:18). Intoxicating wine is contrasted with the filling of the Spirit. Paul warns against the spirits of the bottle, which intoxicate man and affect his walk, talk, and outlook on life.

God warns, "Do not look on the wine when it is red, when it sparkles in the cup, when it swirls around smoothly; at the last it bites like a serpent, and stings like a viper" (Prov. 23:31–32). The Bible likens alcohol that makes one drunk to poison: "Their wine is the poison of serpents, and the cruel venom of cobras" (Deut. 32:33). Because of its danger, God gives the warning, "Woe to him who gives drink to his neighbor, pressing him to your bottle" (Hab. 2:15). Again the Bible warns against drunkenness when it commands, "Let us walk properly, as in the day, not in revelry and drunkenness, not in lewdness and lust, not in strife and envy" (Rom. 13:13). Drunkenness was common in Rome, and Paul wisely exhorts Christians to avoid it.

Paul says drunkenness is a characteristic of the unsaved. Any person who drinks liquor should examine his soul, "Nor drunkards . . . will inherit the kingdom of God" (1 Cor. 6:10).

2. Drunkenness destroys the body. The Bible teaches that God made our bodies and He dwells in us (1 Cor. 6:19). Therefore, we sin against God when we harm our bodies with alcohol.

3. Drunkenness destroys the morals and integrity of our nation. Anything

that destroys our nation's righteousness is sin, and alcohol is an evil that has done much to erode our Christian heritage. Drunkenness leads to lawlessness and disrespect for our national goals.

If we continue on our present course, more of our young will become alcoholics and more of our tax money will be spent on correcting the problems caused by alcohol. Our nation will lose its Christian influence.

4. Drunkenness is contrary to the example set by Christ. Christians are to follow the example of Jesus Christ (1 Pet. 2:21). He never gave himself to drunkenness. The Bible tells us He did not sin (2 Cor. 5:21; 1 Pet. 2:22; Heb. 4:15). He always did the will of God. Therefore, we can say that Christ would not disobey the command of Proverbs, "Look not thou upon the wine . . ." (Prov. 23:31 KJV).

5. Drunkenness opens the door to other sins. Alcohol is an anesthetic. It kills pain by producing a state of tranquilization. Drunkenness releases a person's inhibitions and destroys his self-control. Hence, the drunken person, because his self-discipline is gone, will commit acts that he would never consider doing otherwise, that would embarrass him if he were sober. Drunkenness is not only a sin for what it is, but for what it allows us to do.

Did Jesus create or drink intoxicating wine?

Some Christians use Jesus' example to justify their drinking alcohol. Those who justify drinking alcohol point to three incidences in the life of Jesus for proof for their position.

First, they attest, Jesus served wine to His disciples at the Last Supper. But the wine at the Last Supper could not have been intoxicating because if a Jew ate leaven before the Passover, he could not participate (Ex. 23:18; Lev. 6:17; 7:12; 10:12). Leaven was a sign or picture of sin. Jesus, having never broken the ceremonial law, could have not participated in anything identified with sin—including intoxicating wine—immediately prior to the Passover. Second, Jesus Christ would not contradict Himself when the Bible said, "Woe to him who gives drink to his neighbor" (Hab. 2:15). Finally, the argument of silence: The drink at the Lord's Supper is never called wine. It is referred to as "the cup" or "the fruit of the vine." God knows all things and kept the Holy Spirit from using the word *wine* in relationship to our communion service because it would have complicated the interpretation. This builds a strong argument for teetotalism.

A second argument by social drinkers is that Jesus created wine at the wedding in Cana of Galilee. But get the whole picture. This first miracle in the New Testament was an act of creation to bring joy to the wedding guests, just as His first miracle in the Old Testament was an act of creation bringing joy to all those involved (Col. 1:16-17). Nature's process to make wine (sweet) is by bringing water from the clouds into the earth, up through the vine into the grape, finally to be crushed into a juice. The miracle followed this process at the wedding although the process was speeded up into an instantaneous act. Making intoxicating wine involves allowing the grape to rot and adding man's creative elements (leaven) to produce alcohol. Intoxication is not the process of God; it is man's addition. God said, "Do not look on the wine when it is red, when it sparkles in the cup, when it swirls around smoothly" (Prov. 23:31). As God, Jesus could not have contradicted this command from Proverbs and provided wine for the guests at the wedding meal.

Many of the commentators look at this verse to prove Jesus created intoxicating wine: "Every man at the beginning sets out the good wine, and when the guests have well drunk, then the inferior. You have kept the good wine until now!" (John 2:10) They interpret "good wine" to mean that the created wine (last) was fermented wine. However, fresh-crushed juice is a better interpretation. This was sweet grape juice, the kind that gave joy from the Lord.

The third attack is against Jesus' abstinence. Some point to the verse that John the Baptist was a teetotaler but Jesus was a "winebibber" (Matt. 11:19 KJV), implying John could not take strong drink whatsoever, but Jesus must have taken a social cocktail. First, we have no record of Jesus ever tasting wine, not even sweet wine, although He probably enjoyed sweet wine. Second, the verse does not state Jesus was a "winebibber." The verse repeats a claim by His enemies that Jesus drank. Read the verse carefully, "The Son of Man came eating and drinking, and they say, 'Look, a glutton and a winebibber'" (Matt. 11:19). Because Jesus went to a feast where sinners got drunk, the enemies of Jesus claim He was a "winebibber." The truth is Jesus went to their feast to preach the gospel to them and deliver them from sin, including the sin of drunkenness.

The Bible never teaches that happiness is the result of an artificial stimulant such as alcohol. True happiness comes from enjoying the provisions of God, such as the beauty of nature, doing God's will, or partaking of the fruit He has provided, that is, the fruit of the vine, the crushed grape.

QUESTIONS
ABOUT
POLITICAL MATTERS

What are the arguments against abortion?

For hundreds of years our Western culture has specifically protected the right of every individual to life, and has included the unborn child in that protection. Western civilization has historically been against abortion.

Human life begins at conception. The fetus is a new being entirely separate from its parents because it has a different chromosomal makeup.

The fetus is alive at conception because it has the capacity to replace its own dying cells.

The fetus needs food and time to grow into an adult human.

The fetus is just as much alive and human "before birth" as it is "after birth"; it is not a different life.

The human heart begins to beat at eighteen days.

At six weeks, an electrical impulse begins in the human brain. Activity can be recorded on an electroencephalogram.

Children have been born prematurely at nineteen weeks and six days after the mother's menstrual period and have become perfectly healthy children. Therefore, if some children can survive at this premature age, why can we not attempt to save all fetuses/children at this age, rather than terminating their lives?

The body of the child belongs to the child, just as the body of the mother belongs to the mother. The mother is not aborting a part of her anatomy; she is aborting a life, which she and a man have created and placed in her.

Since we have not given the right of a mother to terminate a child's life after birth, why should she have the right to terminate the child's life before birth?

Should a Christian defend himself when attacked?

The question of no retaliation or nonviolence is often raised about Christians. This question comes from the following verse by Jesus: "You have heard that it was said, 'An eye for an eye and a tooth for a tooth.' But I tell you not to resist an evil person. But whoever slaps you on your right cheek, turn the other to him also. If anyone wants to sue you and take away your tunic, let him have your cloak also. And whoever compels you to go one mile, go with him two" (Matt. 5:38–41).

In these verses Jesus was referring to the Christian's response to actions of evil or malicious persons. The principle of retaliation *(lex talionis)* is common in both Jewish and other ancient Near Eastern law codes, especially in the code of Hammurabi. However, Jesus is clearly saying the Christian should not seek vengeance when attacked. Many times an offended person will overreact to an attack and retaliate in such a way as to return in like manner (i.e., an injury for an injury; an insult for an insult). These verses serve to drive home the point that a Christian, rather than avenging himself upon a brother who has done him a *personal* wrong, should go to the opposite extreme.

Jesus' point in verse 39 is that we (as individuals) should "resist not evil." Evil is seen here not as a state, but rather as actions of the evil ones. It represents the evil and sinful element in man that provokes him to an act of evil. Jesus shows in this verse how the individual believer should respond to personal injury: Don't give evil for evil.

These verses do not mean that a man should not defend his family or his country, but rather that he should not attempt personal vengeance to compensate for personal injury.

Jesus told His disciples not to expect divine justice from an unregenerate society. All justice ultimately is in the hand and the heart of God. As long as human governments prevail, justice will be limited by man's finite abilities. The believer is to place his total confidence in the ultimate sovereignty of God over the affairs of his individual life.

Why is cloning wrong?

The body is made of microscopic cells, each one containing a nucleus. Every nucleus has a chain of chromosomes that determine, among other things, the color of skin and eyes. A new baby at conception gets half of the genes from the father, the other half from the mother. The blending process involved ensures that no two children of the same parents have the same combination of genes. Every child is absolutely unique!

The cloning process involves removing the nucleus of a fertilized human egg and replacing it with a nucleus from a person to be cloned. The egg is allowed to grow, then implanted into the womb of a mother.

Cloning is wrong because the "engineer" or scientist elevates himself to the level of God. He is trying to do what God does by attempting to determine what people should be like, and is entering into the realm that God has reserved for Himself. If an engineer could clone a person, then he or she could disprove that there ever was a God, or a Creator, and could refute the "need" for God to guide, protect, or even save us.

Second, the engineer now becomes the decision maker on who should live, when they should live, and how they should live. If the engineer is allowed to determine which "fertilized egg-person" lives, then eventually he or she will also be allowed to determine who will die.

Part of the motivation behind cloning is "selective breeding." Why? Because humans are not satisfied with the children that are born (or are to be born)—their sexes, quality of life, and so on. The engineer wants selective breeding to improve the human race.

People ask three basic questions: "Where did I come from?" "Who am I?" and "Where am I going?" If people became able to clone humans, then they would be able to answer these questions apart from God. "Where did I come from?" could be answered by evolution. "Who am I?" would be answered by cloning. "Where am I going?" would be answered by humanism.

God's plan for procreation was a human producing a human. In the beginning God told Adam and Eve, "Be fruitful and multiply" (Gen. 1:28). When someone attempts cloning, he or she is supplanting God both in desire and destiny.

Another thing about cloning: The scientist, like Ponce DeLeón, is looking for the eternal fountain of youth. Because there is a yearning in man to live forever, and the "engineer" rejects God's plan of eternal life, people want to clone themselves so they may live after they die—in the lives of the next persons cloned from their genes.

What about cloning for reproduction of body parts?

Some scientific engineers say that a person could be cloned exactly like you, having identical DNA, blood type, and so forth. At present, transplanting a heart or kidney is often hampered by the rejection of the new organ because it is *not* genetically identical to the recipient's. If, however, cloning could produce embryos with the identical genetic makeup of the sick person, then the possibility of "perfect spare parts" could be a reality. This perfect clone could supply body parts for you as needed (for example, a new liver, eyes, and so on). If the clone does not have a soul in the view of the "engineer," then the engineer does not have to worry about destroying the created body, and those body parts can become replacements for the sick person. However, it would involve the destruction of embryos to produce clones, and then the clones would be destroyed after they were no longer of use. The world uses the term *cannibalized* when parts are taken from one automobile to repair another one. Cloning would lead to cannibalization of the clone for spare parts. Then other issues would be faced: "Where is the soul?" and "Is this murder?"

Is stem cell research acceptable to Christians?

Many have suggested the great benefits of using stem cells to find cures for diseases. They argue that it's humanitarian to use medical research to discover cures for otherwise fatal or debilitating diseases. However, a stem cell is a human embryo in the early stages of development. This is wrong because the embryonic child is destroyed in the process.

What does Jesus say about divorce?

"It hath been said, Whosoever shall put away his wife, let him give her a writing of divorcement: But I say unto you, That whosoever shall put away his wife, saving for the cause of fornication, causeth her to commit adultery: and whosoever shall marry her that is divorced committeth adultery" (Matt. 5:31–32 KJV). "It hath been said" is a reference to the Old Testament commandment of the Mosaic regulation found in Deuteronomy 24:1. The normal custom of the ancient Near East was for a man to verbally divorce his wife. The Arab custom was to say "I divorce you" three times and the divorce was consummated without any legal protection of any kind to the wife. In contrast, the ancient law of Israel insisted on a *writing of divorcement* or certificate of divorce. This written statement gave legal protection to both the wife and the husband. Jesus explained elsewhere (Matt. 19:8) that Moses' concession was not intended to be taken as license. In ancient rabbinic Judaism, Moses' statement had been variously interpreted from meaning adultery *(shamai)* to the trivial matters of personal preference *(hillel)*. The only legitimate exception for divorce allowed by Christ is for *the cause of fornication* (Greek *porneia*), meaning sexual unfaithfulness. Fornication may mean adultery prior to or after marriage, as well as unfaithfulness during the period of betrothal.

"They said to Him, 'Why then did Moses command to give a certificate of divorce, and to put her away?' He said to them, 'Moses, because of the hardness of your hearts, permitted you to divorce your wives, but from the beginning it was not so. And I say to you, whoever divorces his wife, except for sexual immorality, and marries another, commits adultery; and whoever marries her who is divorced commits adultery'" (Matt. 19:7–9).

The question "Why then did Moses command . . .?" revealed the misuse of Deuteronomy 24 by the Jews of Jesus' day. Moses did not *command;* he *permitted* divorce. God had instituted marriage in the Garden of Eden. He is not the author of divorce; man is its originator. However, to protect the Hebrew woman from being taken advantage of by a verbal divorce, Moses commanded that it be done with a *writing of divorcement,* an official written contract, permitting remarriage. The Jews tended to take this as an excuse or license to get divorced whenever they pleased. The original provision was for the protection of the wife from an evil husband, not an authorization for him to divorce her at will. Therefore, Jesus gave one exception to the no-divorce intention of God: *fornication* (Greek *porneia*) "sexual sins," not to be limited to premarital sex only. It includes all types of sexual sin: adultery, homosexuality, bestiality, and so forth. Among the Jews, only the male could divorce, so Mark 10:12 reverses the statement for His Gentile audience.

"His disciples said to Him, 'If such is the case of the man with his wife, it is better not to marry.' But He said to them, 'All cannot accept this saying, but only those to whom it has been given: For there are eunuchs who were born thus from their mother's womb, and there are eunuchs who were made eunuchs by men, and there are eunuchs who have made themselves eunuchs for the kingdom of heaven's sake. He who is able to accept it, let him accept it'" (Matt. 19:10–12).

Since divorce, on any grounds, was common in those days, the disciples felt *it is not good to marry.* The severity of Jesus' statement was in total contrast to the society of that day and represented the true intention of God. While divorce appears to be allowed in both Testaments (Deut. 24:1–5; 1 Cor. 7:15, 27–28), it is never encouraged because it always violates God's original intention in marriage.

Does the Bible say a divorced person can remarry?

"Are you bound to a wife? Do not seek to be loosed. Are you loosed from a wife? Do not seek a wife" (1 Cor. 7:27). Although what Paul has said can never justify the dissolution of a marriage, hopefully it will discourage some from getting married to the wrong person. Notice that "bound" refers to marriage and "loosed" to divorce. This verse warns the divorced about remarriage, but also states that it is not a sin to do so. If God permits a divorce, then He permits a remarriage.

I got a divorce before I was converted; do I have to go back and correct it?

We serve a God who is forgiving, and who takes you as you are. Therefore, He takes you from a divorced condition and forgives "all your sin" (1 John 1:7). Paul gave us the principle of serving Christ in the circumstances in which we are called. First Corinthians 7:20 says, "Let every man abide in the same calling wherein he was called" (KJV). Therefore, if you were divorced before you were saved, do not try to revisit your previous marriage or reconcile yourself to a previous spouse. Neither should you divorce your present spouse: "Brethren let each one remain with God in that state in which he was called" (1 Cor. 7:24). Paul also tells us, "Are you bound to a wife? Do not seek to be loosed" (1 Cor. 7:27). In other words, do not seek release from your current spouse.

What does the Bible teach concerning homosexuality?

The Bible condemns homosexuality as a sin. However, it also tells us that if these people will repent of their sins and trust Jesus as their Savior, they can be saved. Romans 1:18–32 describes the sins of homosexuality and lesbianism, then concludes God has to give them up to uncleanness because they are stubborn and willful in their sins.

"For this reason God gave them up to vile passions. For even their women exchanged the natural use for what is against nature. Likewise also the men, leaving the natural use of the woman, burned in their lust for one another, men with men committing what is shameful, and receiving in themselves the penalty of their error which was due. And even as they did not like to retain God in their knowledge, God gave them over to a debased mind, to do those things which are not fitting." (Romans 1:26–28)

Genesis 19:1–28 describes the destruction of Sodom and Gomorrah because of the sin of homosexuality. The men of the city desired that Lot send his two guests out to them that they might "know" them. The word *know* has been consistently translated by Christian scholars over the centuries as "to have sexual relations, that is, intercourse" with them. One of the many reasons God destroyed these two cities was because of homosexuality.

Deuteronomy 23:17–18 teaches that no whore or sodomite can be accepted among the children of Israel because all who do so are an abomination to Him. Throughout the books of the Kings there are references to the people sinning by turning to sodomy and other references to kings who, in obedience to the Lord God, drove the sodomites out of their lands (see 1 Kings 14:24; 15:12, 22:46; 2 Kings 23:7).

First Corinthians 6:9–10 KJV tells us that those who are effeminate or who are "abusers of themselves with mankind" will not inherit the kingdom of God. But the Bible holds out hope for the homosexual becoming a Christian because it says, "And such were some of you. But you were washed, but you were sanctified, but you were justified in the name of the Lord Jesus and by the Spirit of our God" (1 Cor. 6:11).

Are homosexuals born with their sexual preference?

If you say that homosexuals are born with a sexual preference, then you imply that God created them that way. But they are *not* born with that sexual preference, because God condemns the sin of homosexuality (1 Cor. 6:9; Lev. 20:13; Rom. 1:26–31). God, being righteous, could not condemn an unnatural appetite or sinful desire in a person and at the same time create a person *with* that desire.

Some believe that homosexual expression may be tied to the influence of demonism. Inasmuch as demonism can be transferred from parent to the child, the demonic influences can enter the child from the parents who have given themselves to that influence. Other Christians believe that homosexuality could be a disorder in the genes, and a person could physically be born with a disorder in the genes—homosexual desires. Neither belief excuses homosexual activity.

Though homosexuals are not born homosexuals, *all* people are born with a sin nature and have a desire (lust) to sin. Most childhood training teaches children to control their desires. Since homosexuality is only one of the expressions of lust, then the homosexual who says he or she was born into that desire is correct inasmuch as that individual was born with an appetite for sin; he or she just happens to express that appetite toward someone of their same sex. Homosexuals, who are born in sin, just as each person has to deal with his or her sin, must bring it to Jesus Christ for forgiveness by His blood (John 1:29). The difference is that Christians, who are born in sin, repent of that sin and seek forgiveness. Some homosexuals refuse to admit that their lifestyle is sin and will not ask for God's forgiveness, but justify themselves by claiming that they were born that way.

Are Christians obliged to obey the human government over them?

The Bible gives us several commands to obey the political rulers over us:

"Let every soul be subject to the governing authorities. For there is no authority except from God, and the authorities that exist are appointed by God" (Rom. 13:1).

"Remind them to be subject to rulers and authorities, to obey, to be ready for every good work" (Titus 3:1).

"Therefore submit yourselves to every ordinance of man for the Lord's sake, whether to the king as supreme, or to governors, as to those who are sent by him for the punishment of evildoers and for the praise of those who do good" (1 Peter 2:13–14).

Of course, there may be times when government leaders violate the power and authority given them by God and issue laws or acts contrary to Scripture. In these situations the Christian must not submit but obey God. An example of this principle is found in Acts 5:29, where the apostles boldly refused to submit to governing authority on the grounds that it was contrary to the will of God (Acts 4:19).

A Christian should support his government leaders by earnest prayer for them to be saved and for them to be filled with divine wisdom to guide them in the affairs of governing the people (1 Tim. 2:1). However, if the leaders are wicked and are doing contrary to God's Word, then as a Christian you should pray for their removal from office and exercise your right as a citizen to vote them out of office.

Are Jewish people who reject Christ going to heaven?

The Jews are very special to God—they always have been. They have a unique place in His program for this world. The Bible says that the Jews are "the apple of His eye" (Deut. 32:10). The Jews are in the line of Abraham, Isaac, and Jacob and in the line through which Christ was born. Jesus was a Jew. Christians should love Jews because "to them were committed the oracles of God" (Rom. 3:2). Through the Jews God revealed Himself in the Holy Scriptures and gave the message of redemption. In the Abrahamic covenant, the Lord told Abraham: "I will bless those who bless you, and I will curse him who curses you" (Gen. 12:3).

The nation of Israel is still God's chosen people. His covenant with Israel is an everlasting covenant. Even though a majority of the nation rejects Jesus Christ as Savior and as Messiah, many of the members of the nation of Israel who have accepted Jesus as Savior and Messiah will be saved (Rom. 10:9–13). One day the nation as a whole will turn to Christ and will know He is indeed the only begotten Son of God, the true Messiah of Israel, the only Savior and hope for a lost and dying world.

The Jews who reject Jesus as Messiah are missing the joy and peace of having their sins freely forgiven and of knowing they are fully accepted by God. In the words of our Savior Jesus Christ with regard to whether or not a Jew would go to heaven or hell, He made the statement, "Unless one is born again, he cannot see the kingdom of God" (John 3:3). This statement was made to a Jewish Pharisee named Nicodemus, a ruler of the Jews. Thus, Jesus Christ Himself uttered the statement of utmost eternal importance for all men to consider: "He who believes in the Son has everlasting life; and he who does not believe the Son shall not see life, but the wrath of God abides on him" (John 3:36).

Should Christians swear or take an oath in court?

There are some Christians and some churches that teach their members not to swear or take an oath in court. They base their conclusions on the following verses:

"Again you have heard that it was said to those of old, 'You shall not swear falsely, but shall perform your oaths to the Lord.' But I say to you, do not swear at all: neither by heaven, for it is God's throne; nor by the earth, for it is His footstool; nor by Jerusalem, for it is the city of the great King. Nor shall you swear by your head, because you cannot make one hair white or black. But let your 'Yes' be 'Yes,' and your 'No,' 'No.' For whatever is more than these is from the evil one" (Matt. 5:33–37).

During the time of Christ's earthly ministry, many Jews had developed an elaborate system of oath taking, which often shielded them from telling the truth. For example, one might swear that he had told the truth according to the dome of the temple, while another might swear by the gold on the dome of the temple! In other words, there were stages of truth and thus stages of falsehood within their system of taking oaths. In our time this custom is found in phrases such as, "I swear to God," "Cross my heart and hope to die," or "on my mother's grave." All such oath taking, Jesus would announce, was unnecessary. He taught His followers to habitually tell the truth.

According to Jesus, the Christian is not to take an oath by heaven, earth, nor the city of Jerusalem. He is not to swear on the basis of his own head or any other physical feature. He is to speak the truth in such a way that his "yes" means *yes* and his "no" means *no*. This does not necessarily mean that it is wrong to "swear to tell the truth" in a court of law. The point is that it should be unnecessary to ask a true Christian to swear to tell the truth.

However, the Christian lives under laws requiring him to swear to tell the truth. The Christian is then only affirming what he purposes in his heart to do. To get away from the term *swear,* it is legally permissible for the witness to "affirm to tell the truth" without his or her having to repeat the standard court oath.

What does the Bible teach about war and the military preparedness of a nation?

In the Old Testament the Hebrew word *milhamah* (translated "war") occurs more than three hundred times. *Milhamah* is only one of several Hebrew words associated with the various facets of war. More than three hundred times in the Old Testament, God is called "the Lord of hosts" (armies). The song of victory sung by Moses and the children of Israel after they escaped Pharaoh (Ex. 15:3–4) was, "The LORD is a man of war; the LORD is His name. Pharaoh's chariots and his army He has cast into the sea."

Many of God's great leaders were military men (Saul, David, Moses, Gideon, Joshua, and others). Abraham went to war and rescued Lot. The Bible says, "He armed his trained servants . . . and attacked them" (Gen. 14:14–15). The Lord chose Joshua to be Moses' successor to lead the Israelites into the land of Canaan. In order to do this, Joshua was commanded to exterminate all of the inhabitants of Canaan and was promised God's help (Deut. 7:17–24). Then God helped Joshua in the battle of Jericho (Josh. 6:1–27).

The Lord uses government officials as vehicles to convey judgment upon nations that need it: "He is God's minister, an avenger to execute wrath on him who practices evil" (Rom. 13:4). The Old and New Testaments are full of examples of human governments being ordained of God (Dan. 2:37–38; John 19:10–11).

In summary, a nation must realize that while building a strong military defense, their trust must ultimately be in God. The danger of total faith in a military defense apart from God is as great as the danger of a second-rate military defense. Americans and Christians must work hard for a strong country, capable of defending itself against military aggression. At the same time we must pray for peace that can be won without compromising the principles upon which America was founded—principles for which our forefathers fought. Finally, we must realize that the only real and lasting peace will come when the Prince of Peace returns to set up his millennial kingdom.

QUESTIONS ABOUT ANGELS

What is an angel?

An angel is a living being who has a personality (intellect, emotion, and will). Angels do not have physical bodies, but can manifest themselves physically. Angels are powerful, but they are not omnipotent; wise, but not omniscient. There are great numbers of them, but they are not limitless. An angel's main task is to minister to God or for God (Heb. 1:13).

Which angels have names?

Though it is likely that all angels have names, only three angels' names are recorded in Scripture: *Lucifer*, whose name means "bearer of light"; *Michael*, whose name means "who is like God"; and *Gabriel*, whose name means "man of God."

Who was the highest angel?

Lucifer was the highest angel (Ezek. 28:1–17). The Bible says he was full of wisdom (v. 17), perfect in beauty (v. 12), was the angel who "covered" God (vv. 14, 16), was perfect in all of his ways (v.15), and was anointed for service to God (v. 14).

Why did Lucifer fall?

The Bible says he left his first estate (Isa. 14:12–14). First he ascended into heaven (to possess it). Then he exalted his throne (which means he desired to rule or have power over the other angels). Third, he wanted to sit on the mount of the congregation (to govern heaven). He wanted to ascend above the highest of the clouds (he wanted the glory of heaven), and finally, he wished to be like the Most High (the Lord Most High, Possessor of heaven and earth).

Are angels male or female?

While many statues and artwork seem to depict angels as female, the word *angel* is always used in the masculine gender in the Scriptures (both Hebrew and Greek). However, sex in a human sense is never ascribed to them.

When were angels created?

Most people feel that angels were created in eternity past; God speaks, "Where were you when I laid the foundations of the earth . . . when the morning stars sang together, and all the sons of God shouted for joy?" (Job 38:4, 7). This seems to indicate that at Creation, angels were shouting for joy when they saw what God was doing.

However, some people feel angels were created during the creative week because the Bible says, "For in six days the Lord made heaven and earth, the sea, and all that in them is" (Ex. 20:11 KJV). Since angels are a part of the heavens, these people believe, they were created during these six days.

Will more angels be created?

Apparently Colossians 1:16–17 says that all angels were created simultaneously, and that the act of Creation was complete. This means none will be added in the future.

Can angels die?

The Bible says they cannot: "Nor can they die anymore, for they are equal to the angels and are sons of God, being sons of the resurrection" (Luke 20:36).

Can we see angels today?

Angels remain unseen by humans until they choose to appear in some physical manifestation. However, the Bible teaches, "Do not forget to entertain strangers, for by so doing some have unwittingly entertained angels" (Heb. 13:2). That means we might have talked to someone who blessed our lives, not knowing he was an angel.

Why do angels not remain visible at all times?

Perhaps people would worship them if they could see them. Remember, humans are prone to idolatry. They probably could not resist worshiping angels.

How many angels are there?

At one place Jesus said, "Or do you think that I cannot now pray to My Father, and He will provide Me with more than twelve legions of angels?" (Matt. 26:53). At another place the Bible says, "An innumerable company of angels" (Heb. 12:22 KJV). There are so many we cannot number them, but it does not mean that they are limitless. Only God is limitless. The Bible seems to teach that there is a guardian angel for each person on earth (Matt. 18:10, Acts 12:15). If that is true, there must be at least six billion angels, because that's how many souls there are on earth.

What is an elect angel?

Paul told Timothy, "I charge you before God and the Lord Jesus Christ and the elect angels . . ." (1 Tim. 5:21). Elect angels seem to be those who chose righteousness and followed God, as opposed to those who chose unrighteousness and followed Lucifer. Afterwards those were called fallen angels, unclean spirits, or demons.

What are cherubim?

This is a special group of angels attached to the throne of God whose task is to guard the holiness of God. Remember, a cherub was placed at the gate to Eden so that people might not enter after Adam and Eve were cast out. Also, the two likenesses of angels that were placed on the ark of the covenant (Ex. 25:18–22) were cherubim.

What are seraphim?

The word *seraphim* means "burners." These are angels who are concerned with the holiness of God. They cry out continually, "Holy, holy, holy" (Isa. 6:3). Most people feel the seraphim probably relate to sacrifice and cleansing.

What are other names assigned to angels?

They are called the *sons of God* (Job 38:7), *sons of the Mighty* (Ps. 29:1 NASB), *watchers* (Dan. 4:13–14), *holy ones* (Matt. 25:31), *princes* (Dan. 10:13, 20, 21), *thrones* (rulership) (Col. 1:16), *dominions* (Col. 1:16), *principalities, powers* (Col. 1:16), *morning stars* (Job 38:7), *beasts* (Rev. 4:6–8 KJV), and *the elect* (1 Tim. 5:21).

How strong are angels?

They have vast power, but they are not omnipotent, meaning they are not all-powerful.

How smart are angels?

Angels are exceedingly wise and knowledgeable, but not omniscient, meaning they do not know all things at all times. Only God knows all things at all times. The knowledge of angels is limited, as Jesus said, "But of that day and hour no one knows, not even the angels of heaven, but My Father only" (Matt. 24:36). However, angels can learn new things. Notice what Peter said: "Things which angels desire to look into" (1 Pet. 1:12). The angels do not understand all of the ramifications of the gospel, but according to Peter they are learning from us.

Can angels sin?

When Lucifer fell, apparently a group of angels fell with him. Many teach that one-third of all the angels fell with Lucifer (Rev. 12:4). Those angels which have fallen into sin are "confirmed in wickedness," meaning they cannot be converted, nor can they do good. Those angels that chose to follow God are "confirmed in holiness," which means they can only do good and cannot be lost in hell.

Some people feel it is wrong to say angels do not have another chance of sinning. However, that will be the condition of every Christian once he dies; when we get to heaven we will lose our sin nature, not being able to sin.

What do angels do for us today?

Angels apparently deliver us at our deaths into the presence of God. Lazarus "was carried by the angels to Abraham's bosom" (Luke 16:22). Angels also deliver messages for God (Rev. 22:8, Luke 1:26–27).

Can angels read our minds?

No. Only God knows the thoughts of all people, because only God knows all things at all times. However, angels can understand our external actions; therefore, they have some understanding of what is going on in our minds.

What do our guardian angels do for us?

Children are described as having "their angels" (Matt. 18:10). When Rhoda was guarding the door while Peter knocked for entrance, the person at the door was described as "his angel" (Acts 12:15). Apparently, some thought Peter might have died and his angel appeared at the house.

God protects His people by angels. The Bible says, "The angel of the LORD encamps all around those who fear Him, and delivers them" (Ps. 34:7) Guardian angels "always see the face of [Jesus'] Father who is in heaven" (Matt. 18:10), implying that God knows when we are in danger, and sends a guardian angel to help us. Origen, one of the early church fathers, said, "We must say that every human soul is under direction of an angel who is like a father." St. Basil said, "An angel is put in charge of every believer, providing we do not drive them out by sin. He guards the soul like an army." The angel protects the physical aspect of our lives, whereas the Holy Spirit protects the spiritual aspect of our lives.

Why is there so much interest in angels in the secular community?

There is a lot of new interest in angels that was not previously evident in the secular world. As an illustration, there are stores selling angel products, Web sites on angels, newsletters on angels, and a total of two thousand books written on angels in the past few years. In 1975, Billy Graham published a hardback book entitled *Angels,* which shocked everyone by selling over one million copies. At that time, it was the largest-selling hardback book ever released. Why so much current interest in angels?

Throughout the Bible, angels did not manifest themselves all the time. There were many times when heaven was silent and there were no manifestations of angels. However, when God plans to intersect history with a new plan or person(s), the Lord usually uses angels to introduce His person or program to mankind. Could the new interest in angels suggest the coming of Christ is close?

Do unsaved people have angels?

Many have said "no" because Hebrews 1:14 indicates, "Are they not all ministering spirits, sent forth to minister for them who shall be heirs of salvation?" (KJV). Notice angels are not sent to everyone, but only to *heirs of salvation.* This would exclude unsaved people.

Are some angels Chinese?

This is like asking, "Are some angels Korean, others Africans, and still others with the bronze skin of the Near East?" When angels appeared to Daniel in Babylon, apparently that angel had the characteristic of a Babylonian or a Jew such as himself. Daniel wasn't surprised by the angel's appearance, implying it had olive skin. Later Cornelius saw an angel and was not surprised by it. Apparently, that angel would have had fair skin like an Anglo-Roman.

If angels are making appearances to people today, and people wouldn't recognize them (Heb. 13:2), doesn't that suggest angels have the appearances of the people to whom they manifest themselves? That means an angel would look Chinese when appearing to a Chinese person. Wouldn't a guardian angel appear in the physical manifestation of the person that angel is guarding?

Is the television show *Touched by an Angel* in keeping with Bible teaching?

The television show *Touched by an Angel* has caused many people to think about the supernatural, and it has made many people sensitive to God's plan in their lives. Because of that, it has a positive value. However, the show portrays an angel as a woman, and angels are never portrayed as women in the Bible. Second, the angel usually appears to a person who is a derelict or has some moral problem. In actuality, angels usually appear to God's people, to "heirs of salvation." Finally, the television show gives credit to angels working out the problems of people. In the Bible, credit or glory always goes to God.

Can we or should we attempt to talk or pray to angels?

Some churches teach their people to pray to angels. However, not once in Scripture are we ever given an illustration of people praying to angels, nor do they use an angel as an intercessor between them and God. The Bible teaches, "For there is one God and one Mediator between God and men, the Man Christ Jesus" (I Tim. 2:5).

The closest we can come to talking to angels is found in a few psalms such as Psalm 103:20 KJV. The psalmist said, "Bless the Lord, ye His angels . . ." This seems to picture the psalmist talking to angels, telling them to bless God. However, this might not be an actual conversation. It could be the psalmist talking to himself, wanting angels to do what God has instructed them to do, to worship Him.

Can angels preach the gospel?

In the case of Cornelius, who was unsaved, the angel did not preach the gospel to him. Rather, the angel instructed Cornelius to send for Peter. It was Peter who preached the gospel to Cornelius, not an angel. The task of preaching or evangelism is given to believers, not angels (Matt. 28:19–20). We cannot assume an angel will fulfill the responsibility of Christians.

Can we see an angel today?

There are some Christians who claim to have seen angels. Most, when asked what the angels looked like, described contemporary adults who reflected their cultures and lifestyles. Most people do not claim that angels have wings, nor have they seen them fly.

The Bible teaches, "Do not forget to entertain strangers, for by so doing some have unwittingly entertained angels" (Heb. 13:2). This verse says that we may have entertained angels, but not known they were angels. This is probably in reference to Abraham, who entertained Jesus (a Christophany) and two angels in Genesis 18. It was not until later that Abraham realized the two were angels.

Have we entertained angels?

If we have entertained angels, we are probably not aware that we did, because the Bible teaches that when we do, we entertain angels "unawares" (Heb. 13:2).

The issue is not, Can we see angels? God can work this out, and angels have appeared in the past. The issue is, Will God manifest angels to us? Probably not, for God wants us to put our trust in Him, and to follow the instructions of the Scripture. God doesn't want us to follow outward symbols or things, or angels.

What is the difference between the ministry of angels and the ministry of the Holy Spirit?

Apparently the main duty of angels is to relate to man's physical or material needs. The main ministry of the Holy Spirit is to relate to man's spiritual life. However, on occasion angels do relate spiritually to people, usually as they minister physically. Likewise, on occasion, the Holy Spirit has answered prayer for physical needs.

Can angels sing?

The vast majority of references to angels describe them as *saying* or *speaking*. Only a few references indicate that angels sing. However, the emphasis is on giving worship and glory to God with their spoken words.

Do angels have wings?

There is no description in the Bible of angels with wings. Every time an angel made an appearance to someone, the person always thought the angel was human. Humans did not observe that angels had wings or could fly.

However, seraphim and cherubim have been described as having wings (Isa. 6:2). So technically angels do not have wings, but cherubim and seraphim have wings. Remember there are many different orders of angels. When Paul describes fallen angels, he calls them "principalities," "powers," "rulers of the darkness of this age," and "spiritual hosts of wickedness in the heavenly places" (Eph. 6:12). Cherubim and seraphim are orders and divisions of "good" angels.

What are ministering angels?

The Bible teaches the existence of ministering angels. "Are they not all ministering spirits sent forth to minister for those who will inherit salvation?" (Heb. 1:14).

The word translated *angels* from the original Greek language is *angelos*, which carries the same meaning as "messenger." Angels apparently assume various forms, sometimes a physical human form (Gen. 18:2; Heb. 13:2). They are called "ministers" (Greek *leitourgous*) of God, i.e., servants of God. Angels are sent forth to minister for God or to serve us, God's people (Heb. 1:14). The use of the present participle here, "being sent forth," emphasizes the continuance of angelic ministry. Ministering angels continue today (Psalm 91). They are sometimes called *guardian angels*.

QUESTIONS
ABOUT
THE BIBLE

What is the Bible?

The Bible is also called the Holy Bible, the Scriptures, the Sacred Scriptures, the Word of God, and the Sacred Writings. The Bible is made up of sixty-six books, thirty-nine in the Old Testament, also called the Old Covenant, and twenty-seven in the New Testament, also called the New Covenant.

Christians believe the Bible is inspired by God. It does not contain errors, being written by holy men who were guided by the Holy Spirit so that they wrote without error. What they wrote is reliable and accurate in every way.

The Bible is the Christian's guide for belief and practice, and contains the truth of God. It tells the story of how God revealed salvation to man, and how Jesus Christ provided salvation for all through His sacrificial death on the cross. One needs only to believe in Jesus Christ to be saved.

The Bible is true; and contains the truth that is revealed by God to us; however, not all truth is revealed in the Bible, for truth is found in history and the natural world. But wherever the Bible has spoken, it is truth.

What is "revelation"?

The Bible is called the "revelation of God." Technically, the word *revelation* is the act of God whereby He gives us knowledge about Himself and His work that we could not otherwise know.

How has God revealed Himself?

God has revealed Himself through visions (Isa. 6), dreams (Dan. 2), poetry (Ps. 139), biographies (the Gospels), sermons (Matt. 5), face-to-face (Deut. 5:4), by writing on stone (Deut. 10:4), through miracles (John 6), in parables (Luke 15), in compulsive desires (Acts 21:10–13), by angels (Luke 1:26–38), through historical research (Luke 1:1–4), and by Jesus Christ (John 1:14).

How much has God revealed to us about Himself?

God has not told us everything there is to know about Himself or His plan. We are *finite,* and God is *infinite*; we can never know everything about God. Deuteronomy 29:29 says, "The secret things belong to the LORD our God, but those things which are revealed belong to us and to our children forever, that we may do all the words of this law." This does not mean the Bible is incomplete or that the task of writing the Bible was poorly done. It means that God's divine revelation is complete concerning the facts of redemption. There's nothing else we need to know to get saved.

What are the different ways God reveals Himself to us?

When the wise men came from the East seeking the newborn king (Matt. 2:1–11), God must have allowed them to understand something of what He was doing. That was, in part, *general revelation* which came to them in nature. Their consciences might have influenced them to seek to worship the newborn King of the Jews. Their examination of *natural revelation* led them to Jerusalem, where they encountered *special revelation*. There they heard a verse of Scripture (Mic. 5:2) that directed them to Bethlehem. In Bethlehem, they had their *fullest revelation of God* as they worshiped the baby King, the Word that became flesh (John 1:14).

How has God used our senses in revelation?

God has communicated to people by sight (Rev. 1:19), hearing (Rev. 1:10), smell (John 11:39), taste (Ezek. 3:3, 4, 9–17), and touch/feel (1 John 1:1). This means God uses all of the senses of a person to speak to them.

Can we use philosophy to find God?

God has not revealed Himself through man's reason. We cannot find God by philosophy or human reason; we find God only through the Bible. "Beware lest anyone cheat you through philosophy and empty deceit, according to the tradition of men . . . and not according to Christ" (Col. 2:8). However, God expects us to use our reason in understanding the messages He has given to us (Isa. 1:18). Correct doctrine will always be reasonable, and it will never contradict itself, because the message of God reflects the mind of God. Hence, reason is not a means of finding truth about God, but when we use our reason we can find how He has revealed Himself to us. God invites us: "Come now, and let us reason together" (Isa. 1:18).

How has God revealed Himself in nature?

All of creation is a "fingerprint" of the Creator God. "God is revealed from heaven . . . because what may be known of God is manifest in them, for God has shown it to them" (Rom. 1:18–19). Because the world is so massive, there must be a greater power to create the world. And second, the Creator had to possess free will to begin and end the creative process. If the Creator didn't have free will, then the power of creation would have continued unabated. The Creation demonstrates there was a powerful Creator who chose to begin the creative process and end it. The Creator is the Lord God (Gen. 1:1).

How do the claims of Jesus Christ prove the Bible is the Word of God?

In the Bible, Jesus claims to be God. If His claims are false, then the Bible is mistaken, is wrong. If His claims are correct, then the Bible is correct and the Word of God is authorative. Consider the alternatives.

If Jesus' claims were false and He *knew* His claims were false, then He made a *deliberate misrepresentation*, which means Jesus was a liar, or hypocrite, or had a demon that was deceiving people. Then Jesus was a *fool* for dying for something He knew was false.

On the other hand, if Jesus made false claims but did not know it, then He was sincerely *deluded*. That means He was a lunatic or mentally deranged.

However, if His claims are true, then Jesus is Lord and people must accept Him and follow Him, or reject Him and be condemned in hell.

Is the Bible the Word of God just because it claims to be?

You cannot prove that the Bible is the Word of God by merely saying, "It claims to be the Word of God." That is a circular argument. However, over three thousand times the authors make various statements such as, "Thus saith the Lord," and, "God spoke." We would expect that if a supernatural God wrote the book, then His truthfulness would demand that He claim to be the author. Also, if God has a message to communicate to mankind, then the uniqueness of the message would demand a unique avenue of communication, that is, the Bible would be a revelation and an inerrant book. Since God demands that people believe His message, then the method of communication must have credibility, some basis for people believing it. Therefore, God not only gave people a message, but He communicated it in a way that was believable and credible. If the Bible is a fraud, people should reject it for its lack of integrity and reliability. However, if the Bible is God's book, we must accept its message and believe in its Author.

How does fulfilled prophecy prove that the Bible is the Word of God?

Only God accurately knows the future. Therefore, when the future is accurately predicted in minute detail, then the message must be from God.

What are some future events that are predicted in the Bible?

The Bible predicted the coming world empires: Babylon, Medo-Persia, Greece, and Rome. It predicted that the Messiah would be born of a virgin in Bethlehem of Judea, and that He would do miracles, preach, and die for the sins of the world. The Bible predicted that the Messiah would ride into Jerusalem upon a donkey, be betrayed for thirty pieces of silver, be buried in a borrowed tomb, and be raised from the dead. These fulfilled prophecies demonstrate that the message of the Bible is from God.

How have the enemies of Scripture tried to explain away fulfilled prophecy?

Usually they claim the books of the Old Testament were written after the predicted events occurred, suggesting that the prophetic predictions are really nothing more than historical accounts. Next, some critics try to spiritualize the prophecies, suggesting that they were not events that were actually fulfilled, but that the predictions are only allegories for today's readers.

How does the converting power of the Bible demonstrate that its message is from God?

When people read or hear the Bible with hearts willing to believe, they are convicted of their sins, converted to Jesus Christ, and their lives are transformed. Because of the vast number of Christians who testify to the transforming power of the Bible, they all demonstrate that the message of the Bible is from God.

How has the unity of the Bible demonstrated that it is a message from God?

The Bible has a message that centers on Jesus Christ, a unified theme that God loves the world, Christ died for all, and that mankind can be saved. Even though there were numerous authors (at least thirty-six) writing over approximately sixteen hundred years and representing fifty-five generations, and even though these authors represent a great diversity of occupations and ethnic/sociological backgrounds, the unified structure and theme of the Bible suggest there is one Mind who put it all together—God Himself, the Author of Scripture.

What is the inspiration of Scripture?

The inspiration is the guidance or influence of the Holy Spirit on the human writers of Scripture so that God controlled them in such a way that they wrote exactly what God wanted them to write without error (2 Tim. 3:15).

What does the word *inspiration* mean?

Inspiration comes from the Greek *theopneustos,* which means "God breathed out." The Bible says, "All Scripture is given by inspiration of God" (2 Tim. 3:16). This means God breathed or put His Spirit into/on the words of Scripture.

How did God put inspiration into Scripture?

God guided the men that wrote the Scriptures. "Holy men of God spoke as they were moved by the Holy Spirit" (2 Pet. 1:21). The word *moved* means "to be borne along." As these human authors wrote the Scriptures, the Holy Spirit was the divine Author guiding them in the process.

Does inspiration apply to each word of the Bible?

Yes, the "words" of the Word of God were put there by God. Paul says, "Now we have received, not the spirit of the world, but the Spirit who is from God, that we might know . . . not in words which man's wisdom teaches but which the Holy Spirit teaches" (1 Cor. 2:12–13). Notice that the Holy Spirit's influence extends to the words of Scripture. The New Testament suggests that God wrote the Scriptures through human authors by such statements as, "For David himself said by the Holy Spirit . . ." (Mark 12:36).

Did Jesus believe in the authority and inspiration of Scripture?

Yes, Jesus appealed to the Scriptures as His authority each time He said, "It is written" (Matt. 4:1–11). When Jesus said, "The Scripture cannot be broken" (John 10:35), He was saying a person cannot treat a historical event in the Bible as though it never happened. Then Jesus said there was accuracy in the letters of the words: "For assuredly, I say to you, till heaven and earth pass away, one jot or one tittle will by no means pass from the law till all is fulfilled" (Matt. 5:18). The jot and tittle were parts of a word, such as the dot of an *i* or the crossing bar on a *t.* Jesus was suggesting that even letters in words were accurate and authoritative.

How did God inspire the Bible?

The Hebrew Christians were told, "God, who at various times and in various ways spoke in time past to the fathers by the prophets, has in these last days spoken to us by His Son" (Heb. 1:1–2). God used a variety of ways to reveal His inspired Word to the chosen writers, who then wrote it down for us. Sometimes these writers were aware of the significance of what they were recording and why they were writing (John 20:30–31; Rev. 1:1–3), but on other occasions, they did not realize the full truth they were communicating. Concerning those who wrote the messianic prophecy, Peter said, "To them it was revealed that, not to themselves, but to us they were ministering the things which now have been reported to you through those who have preached the gospel to you by the Holy Spirit sent from heaven— things which angels desire to look into" (1 Pet. 1:12). Peter was saying that some authors did not fully understand the message they wrote, but today we can examine its content to understand its meaning. The following chart compares some of the different ways God has used to reveal His inspired Word.

THE MANNERS OF INSPIRATION/REVELATION (Heb. 1:1)
        Dreams – Dan. 7:1
        Visions – Ezek. 1:1
        The actual voice of God – Lev. 1:1
        Symbols/object lessons – Jer. 19:1–15
        Dictation – Rev. 2:1–3:22
        Eyewitness reports – 1 John 1:1–3; Rev. 1:2
        Guidance of the Holy Spirit – 2 Peter 1:21
        Experience of men/testimony – Ps. 23; 51
        Historical research – Luke 1:1–4
        Jesus Christ – John 1:14; Heb. 1:2

Even though God used a variety of different methods to produce the Bible, each verse is as inspired as the next. Every verse of Scripture is authoritative. Jesus acknowledged that not one letter or even one part of a letter would be changed until all Scripture was fulfilled (Matt. 5:18). There is no such thing as a degree of inspiration on a particular part of Scripture, so that one verse is greater or lesser than another part of Scripture. Although there were varying degrees of knowledge about the subjects on which they wrote, the authors wrote exactly what God wanted written. God used a variety of ways to give us His Word (poetry, history, testimony, law, epistles, or biography), yet every word is His Word, complete and inerrant as a result of the inspiration of the Holy Spirit (2 Tim. 3:16; 2 Peter 1:21).

What does *inerrancy* mean?

Inerrancy means that what is inspired is also authoritative.

Does the Bible teach inerrancy about itself?

The Bible teaches inerrancy. Paul wrote, "All scripture is given by inspiration of God" (2 Tim. 3:16 KJV). Peter claimed, "Holy men of God spoke as they were moved by the Holy Spirit" (2 Pet. 1:21). When New Testament writers quoted from the Old Testament, they considered themselves to be quoting God. This is seen in one of the prayers of the early church: "Lord, thou art God, which hast made heaven, and earth, and the sea, and all that in them is; who by the mouth of thy servant David hast said . . ." (Acts 4:24–25 KJV). The writer to the Hebrews wrote, "As the Holy Spirit says . . ." (Heb. 3:7) and then went on to quote David.

Even while some New Testament books were being written, other New Testament books were already recognized as Scripture. Peter wrote, "Our beloved brother Paul . . . has written to you, as also in all his epistles, speaking in them of these things, in which are some things hard to understand, which untaught and unstable people twist to their own destruction, as they do also the rest of the Scriptures" (2 Peter 3:15–16). Peter classified Paul's writings with the other Scriptures and was in fact saying Paul's writings were Scripture.

Did Jesus believe every word in the Bible was accurate?

Jesus testified to biblical inerrancy. He used the Bible authoritatively during His ministry. When He was tempted by Satan to sin, three times He said, "It is written" (Matt. 4:1–11). He appealed to the Scriptures to defend His actions (Matt. 26:54–56; Mark 11:15–17). He also claimed the "Scripture cannot be broken" (John 10:35). What He was saying was that the Scriptures cannot be treated as if events never happened.

Jesus believed every letter of Scripture was accurate. He taught, "Till heaven and earth pass away, one jot or one tittle will by no means pass from the law till all is fulfilled" (Matt. 5:18).

Most of the Old Testament was originally written in Hebrew. The *yod* was the smallest letter of the Hebrew alphabet. *Caph* and *beth* were very similar letters, distinguished only by an extended line at the base of the letter *beth*. Many Bible commentators believe that Jesus was referring to word-perfect inerrancy when He said not one "jot or tittle" would pass from the law until all was fulfilled. As far as Jesus was concerned, even the smallest letter of the alphabet or an otherwise insignificant mark distinguishing two letters would "in no wise pass from the law till all be fulfilled." Had the Bible been originally written in English, Jesus might have said, "Not one dot over an *i* or one crossing of the *t* will pass from the law." Jesus obviously believed in inerrancy.

Did Paul and the other apostles teach inerrancy?

Paul had no question that he was proclaiming the Word of God as he wrote. He told the Corinthians, "If anyone thinks himself to be a prophet or spiritual, let him acknowledge that the things which I write to you are the commandments of the Lord" (1 Cor. 14:37). John referred to his writings as "the record that God gave of his Son" (1 John 5:10 KJV).

Concerning the Old Testament authors, Peter wrote, "To them it was revealed that, not to themselves, but to us they were ministering the things which now have been reported to you through those who have preached the gospel to you by the Holy Spirit sent from heaven—things which angels desire to look into" (1 Peter 1:12).

The writers of the New Testament claimed to be speaking by the Holy Spirit. This was in fulfillment of Jesus' promise to his Disciples, "The Holy Spirit . . . will teach you all things" (John 14:26). When these men wrote, they were aware that they were speaking God's message, not that which they had themselves developed (Acts 2:4; 4:3, 31; 13:9; Gal. 1:1, 12; 1 Thess. 2:13; 4:28; Rev. 21:5, 22:6, 18–19).

Could a perfect God write an imperfect book?

The real issue of inerrancy is centered in the character of God. Some who deny inerrancy will eagerly point out that the Bible is God's revelation, but that they do not necessarily believe the Bible is completely accurate. We recognize that the Bible comes from God, and the perfect nature of God would make it impossible for Him to write a book that was not perfect. God, because He is God, could not have produced other than an inerrant revelation of Himself. If a choice is to be made, the Bible says, "Let God be true, but every man a liar" (Rom. 3:4 KJV). Twice the Bible says it is impossible for God to lie (Titus 1:2; Heb. 6:18). The divine attribute of truth is also ascribed to the Bible (Ps. 119:160; John 17:17).

Does God ever accommodate Himself to man's limited knowledge?

There were times when God responded on the basis of man's understanding of nature. When Joshua prayed for the sun and moon to stand still (Josh. 10:12), he evidently didn't understand what caused the sun and moon to move across the sky. Obviously, it was the earth's turning that God stopped, which gave the appearance of the sun and moon standing still, to give Joshua a longer day to finish the battle. But this accommodation of God to man's understanding in no way lessens the inerrancy of God's Word.

Did the church fathers believe in inspiration?

Clement of Rome (A.D. 80–100) suggested, "You have looked closely into the holy Scriptures, which are given to the Holy Spirit. You know that nothing unrighteous or falsified has been written in them."

What does the character of God teach us about inspiration?

Since God wrote the Bible, we would expect that a God who is Truth would not and cannot tell a lie; nor would He take credit for a lie. If the Scriptures were not accurate, then God would not have inspired them, and if the Scriptures had errors in them, God could not have written the Scriptures because He would be guilty of misleading readers.

What do we know about the Hebrew language?

The Old Testament was written in Hebrew, except a few passages in Daniel, written in Chaldean. Hebrew is a simple, solitary, straightforward language. It is a bold, beautiful language with descriptive words and idiomatic expressions. It has twenty-four letters, and was one of the first phonetic languages.

What do we know about the Greek language?

Of all the languages on earth, Greek is one of the most exact languages to express the minute thinking of authors. The Greek of the Bible was originally called "the Holy Spirit language," but with the discovery of a number of texts by archaeologists, the New Testament Greek was found to be the *Koine* Greek which means the common language of everyday people. God did not write the New Testament in classical Greek, which only the elite could read; God wrote it in the language of everyday people.

What do we call the original manuscripts?

They were called the *autographs,* because they were actually written by the people who claimed to be the authors.

Why were the autographs lost?

God has allowed the autographs to be lost because, like relics from the Holy Land, they would have been venerated and worshiped. So when the church was persecuted, especially during the time of Dioclesian, many autographs were destroyed. Dioclesian thought that if he could eliminate the writings of Christians, he could eliminate Christianity. Later, some autographs were lost due to the wear and tear of much use by the early church. There was a practice during the early church of copying Scriptures to be distributed to every church established throughout the Mediterranean world. When many copies were made, they didn't keep the original.

On what were the actual New Testament pages written?

Some books were written on parchment, which is a specially prepared skin of an animal. Other books were written on papyrus, a type of "paper" that was prepared from a reed that grows in marshy areas. Papyrus is also called *chartas,* a word from which we get our word *charter.*

The word *bible* does not occur in the Bible, so where did we get the word?

The word *Bible* comes from *Ta biblia,* which means "a collection of little books." Technically, the Bible is a collection of sixty-six books.

How were the pages of the Bible stored?

The Old Testament books were written on the skins of animals and rolled into a scroll. The scrolls were kept in jars to keep them dry. Some of the New Testament books were also kept in scrolls. In time, though, collections of papyrus sheets (paper) were sewn together in book form, much like we use today. Each of these was called a *codex*, which was a book in which the pages were sewn, not rolled, together.

Why did the New Testament church combine the twenty-seven individual books into one?

Because the Old Testament had been collected from thirty-nine individual books, the church did the same with the New Testament. Also, because all of the New Testament books were written by apostles and prophets, everyone wanted a copy. They were collected together and usually kept in the libraries of rich Christians or by a church. But then too, the books were about Jesus Christ, and every Christian wanted a copy because of their love for Him. Since they wanted to know everything about Jesus, they collected as many New Testament books about Him as possible. Then, as the apostles began to die, people wanted a collection of their teachings for themselves, and to pass on to others. As the churches began using the various New Testament books for public worship, they collected them together for reading in church services (Col. 4:16). As false doctrine and controversy arose, churches brought Scripture together into a collection to answer heresy. When Dioclesian (A.D. 303) ordered the destruction of all sacred books, Christians gathered them, cataloged them, and hid them for posterity.

What early manuscripts have existed until today?

First, *unical manuscripts* were those written in capital letters. Some date back as early as A.D. 200. Next, the *minuscule manuscripts* were written in small letters. Today we have over eight thousand copies of the *Latin Vulgate*, which was translated from the Greek and other early manuscripts into Latin. Scholars have gathered the *patristic citations*, which are quotations of every Scripture by the early-church fathers, demonstrating that every New Testament verse has been quoted at least once by church fathers. Over fifteen hundred *lectionaries* have been found, which are early books used for public reading and worship.

Finally from the garbage pits of the Mediterranean world, archaeologists have found a multitude of *ostraca,* which were broken pieces of pottery on which average people wrote the Scriptures. The entire Bible can be reconstructed from pieces of ostraca that were found.

What does the word *canon* mean?

The word *canon* comes from the Greek root meaning "rod," which was a measuring reed and eventually became a standard of measurement, such as our yardstick. Today, the Bible is called the *Canon.*

What is the Canon?

The Canon is the set of books that were officially recognized by the church or various church councils as Scripture.

What did "recognition of Scripture" mean?

When a church or church council recognized Scripture, that did not make that Scripture the Word of God. The church simply recognized the authority that God had *already* put in the books.

On what basis did the church or councils recognize that certain books belong in the Canon?

The councils accepted books that were written by apostles or those close to apostles as authoritative books of Scripture. Also, when Christians recognized that God spoke to them through certain books, and that those books had certain spiritual power, they concluded that those books were written under the influence of God (inspiration). These were then accepted as Scripture. Another test was whether or not the authors claimed that their writings were actually the words of God. If they made this claim, the church accepted their testimonies and recognized the books as Scripture.

What is the logical argument for the development of the Canon?

Since God had a message He wanted to reveal and chose to use multiple authors to write it, and since God knew His message would be attacked by critics and that the people who would read His message were not scholars, but average people who needed direction in life, God personally guaranteed the contents of His message and made sure that His words were accurately recorded (inspiration). The different books were compiled into one coherent unit (canon) to be transmitted to future generations, and God protected them so there would be no corruption, alteration, deletion, and/or addition to the Word of God.

Will there be new books found in the future that should be added to the Bible?

The New Testament ends with a warning against taking away or adding anything to the Word of God (Rev. 22:18–19). The book of James describes the Bible as the "complete [or perfect] law of liberty" (1:25). If God were to allow a new book to be added, that would suggest that the Bible was incomplete before, and that God did not supply to those in the past everything they needed to know. It could also suggest that God has a new revelation. Yet the book of Jude describes the Bible as "the faith which was once for all delivered" (Jude 3). This means the faith or Scriptures were once and for all delivered to the saints. We do not need an additional book of the Bible, because we do not need an additional message from God.

Why doesn't the Bible make sense to some people?

Some people look at the Bible and think they're reading a government code-book, because it doesn't make any sense at all. Why? Some people don't understand the Bible because they don't know the Author who has written the Bible. Other people are spiritually blinded so that when they read the words of the Bible on a page, they do not understand the spiritual message God has for them. Some people are too lazy to study the Bible diligently (2 Tim. 2:15), so they miss what God is saying. Finally, some haven't read enough to understand the background of the passages they are reading.

Why do some good people miss the message of the Bible?

Admittedly, some parts of the Bible are harder to understand than others. Even Peter had difficulty understanding what Paul had written (2 Peter 3:15). But some people miss the message because they have a "critical attitude." Others miss the Bible's message because they think the Bible is filled with myths, errors, and misleading statements. Other people have a "romantic attitude," looking only for words to leap off the page and make them love God more deeply. A third group has a "mystical attitude," looking for some esoteric or deeper meaning in the Bible. They do not take the words at face value, unable to interpret the Bible and apply it to their lives.

Why did God veil His message spiritually?

When unsaved people read the Bible, they cannot understand the spiritual nature of its message (2 Cor. 4:3–4). That's because they do not come to the

Bible with their hearts yielded to God. They do not want to hear what God is saying. The Scriptures are spiritually discerned, so they cannot understand it. Paul told the Jewish leaders, "Go to this people and say: 'Hearing you will hear, and shall not understand; and seeing you will see, and not perceive'" (Acts 28:26). People like this are ever hearing, but never understanding; ever seeing but never perceiving.

Some people trivialize the Scriptures and do not take them seriously. God doesn't want people to "play" with the Bible. There is a close relationship between faith and understanding the Scriptures. The Bible is called "the Word of faith," which means proper faith in God will help you understand the Bible.

What is the *King James Version* of the Bible?

The *King James Version* of 1611 and the *Authorized Version* are actually the same Bible. Translation on the King James Version was begun in 1607 and completed in 1610. The Bible did not appear in public until 1611 and was actually called "The Authorized Version," though no act of the English Parliament was ever passed approving it.

During recent decades, the spelling of the King James Version has been modernized, other misprints have been corrected, and the references in the margins have been reexamined. Recent editions have inserted an English word in the text or substituted a different English word that more closely parallels the meaning of the original Greek or Hebrew word.

The King James Version is one of the most reliable of all the versions. It reflects great faithfulness to the grammar and syntax of the Greek and Hebrew in the Old and New Testaments.

What does the Bible teach about the old covenant?

The Old Covenant was to prepare the children of Israel (Jews) for the Mediator of a better covenant (Jesus Christ, Gal. 3:24), which was established upon better promises (Heb. 8:6; Jer. 31:31). The apostle Paul noted that the law "engraved in stones . . . was to be done away" (2 Cor. 3:7 KJV). The New Covenant was new because it replaced the old (Matt. 26:28; Luke 22:7–23; 1 Cor. 11:25; Heb. 8:8–9:15). The Old Covenant law was holy, just, and good (Rom. 7:21), but the best it could do was condemn the sinner. "The letter killeth," but the "spirit giveth life" (2 Cor. 3:6–7 KJV). Sometimes the phrase *Old Covenant* is translated *Old Testament*.

The Old Covenant

a. It was mediated by Moses (Ex. 19; John 1:17; Gal. 3:19).

b. It was conditional (Deut. 28).

c. It could not produce the necessary righteousness (Heb. 8:8).

d. It was written on dead stones (Ex. 32:15).

What does the Bible teach about the new covenant?

The New Covenant is based upon an inner, spiritual change within people (salvation). This covenant is written in their hearts (Ezek. 36:26–27; 2 Cor. 3:6–18). The New Covenant is spiritually superior to the Old Covenant. All who are involved in the New Covenant know the Lord personally. The Old Covenant included a physical and national qualification (given only to Israel). The New Covenant involves complete forgiveness for all its people (all saved) (Heb. 8:12).

The New Covenant

a. It is mediated by Christ (Heb. 9:15; John 1:17).

b. It is unconditional (Heb. 8:9).

c. It can produce the necessary righteousness (Heb. 8:11).

d. It is written on living hearts (Heb. 8:10).

QUESTIONS
ABOUT
CHRISTIAN LIFE

What does the name *Christian* mean?

The name *Christian* designates those who belong to Jesus Christ, who have been saved or born again. The term *Christian* appears in the Bible three times:

"And the disciples were first called Christians in Antioch" (Acts 11:26).

"Then Agrippa said to Paul, 'You almost persuade me to become a Christian'" (Acts 26:28).

"Yet if anyone suffers as a Christian, let him not be ashamed" (1 Peter 4:16).

The term *Christian* was originally a derogatory designation for believers, given to them by unbelievers. The word *Christ*, upon which this title was constructed, suggests the most important thing about believers: They belong to Christ.

Should we as Christians expect the lost to understand why we are different?

We should not expect unsaved people to understand us. God has said, "The natural man does not receive the things of the Spirit of God, for they are foolishness to him; nor can he know them, because they are spiritually discerned" (1 Cor. 2:14). The "natural" person is a lost person, who is spiritually blinded and cannot understand the spiritual motives, values, or insights of the Christian life. No, the unsaved cannot understand the Christian and will not understand him or her apart from the aid of the Holy Spirit.

Can living people be baptized for the dead?

Those who believe this use the following verse for their proof: "Otherwise, what will they do who are baptized for the dead, if the dead do not rise at all? Why then are they baptized for the dead?" (1 Cor. 15:29).

The practice of vicarious baptism such as that which is practiced by some cults today appeared as early as the second century. It should be noted that a biblical doctrine should not be built on any verse as obscure as this one in 1 Corinthians. Since the Bible clearly teaches that baptism does not save an individual, then being baptized in the place of those who are already dead cannot benefit anyone. The interpretation of this difficult verse yields to an understanding of the Greek preposition *hyper*. Usually the word means "over" or "instead of." But there are times when the only translation possible is "concerning." The translation should be "concerning the dead." The idea is that Christian baptism concerning death and the promise of resurrection is a meaningless ordinance unless the resurrection is a reality. Paul was questioning why they were continuing to baptize new converts if there was no resurrection, since baptism symbolizes our death and resurrection.

A second interpretation of the passage is that the expression is to be taken synonymously with the meaning found in verse 30, thus being rendered "baptized with reference to the dead." This would be a *nonsacerdotal* use of the term "baptism." That is, the people of whom Paul was speaking were being literally immersed in such severe persecution that they were dying for their faith.

Is body piercing wrong?

First realize that the body of a Christian is a sanctuary, where the presence of God dwells. First Corinthians 3:16 says, "Do you not know that you are the temple of God and that the Spirit of God dwells in you?" God's purpose for your body is to glorify Him. Notice what God says about those who do not glorify Him: "If anyone defiles the temple of God, God will destroy him. For the temple of God is holy, which temple you are" (1 Cor. 3:17).

In the Old Testament, body piercing and cuttings were associated with heathen worship. "You shall not make any cuttings in your flesh for the dead, nor tattoo any marks on you: I am the LORD" (Lev. 19:28). This is technically called *markings for the dead*. It was to honor the dead, worship the dead, or for salvation of the dead. As an example, when the priests of Baal were praying for their heathen god to send fire from heaven, "They cried aloud, and cut themselves, as was their custom, with knives and lances, until the blood gushed out on them" (1 Kings 18:28). Body markings were a part of their worship to Baal, perhaps the most "sanctified" part of Baal worship, because the priests were pleading for Baal to hear their requests.

Today, it is very popular for young people to participate in body piercings, i.e., earrings on boys, nose piercing, tongue piercing, navel piercing, etc. While this social pressure may force young people to follow the example of body piercing, they must answer the question, why? The dominant practice of body piercing was introduced by rock groups, and was identified with those who were rebellious against God.

How has demonism been associated with body piercing?

On some occasions demon possession has been associated with body piercing. The place where the demon supposedly entered the body is the place where it has been pierced. Occasionally the marking on the physical body is the seal of the demon's possession. Body piercing shows ownership or association. This does not say that everyone who has body piercing is associated with demons, but many who have been demon possessed have practiced body piercing (see the following questions concerning tattoos).

Should a Christian get tattoos or support others who get tattoos?

In the Old Testament the Lord commanded His people, "You shall not make any cuttings in your flesh for the dead, nor tattoo any marks on you: I am the LORD" (Lev. 19:28). The marks that God prohibited were actually identification with the heathen religion, tribe, and/or god; acts of worshiping a heathen god; or other forms of rebellion against God. God did not want His people to identify with heathen cultures, religions, or gods. Therefore, God demanded no compromise with heathen practices. Markings in reverse indicated that the person was not a part of God's people. When a person became a follower of God, he would cover his markings out of repentance from the old, but also out of embarrassment for his former rebellion against God. The new follower wanted to be identified with God, not with the former style of life.

Should a Christian have a tattoo today?

Tattoos are also called *body art*, suggesting that God's creation of the body was not beautiful, nor was it perfect. Does a person have to add art to the body to complete the design?

The Christian should realize that his or her body is the temple of the Holy Spirit. "Do you not know that your body is the temple of the Holy Spirit who is in you . . . and you are not your own?" (1 Cor. 6:19). Since your body is God's sanctuary, where His presence dwells, many feel that putting tattoos on the human body is like putting graffiti on the church building.

In the Old Testament, when a person bought a slave, he took an awl and bored a hole in the slave's earlobe, indicating ownership. In the same way, tribes tattooed, or marked, their young for ownership. A Christian should not have tattoos because they send a mixed message. They are not telling people "God owns him." God says, "Know that your body is the temple of the Holy Spirit who is in you . . . For you were bought at a price; therefore glorify God in your body and in your spirit, which are God's" (1 Cor. 6:19–20).

What if a person already has a tattoo?

The answer is not removing the physical marks on a body; the answer is knowing God and becoming His follower. Jesus received the marks on His body (beatings, spike marks, and so forth) to become sin for us. We are cleansed by the blood of Jesus Christ (1 John 1:7). "And by His stripes we are healed" (Isa. 53:5).

Should I confess to another person after I've sinned against him or her?

When we have sinned against a brother, we should confess our sins to him. One of the recipes for confession reads, "If you hide your sin, God will reveal it; but if you confess your sins openly, God will hide it and remember it no more."

If you have sinned against a brother, you ought to confess it to him because you have wronged him. Just confessing it to God will never make it right between the two of you (Matt. 6:12). If you have sinned against God, you cannot slip back into fellowship with Him through the back door; you must come openly. The same goes for sinning against your brother. If you have sinned against him, you must come openly. Jesus said, "Therefore if you bring your gift to the altar, and there remember that your brother has something against you, leave your gift there before the altar, and go your way. First be reconciled to your brother, and then come and offer your gift" (Matt. 5:23, 24).

How wide should public confession of sin be made?

At times great revivals have been stunted because people have confessed too many sins too openly. A man had lust in his heart toward an attractive woman in the church. Both the man and the woman were married to other partners at the time. After he confessed his sin to the woman and asked her forgiveness, it opened the door for them to discuss sex. Eventually, they both divorced their mates and married each other. You shouldn't confess all sins to the public, because the public doesn't have a right to know everything that you have done. Also, the public can't handle all of the sins you have done and cannot easily forgive you. So follow this formula: *The circle of the sin determines the circle of confession.* If you have only sinned against one, confess to that person. If you have sinned to a small group, confess to them. If your sin is open and known by the whole church, confess to the whole church.

Sometimes your confession may hurt other people. The private sins of a father and husband, when openly known, may hurt the children and wife. But confessing your sins before the church can restore some of the damage done to the church. Your confession of sin demonstrates your earnest desire to be right with God and to walk with Him.

Remember, your public confession does not get you forgiveness with God. But if you are truly forgiven by God, you will want to confess your sins publicly.

If I have confessed my sins and been forgiven by God, will I be judged for them when I get to heaven?

Some feel that even though their sins are forgiven, they will still be punished for them when they get to heaven. They might quote a verse such as, "For if we would judge ourselves, we would not be judged" (1 Cor. 11:31). They believe that we need to straighten up our acts here on earth so we won't be judged in the future. But that verse does not describe our punishment at the future Great White Throne Judgment in heaven, but our being judged of Christ here on this earth. If we take care of our sins on this earth, God will not punish us on this earth.

God's future punishment in hell is not expressed against any individual who is born again. There is only one question all must answer: "Have you received My Son, Jesus Christ?" If a person is born-again, then he or she will go to heaven.

"And anyone not found written in the Book of Life was cast into the lake of fire" (Rev. 20:15). The unsaved face future punishment when God will cast the wicked into hell. Their sins will determine the severity of their punishment in hell. "And I saw the dead, small and great, standing before God, and books were opened. And another book was opened, which is the Book of Life. And the dead were judged according to their works, by the things which were written in the books" (Rev. 20:12). There are two books, or sets of books, that will be examined in judgment. First, there is *the Lamb's Book of Life.* All whose names are there will go into heaven. Those whose names are not will go to hell (Rev. 20:15). The second book(s) is the *book of works,* which determines an unsaved person's punishment in hell.

Christians will not have to answer for their sins in the future. God has separated our sins from us. "As far as the east is from the west, so far has He removed our transgressions from us" (Ps. 103:12).

Is it possible for a child of God to live in gross sin?

Yes, it is. Think of David committing adultery and murder, Samson continually committing adultery, and Ananias and Sapphira stealing, and then lying to God. By men's standards these are terrible, gross sins. However, one of the worst sins of all is to deny Jesus Christ. Perhaps Peter's denial of the Lord, accompanied by cursing, was the worst sin of all. Some would mistakenly conclude that Judas's sin was the worst of all, but remember that Judas was not a child of God.

If a person is truly born-again, he will repent after he has sinned and turn again to God. Ananias and Sapphira lied to the Holy Spirit and were struck dead. Some feel they were not saved, and that's why God took their lives. Notice that David cried out in anguish when his sin was revealed (Ps. 51). Only after Samson was put in bondage in the granary did he repent and ask God for a second chance.

Peter's denial of the Lord was followed by Jesus' question, asked three times, "Do you love Me?" (John 21:15–17). If Peter could come back from his gross sin, any Christian living today can confess his sin, repent, and come back to the Lord.

Are there degrees of sin (greater and lesser sins)?

Yes, Jesus said there was a greater sin. "Jesus answered, 'You could have no power at all against Me unless it had been given you from above. Therefore the one who delivered Me to you has the greater sin'" (John 19:11). It was a great sin for Pilate to allow Jesus to be crucified, but the religious leaders and Judas, who delivered Jesus to death, committed a greater sin than Pilate.

Even the law in the Old Testament recognizes the difference between murder and manslaughter. Manslaughter was a person unintentionally killing another. But murder was premeditated and intentional.

In the last judgment of the unsaved, they will be judged out of *the books of works.* "And I saw the dead, small and great, standing before God, and books were opened. And another book was opened, which is the Book of Life. And the dead were judged according to their works, by the things which were written in the books" (Rev. 20:12).

Two things happen at this last judgment. First, if a person's name is not found in *the Lamb's Book of Life,* he or she is condemned to hell. Then *the books of works* will be opened; that determines the individual's punishment in hell.

No matter what sin you have committed, if you turn to Jesus Christ for salvation, confessing your sin and asking for forgiveness, He can forgive every sin. If you call upon God for pardon, He will not send you to hell. Rather, eternal life will be given to you.

Is it normal to have doubts about salvation?

Yes, it is quite normal to have doubts because that is one of the devil's tools to discourage you and to motivate you to give up living for God. "But as many as received Him, to them He gave the right to become children of God, to those who believe in His name" (John 1:12). This verse says that if you receive Jesus, God will receive you. If you do one thing—accept Jesus into your heart as Savior and Master—He will do one thing: give you the privilege of becoming one of His dear children. If an individual truly repents of his sin and accepts Jesus into his heart, God says that He will accept that person (John 6:37).

Some people wait for some strange sort of feeling about salvation. Some may have a feeling of joy or a guilty feeling that produces tears. But the main feeling God wants is *sincerity*. Just be sure that you sincerely accept Jesus as your Savior.

After salvation, make public your profession of faith in Jesus Christ. Follow Jesus' example in being baptized, buried in the water and raised again, symbolically. Baptism is not a part of your salvation, but it is an act of obedience as a child of God.

Then set out to read your Bible every day. Pray. Try to witness to others, and go to church regularly so that you will keep your own heart warm and closer to the Lord. Make up your mind that you will go all out for Christ, putting Him first in your life. Try to please Him above self, all others, or above anything else. Make up your mind that you will do this for the rest of your life.

The book of 1 John is filled with practical things that Christians do. These things do not save a person, but they are good indicators that a person really is saved. So read through 1 John and circle the verses that tell things that Christians do. For example, 1 John 1:7 says, "Walk in the light as He is in the light." First John 1:9 says Christians confess their sins. First John 2:5 says Christians keep God's Word. Christians abide in God (1 John 3:6). They overcome the world (1 John 4:4). And 1 John 5:1 says Christians believe that Jesus is the Christ.

If you stumble and fall, repent and confess your sin(s) and ask God to forgive you. You can never lose your salvation, but if you have unconfessed sin, you will lose close fellowship with God.

What about people who claim to have seen Jesus?

The majority of conservative Christians say that the physical Jesus would not manifest Himself to people today, as He did in His postresurrection appearances. Since Jesus returned to heaven in the flesh, it is not necessary for people to see Jesus to understand Him, or to do His will, or to get a new message or revelation from Him. Many evangelical Christians believe that the day of revelations and visions has passed, so the day when Jesus would manifest Himself physically has passed.

Yet in every generation there are people who have claimed to have seen the physical Jesus and/or claimed Jesus has appeared to them. How can this be? First, people see in life what they want to see, and those who have a deep love and desire to see the physical Jesus may be seeing something that is not there. They see Jesus in their minds. Also, some people with mental problems may claim to see something, but what they see is an extension of their mental problems.

But can anyone say categorically that Jesus would not appear to him or her today? Jesus can do anything He wants to do, and He can appear if He chooses to do so. However, would He *choose* to appear, and is an appearance of Jesus to any person today within His plan? Probably not.

What is a miracle?

One of the best definitions of a miracle was given by C. S. Lewis: "A miracle is an interference with nature by a supernatural power." Most people today use the term *miracle* loosely. They say many things are miraculous that may be coincidental or unusual. The New Testament uses three words to describe miracles. The first word is *signs,* which are miraculous interferences with nature to authenticate a message. Second is the word *miracle,* which is a work of God that is motivated by His compassion or that demonstrates His love for people. Third is the term *wonder,* which is a demonstration of the power of God.

Is belief in eternal security necessary for a person to be saved?

No, the doctrine of eternal security does not save anyone. It is Jesus Christ that saves. A person must know the plan of salvation: (1) that the person is a sinner (Rom. 3:23), (2) that sin will be judged (Rom. 6:23), (3) that Jesus has paid the price for that sin (Rom. 5:8), and (4) that believing in Jesus Christ actually saves a person (Rom. 10:9). The book of Romans declares, "Whoever calls on the name of the LORD shall be saved" (Rom. 10:13). Therefore, *anyone* who calls upon the name of the Lord shall be saved.

The phrase *eternal security* is not in the Bible, and yet it is a point of controversy. Many Christians "fight" over it because some believe in it and others completely reject it. However, those who understand that being in Jesus Christ makes them secure have wonderful confidence and assurance. Those who do not understand that Jesus gives eternal life, which lasts forever, have missed a great joy in life. They are saved; however, they may be missing a great joy or may allow tension and doubt to take away their peace. All people who trust in Jesus Christ are saved and saved forever whether they believe in eternal security or deny it.

Does believing in eternal security give people a license to sin?

Some people say that those who believe in eternal security have a license to sin. That is, since they know they are going to heaven they don't have to live a holy and pure life here on this earth. While that may be true in someone's experience, that is not the teaching of the Bible. A person who is saved by the blood of Jesus Christ has not done any "good works" to merit salvation. His salvation is not based on works (Eph. 2: 8–9). Also, that person does not have a "right to sin." The Bible says, "These things I write to you, so that you may not sin" (1 John 2:1). And if anyone persists in sinning, the same Scripture says, "He who says, 'I know Him,' and does not keep His commandments, is a liar, and the truth is not in him" (1 John 2:4). If a person is really born-again, he will have a new desire to please God. "He who says he abides in Him ought himself also to walk just as He walked" (1 John 2:6).

A Christian should not plan on sinning, nor use any doctrine as an excuse to sin, but should plan to keep the words of Jesus: "Be perfect, just as your Father in heaven is perfect" (Matthew 5:48). But if a Christian does sin, the Bible promises, "If we confess our sins, He is faithful and just to forgive us our sins and to cleanse us from all unrighteousness" (1 John 1:9).

Is there any biblical basis for losing one's salvation?

Those who believe you can lose your salvation point to certain verses that say persistent and continual sin will lead to the judgment of God. "'Now the just shall live by faith; but if anyone draws back, My soul has no pleasure in him.' But we are not of those who draw back to perdition, but of those who believe to the saving of the soul" (Heb. 10:38–39). This verse seems to say that a person can draw back from God and go to hell.

Again, "For if you live according to the flesh you will die; but if by the Spirit you put to death the deeds of the body, you will live" (Rom. 8:13). Some believe that any Christian who follows the flesh will die, that is, will be lost forever. However, those who believe in eternal security teach that this verse means they will die physically, a premature death, because they deny the will of God for their lives.

Again, "For if we sin willfully after we have received the knowledge of the truth, there no longer remains a sacrifice for sins, but a certain fearful expectation of judgment, and fiery indignation" (Heb. 10:26–27). Some teach that those who sin after they have been saved, will end up in hell.

How do believers in eternal security respond to the statement in Hebrews 10:26–27?

Those who believe in eternal security believe that this verse is a reference to Jews in the first century who attempted to go back to the Old Testament temple in Jerusalem to sacrifice a lamb to get forgiveness of sins. If they did that, "there no longer remains a sacrifice for sins."

Again, Hebrews 6:4–6 says, "For it is impossible for those who were once enlightened, and have tasted the heavenly gift, and have become partakers of the Holy Spirit, and have tasted the good word of God and the powers of the age to come, if they fall away, to renew them again to repentance, since they crucify again for themselves the Son of God, and put Him to an open shame." Some believe that if you are once saved but turn your back on Jesus Christ, it is impossible to be saved a second time. Those who believe in eternal security teach that this is an exhortation to the Jews in Jerusalem to not return to the temple to sacrifice a lamb for the forgiveness of sins. Since Christ has taken away all sin, there is no longer the need for animal sacrifices to take away sins.

Is it possible that my name could be blotted out of the Book of Life?

The concept of having one's name blotted out of the Book of Life appears in this verse: "He who overcomes shall be clothed in white garments, and I will not blot out his name from the Book of Life; but I will confess his name before My Father and before His angels" (Rev. 3:5). This is a warning to live for God because no one knows what hour or date Jesus Christ may return. This is not a warning that your name will be blotted out of the Book of Life, or that a Christian can lose his salvation. Look at the context carefully. This is an encouragement for believers to continue serving Jesus Christ to the end. This verse does not have a *negation*, for example, "If you sin you will be blotted out." Rather, this verse has only a *positive* affirmation; Jesus says, "I will not blot out his name from the Book of Lfe, but I will confess his name before My Father."

Why do we know this? Because Jesus promised before He returned to heaven, "'Lo, I am with you always, even to the end of the age.' Amen" (Matt. 28:20).

Does the last chapter of the Bible teach that you can have your name blotted out of the Book of Life?

In the last book of the Bible, John, the writer, suggests that you cannot add to this book, nor can you take away from it. "For I testify to everyone who hears the words of the prophecy of this book: If anyone adds to these things, God will add to him the plagues that are written in this book; and if anyone takes away from the words of the book of this prophecy, God shall take away his part from the Book of Life, from the holy city, and from the things which are written in this book" (Rev. 22:18–19). These verses do not discuss whether a person can lose eternal life after he has it. Rather, they are discussing the fact that the Bible contains the only way of salvation that is available to all. If anyone adds to the gospel, or the way of salvation, that person does not understand salvation and is not saved. If a person knows the plan of salvation but adds something, like works, that person will be judged more severely by God. Those who add to the gospel are part of religions that add works, sacraments, baptism, and the like.

Those who take away from the gospel do not possess salvation (Acts 4:12). Those people who apparently know the gospel but minimize it are not saved. People who deny the Bible, question its inspiration and authority, make Jesus less than God, or make His death on Calvary less than propitious for the sins of the world will not enter heaven. Their names are "blotted out."

Will a Christian go to hell if he commits a sin that leads to his death?

No one is saved because of what he or she does in this life, nor is a person lost because of the lack of good works done in this life. Salvation is not of works (Eph. 2:8–9). A person is saved because he or she trusts in Jesus Christ for forgiveness of sin. The individual is declared righteous before God. If the person who has committed suicide trusted in Christ before he or she died, that person would obviously go to be with the Lord at death.

You do not have to wait until you die to find out if you will go to be with the Lord after death. Jesus said, "Most assuredly, I say to you, he who hears

My word and believes in Him who sent Me has everlasting life, and shall not come into judgment, but has passed from death into life" (John 5:24). This Scripture teaches that a believer "has everlasting life" while he lives. The moment a person trusts in Jesus Christ, he or she passes from death to life and has eternal life forever. So, will a rebellious Christian who gets drunk and kills himself in an automobile accident go to heaven, even though he is responsible for self-murder? Yes, because he once trusted in Jesus, and therefore "passed from death into life." The same will be true of the Christian who kills himself by chain-smoking, taking illegal drugs, contracting AIDS through illicit sex, or by any other of a dozen ways to shorten one's life.

If a Christian commits suicide, will he/she still go to heaven?

Some in the Roman Catholic Church teach that if a person commits suicide, extreme unction is not administered; hence, his sins are not pardoned (he has committed unpardonable sin). Some Protestants have been influenced by this Roman Catholic view. However, though Samson took his own life by bringing the temple of Dagon down upon himself, thus committing suicide, he is still listed in the Christian "Hall of Fame" (Hebrews 11:32). Saul is also mentioned as one who committed suicide (1 Sam. 31:1–13). Christians debate whether Saul was saved or unsaved. If King Saul was saved, then he is another who committed suicide and apparently went to heaven. So yes, a saved person who commits suicide will go to heaven.

Can a Christian live in sin all his life, die in sin, yet still go to heaven?

Some Christians believe that if you are genuinely saved, you are forgiven, and what you do in life makes no difference. Therefore, a Christian can continue in sin and go to heaven when he dies because "the blood of Jesus Christ His Son cleanses us from all sin" (1 John 1:7). Some can be turned over to Satan for the destruction of the body, that the soul may be saved (1 Cor. 5:5). This verse seems to imply that these people lived in sin, or committed a great sin, but went to heaven after they died.

Is it possible for a born-again believer to fall into sin?

John writes to believers, "My little children, these things I write to you, so that you may not sin" (1 John 2:1); he exhorts them not to sin. But he goes on to say, "If we say that we have no sin, we deceive ourselves, and the truth is not in us" (1 John 1:8). The word *sin* is singular, suggesting the sin nature. This means that if we say that we do not have a sin nature, or the ability to sin, we deceive ourselves.

Next the Bible says, "If we say that we have not sinned, we make Him a liar, and His word is not in us" (1 John 1:10). This verse says that if we claim that we do not sin at all (acts of sin), we are wrong.

God tells His children not to sin, but knows they will do so. The remedy? "If we confess our sins, He is faithful and just to forgive us our sins and to cleanse us from all unrighteousness" (1 John 1:9). God has provided forgiveness for His children who confess their sin.

Does the Bible teach sinless perfection?

One verse seems to teach sinless perfection: "Whoever has been born of God does not sin, for His seed remains in him; and he cannot sin, because he has been born of God" (1 John 3:9). In this passage the usage of the word *sin* does not mean that once a person is saved he never sins again. This verse does mean, however, that once a person is saved he no longer lives in a continual, habitual state of sin. The verb employed in the Greek for sin *(hamartian)* is in the present tense, which indicates continual action. These verses do not claim that a Christian never sins after conversion nor, for that matter, that a believer ever reaches perfection in this life. The present tense indicates the breaking of the perpetual hold of sin in the life of the believer. A better English translation is, "Whoever is born of God does not continually and habitually sin." The expression *his seed* is a reference to the divine principle of life that abides in a believer after regeneration in Christ.

Are faith healers legitimate?

The term *faith healer* is a modern invention. Some faith healers who have followed the biblical pattern of praying for the sick have in fact healed the sick. Other faith healers who claimed to have the gift of healing and attached it to prayer have healed individuals through prayer. Many evangelicals do not believe the gift of healing is given to individuals today, but they believe God heals, even using people who call themselves faith healers.

Unfortunately, there are charlatans who portray themselves as faith healers. Their purpose is probably money, power, or some other nonbiblical motive. However, some people, because of their own prayers, have been healed in meetings held by these purported faith healers, thus making an examination of anyone claiming to be a faith healer more difficult.

Is the gift of healing operative today?

Conservative Christians disagree on this topic. Most Christians would say that God heals in answer to prayer, and to take away the power of God to heal is to limit God. They would say that anything that prayer can accomplish, including healing, can be accomplished today. Therefore, the majority of evangelicals say God heals in answer to prayer.

However, many conservative Christians would say that the "gift of healing" is not operative today. They would say that a person does not have a unique gift of healing, but those who do heal do so through the power of prayer, not a personal "giftedness" that God has given to them to heal. What does this mean? Don't deny healing, but look to God through prayer for healing (James 5:14–16).

Does God heal today?

If we were to take healing out of Christianity, we would deny the essence of the Scriptures and what God has promised. The Scriptures say, "Pray one for another, that you may be healed" (James 5:16). In the same context James says, "The prayer of faith will save the sick, and the Lord will raise him up" (v. 15).

There are different responses to healing. Some have claimed to be healed, but they know their claims are misleading. Either they were never sick or were never healed. Second, some are healed psychosomatically; in other words, they thought they were sick, but were not. But when they claimed healing, they in fact were healed of a disease they didn't have. Third, there are actual supernatural answers to prayer when God healed. This third area is where God works when believers follow the principles of healing found in James 5:15–16.

What kind of healings does God do today?

Most conservative Christians feel that God heals by the neutralization of the consequences of disease and/or sin. This means God neutralizes the source of cancer, takes away the symptoms of influenza, or even takes away the symptoms of smallpox. However, conservative Christians have said the body "heals itself," and after the symptoms of the disease are taken away, nature and the body bring the person back to health.

Most conservative Christians do not believe in "miraculous creative healings" such as fingers reappearing that have been eaten off by leprosy. They believe that God may neutralize the cause of leprosy, but not that He miraculously re-creates the fingers or places them back on the hand. Conservative Christians point to Genesis 2:3, when God rested from His work of creation, concluding that God does not create today. This does not say that God could not do it, but that within the self-limitation of God, He does not do it.

God does heal through correct diagnosis and application of medicine and surgery. Since the body heals itself, sometimes God may heal the body by the deletion of food, by changing an unhealthy practice, by healthy exercise, or even through the surgical removal of a diseased organ. God may use a variety of methods, or God may do it directly, but God does heal the body.

Can God heal psychological or mental problems?

Yes, just as God heals the physical body, so can He heal the immaterial aspects of a person. When a person has emotional problems, such as depression, guilt, grief, neurosis, or psychosis, God works with the immaterial the same way He does with the material. God may use diagnosis or the counseling of a specialist, medicine, dilution of practices, and/or food to help restore normality. God may also use understanding by analysis, support groups, or books. However, God may heal a person directly without any of these means. Or God may heal through the use of the Scriptures, the Holy Spirit, and through the power of prayer.

Can God heal addiction?

While we don't say that God heals addiction, we do say that God delivers us from addiction. An addiction is a compulsive power that controls our attitudes, actions, and ultimately our entire lives, that expresses itself as a habit, a compulsive appetite, a predisposition, or a psychological urge that a person cannot control. We normally think of addictions as tobacco, alcohol, or drugs. However, there may be addictions to sexual literature, pornographic films, or good things that a person depends upon and cannot live without, such as television or food. A person may be addicted to gambling, compulsive spending, or a number of other things. These compulsive dependencies are healed through Scripture, prayer, fellowship with Christians who can support the victim to do and think right, acquiring new role models, changing circumstances and lifestyle, medication, professional analysis, and controlled environments, such as hospitals or institutions. In some cases, God "heals" directly without the use of these above-mentioned methods.

How should I get even when someone hurts me?

Jesus gave the proper attitude regarding vengeance when He said, "If anyone wants to sue you and take away your tunic, let him have your cloak also" (Matt. 5:40). This verse does not mean you should not defend your family, your property, or your country, but rather that you should not attempt personal revenge, even though you might use the means of the law to compensate for a personal injury.

Paul reinforces this theme: "Beloved, do not avenge yourselves, but rather give place to wrath; for it is written, 'Vengeance is Mine, I will repay'" (Rom. 12:19; see also verses 20–21).

Self-revenge has no place in the Christian life. We are told to "give place to wrath," which means you allow God to handle the situation, rather than taking revenge yourself.

You should "overcome evil with good" (Rom. 12:21). You must resist the impulse to retaliate, but do good to those who do evil to you.

Should women wear hats to attend church?

"But every woman who prays or prophesies with her head uncovered dishonors her head, for that is one and the same as if her head were shaved. For if a woman is not covered, let her also be shorn. But if it is shameful for a woman to be shorn or shaved, let her be covered. For a man indeed ought not to cover his head, since he is the image and glory of God; but woman is the glory of man" (1 Cor. 11:5–7).

During Bible times, women covered their heads with a cloth, hood, or heavy veil. The head covering was symbolic, indicating the authority that exists over the woman—her husband. During the time of the writing of 1 Corinthians, it was not uncommon for prostitutes to shave their heads and wear wigs, thus signifying their availability. They were not under authority.

Some interpret this verse to mean women should wear hats to attend church. Others interpret this verse to mean women should have longer hair than men. I believe that the long hair of the woman satisfies the requirement for the covering of a woman's head.

What does the Bible say about women wearing jewelry?

The Bible says a woman's attraction should not be her jewelry, her clothes, or her hairdo, but a meek and quiet spirit. Peter wrote in 1 Peter 3:1–4 that women should be in subjection to their husbands and their husbands should love them because of their inner beauty, not because of outer beauty. Many people take 1 Timothy 2:9 and 1 Peter 3:3 to mean one should never wear jewelry. This is not what these verses are saying. They are merely saying jewelry should not be the main attraction of a person. A Christlike image should be that which attracts the attention of other people.

What does the Bible teach about smoking?

It has been proven that using tobacco is harmful to the body, and Christians are exhorted not to harm their bodies. Some Christians use tobacco and harm their bodies because they have not yielded this matter to God, just as other Christians have not surrendered in the matter of eating too much or the matter of eating wrong things.

The Bible teaches that the Christian should take care of his or her body because it is the temple of God, and the Holy Spirit dwells within the heart and body of every child of God: "Do you not know that you are the temple of God and that the Spirit of God dwells in you? If anyone defiles the temple of God, God will destroy him. For the temple of God is holy, which temple you are" (1 Cor. 3:16–17).

Notice from these verses that God insists that we do not defile ourselves in any way (including smoking) because His Holy Spirit lives in us: "Or do you not know that your body is the temple of the Holy Spirit who is in you, whom you have from God, and you are not your own? For you were bought at a price; therefore glorify God in your body and in your spirit, which are God's" (1 Cor. 6:19–20).

Why do innocent people have to suffer?

First of all, no one is completely innocent. We are born into this world sinners (Ps. 51:5), and as sinners, we have a sin nature and are introduced into a world that is infected by sin (Gen. 3:1–21). So at birth we take on the liability of sin and live in an atmosphere of sin, where the consequences of sin (disease, accidents, vicious people, etc.) will affect us. This means people suffer because they live in a sinful world. God is not punishing them. Neither is God the cause of their pain and sufferings.

But God may allow suffering to bring us closer to Him. When people hurt physically, they cry out for God; they do the same with mental and emotional problems.

Look at Jesus. He is the only innocent person to ever live, and look at His suffering. He was Truth, but they accused Him of telling lies. He and the Father were One, yet they accused Him of blasphemy. The Scriptures say, "He was led as a lamb to the slaughter . . . so He opened not His mouth" (Isa. 53:7).

Through our suffering, we are delivered from self-reliance. We think we can solve all our problems until we suffer; then, we learn to pray and ask for God's help.

Does the Bible teach that tongues shall cease? (1 Cor. 13:8)

Paul includes the following statement in the "Love Chapter" (1 Corinthians 13): "Love never fails. But whether there are prophecies, they will fail; whether there are tongues, they will cease; whether there is knowledge, it will vanish away" (v. 8).

Historically, most Christians have taught that this verse means the spiritual gift of tongues will stop sometime after Paul writes this passage.

Charity never faileth (Greek *ekpipto,* means "falls off"; see Luke 16:17). Unlike the leaf of the flower, love never fades and falls off (James 1:11; 1 Peter 1:24). *Prophecies, they shall fail* ("be abolished"). *Tongues, they shall cease.* The significance of the Greek word *pauo* indicates that tongues would soon be "cut off" as a necessity after the New Testament revelation ceased. Those who hold this view teach that tongues are never mentioned again in the New Testament after the warning of 1 Corinthians. *Knowledge, it shall vanish away* ("be abolished"). This is the same word used in reference to prophecy above. Those who think tongues will cease teach that it happens when the miraculous gift of knowledge to write the Scriptures ceases and biblical revelation is complete.

Other Christians (charismatics and pentecostals) do not believe this teaches the cessation of tongues in this life. Rather, these things will cease when the Lord Jesus returns and perfect love is manifested in the world. They teach that prophecies, tongues, and knowledge will not be needed when we are in the presence of God but are needed and beneficial today.

What is the unpardonable sin, and who commits it?

The unpardonable sin was first mentioned by Jesus when the Pharisees rejected the miracles that He did. Jesus knew their thoughts and said, "Therefore I say to you, every sin and blasphemy will be forgiven men, but the blasphemy against the Spirit will not be forgiven men. Anyone who speaks a word against the Son of Man, it will be forgiven him; but whoever speaks against the Holy Spirit, it will not be forgiven him, either in this age or in the age to come" (Matt. 12:31–32).

There are several views concerning this unpardonable sin. First, several in the Roman Catholic Church have taught that the unpardonable sin is suicide. Since a person committing suicide can't take advantage of extreme unction or confess sins to a priest, that person has committed a sin that cannot be pardoned. Suicide is unpardonable because a person cannot take advantage of forgiveness offered by the Church.

Certain Christians believe that when they commit sins of blasphemy, rejection of God, or apostatizing, they lose their salvation. When they commit such sins, "there no longer remains a sacrifice for sins" (Heb. 10:26).

A third view held by dispensationalists is that only those who live in the time of Christ could commit the unpardonable sin. It is attributing to Satan the miracles of God as demonstrated by Jesus Christ. Since Christ no longer lives on earth, people can no longer commit this unpardonable sin.

There is a fourth view that says when people deliberately and in their hearts finally reject Jesus Christ, they are dead while they are living. That means some living people are lost and cannot be saved because they have committed the final act of rejection. Those who hold this view quote such verses as "My Spirit shall not strive with man forever" (Gen. 6:3). People who commit an unpardonable sin cross a point of no return when they reject Jesus Christ one time too many.

A last view is that the only sin God cannot forgive is the sin of unbelief. The very nature of unbelief indicates that God cannot forgive it. But anyone who wants to be saved can be saved. Even Paul the murderer was forgiven, and the thief on the cross was told, "Today you will be with Me in Paradise" (Luke 23:43). The last chapter of the Bible invites "Whoever desires, let him take the water of life freely" (Rev. 22:17). So those who want to be saved have not committed the unpardonable sin. However, if a person dies in unbelief, that person has committed a sin that cannot be pardoned; that person has committed the unpardonable sin. According to this view, no one who is living has committed the unpardonable sin.

So what is the unpardonable sin? The unpardonable sin is simply the final rejection of Jesus Christ at death.

What is a "sin unto death"?

The Bible declares there is "a sin unto death": "If anyone sees his brother sinning a sin which does not lead to death, he will ask, and He will give him life for those who commit sin not leading to death. There is sin leading to death. I do not say that he should pray about that" (1 John 5:16). This sin is committed by a Christian who grieves God by continually sinning in face of Light and the conviction of the Holy Spirit. That Christian's life is cut short; meaning, they die prematurely. It is not a reference to being lost or going to hell. A "sin unto death" is not a reference to the unpardonable sin.

John says that we should not pray for those who sin unto death. What does he mean by this? We have a right to pray for any Christian who is in sin, that God would restore him to fellowship. We also have the right to pray that God would spare him from sickness that comes because of sin (James 5:16, 17). But if God is going to take him home to heaven prematurely because of his sin, then our prayers will have no bearing on the case. We are not to pray for him.

What does the Bible teach about the will of God?

When you talk about the will of God, you must ask, "God's will about what?" God has a will or purpose about many things.

(1) God's Sovereign Will. This means that God is sovereign over His creation—God is the Almighty Ruler/Controller of the universe. In eternity past, God formulated a perfect plan for all history. God is working all things by His will after the counsel of His sovereign will (Acts 2:23; 4:27–28; Rom. 9:6–29; 1 Chron. 29:11–13).

(2) God's Redemptive Will. This involves God's grace and good pleasure for the redemption of fallen man. Jesus emphasized this when He stated, "And this is the will of Him who sent Me, that everyone who sees the Son and believes in Him may have everlasting life" (John 6:40; see also Eph. 1:3–6; 2:8–9).

(3) God's Moral Will. This term involves all the moral commands revealed to us through His commandments. This includes the biblical teachings concerning how we ought to believe and live our daily lives (Deut. 29:29; 1 Thess. 4:3; 5:18; Rom. 12:2).

(4) God's Individual Will. This involves God's will for individual lives. It has been referred to as God's "perfect" or "ideal" will or one's "life-plan."

(5) God's Permissive Will. This term involves what happens to people who step out of God's perfect will for their lives.

(6) God's Circumstantial Will. This term involves that which is not God's best, nor even God's second best for an individual's life.

Does God have a perfect will or perfect plan for each of His children?

Yes! The Bible exhorts Christians to demonstrate God's perfect will for their lives: "And do not be conformed to this world, but be transformed by the renewing of your mind, that you may prove what is that good and acceptable and perfect will of God" (Rom. 12:2).

Can people understand or find God's will for their lives?

God has commanded that we should "understand what the will of the Lord is" (Eph. 5:17). Because God commands us to understand His will, we can discover and know the will of God for our lives. God would not give us the *responsibility* to know His plan for our lives without giving us the *ability* to find and do it.

There are three steps in finding God's will. First, God's will is found through His Word, the Scriptures. God's will never contradicts Scripture. If you think you are doing the will of God, yet your life is contrary to the Bible, somewhere you have misunderstood the will of God.

Second, you can find God's will through circumstances: "And we know that all things work together for good to those who love God, to those who are the called according to His purpose" (Rom. 8:28). As an illustration, the servant Eliezer, in the will of God, found Rebekah to be Isaac's bride. He said, "As for me, being on the way, the LORD led me" (Gen. 24:27).

Third, the will of God can be found through godly counsel. "Where there is no counsel, the people fall; but in the multitude of counselors there is safety" (Prov. 11:14).

How much of your future "will of God" can you know?

Usually the will of God does not include everything that's going to happen in the future. If that were so, then God would take responsibility away from the believer. Instead God usually shows His will to us step by step and day by day. As an example, when Elijah was in the wilderness, God told him to sleep, but didn't tell him what was going to happen. Then God told him to eat, for the journey was long (forty days). Again, God did not tell him what was going to happen. When Elijah arrived at Mt. Horeb, the prophet still didn't see the entire picture. God only revealed a partial view of the future to Elijah (1 Kings 19:4–18). If God gave us His future will at one time, it would overwhelm us. If we knew the sufferings to come, the responsibilities and burdens, we would reject His will. If we knew the miracles God would do through our lives, it would feed our egos.

Is the will of God a predetermined plan for your life?

Some people teach that the will of God has been predetermined by God, right down to the smallest detail. They would say the will of God is like a complete set of blueprints for a building or a jetliner. To make sure the architect and engineers get their will done, they predetermine every aspect of the jet so it will fly. Some feel that God predetermines every part of your life in the same way.

However, this view of the will of God could be interpreted as *fatalism*, that is, the human has no responsibility for what he does, nor accountability to God for his actions. In fatalism, the human just does what is pre-planned for him.

Years ago a young ministerial student walked into a department store to buy shirts for the coming school year. As he looked at a table of shirts for sale, he bowed his head and prayed for God to lead him to the perfect shirt to buy. He wanted to be in the center of God's will. Does God's will entail what size shirt you wear? What style? What design? And what price? Is choosing shirts involved with determining the will of God? God probably does not have a "perfect shirt" for any one person to buy. A Christian should govern his life by biblical principles and make all purchases within those principles; a person should buy a shirt that fits his budget, his size, his purpose, and his wardrobe. If God determines every piece of clothing we buy, then God has determined our wardrobes. But when I look at some Christians, I know God didn't pick out their clothes.

Therefore, the will of God is a *verb*, not a *noun*. If we say the will of God is a *noun*, that means it is a fixed plan, a blueprint. If we say the will of God is a verb, it is a decision that God makes for us at the time. As an example, when it comes to buying shirts, God does not predetermine what shirts you should buy, but a decision needs to be made to determine the best shirt within the budget, style, purpose, and wardrobe. Therefore, the will of God is for you to make the best decision based on biblical principles and circumstances, a decision that will glorify and further the work of God.

Does God have a mate picked out for every person?

Some teach that there is "one man for one woman for one lifetime." By that they teach that God has a specific mate for every person, and the duty of each in life is to find that mate who will be best to carry out the will of God and bring Him glory.

Others teach that the will of God for your mate involves a *decision*, not a predetermined person. They say you must make the best decision based on existing circumstances. You are to find a mate who will be best for you to accomplish God's purpose. Those who hold this position answer that if God has a predetermined mate for you, but something happens that prevents your intersecting with your mate and you marry someone else then you marry outside the will of God. They say you marry in the *permissive will of God*. This means you don't get God's first choice, but His second choice.

The truth is that God leads each person to the best choice for a mate, which leads to the final decision. Will you accept God's choice?

What is the difference between the perfect will of God and the permissive will of God?

The Bible says the *perfect will* of God (Rom. 12:2) is exactly what God wants for your life when you follow His commandments and bring glory to Him. The *permissive will* of God is what God allows to happen, but is not God's perfect will or His *first will*. Sometimes, something you or another person does makes it impossible to carry out the *perfect will* of God. At that time God does not withhold His will from you. Rather, God gives you another chance, another opportunity called the *permissive will* of God. This is what God permits. But remember when you are living within the *permissive will* of God, God at one time had something better for you. Therefore, make sure in the future to find God's *perfect will*.

However, some people do not believe in the *permissive will* of God. They teach that God's perfect will can be done by any person at any time. When you use the word *permissive*, you are saying that God has surrendered to the human will, or to the will of people. As an illustration, when it looked as though Joseph missed the will of God because of the sins of his brothers, he was sold into slavery, and ended up first in Potiphar's house and after that, in prison. But in the *perfect will* of God, Joseph became second in command to Pharaoh in Egypt. Then he could say, "But as for you, you meant evil against me; but God meant it for good, in order to bring it about as it is this day, to save many people alive" (Gen. 50:20). Actually, while Joseph thought he was in the *permissive will* of God, he was actually in the center of God's perfect will.

How can I find God's perfect will?

First you find God's *perfect will* in the Scriptures. While God may not speak to every situation, He gives biblical principles to guide your life so that you may carry out His will. On other occasions God gives you the example of godly people in the Bible or teaches you from the Word of God how to be changed into the image of Christ. Biblical principles help guide you to find His *perfect will*.

Second, the will of God is found through prayer. You must pray and ask God to lead you to His *perfect will*. But at the same time, you must also accept what He brings into your life. Not every prayer you pray will help you find the will of God, but you cannot find it without prayer.

Third, you find the will of God in yieldedness. Some people are rebellious toward God, so He does not show them His will because they are not willing to do it. God tells us, "I beseech you therefore, brethren, by the mercies of God, that ye present your bodies a living sacrifice, holy, acceptable unto God, which is your reasonable service. And be not conformed to this world: but be ye transformed by the renewing of your mind, that ye may prove what is that good, and acceptable, and perfect, will of God" (Rom. 12:1–2 KJV). If you are not yielded to God, He will not show you His will; therefore, you have no chance to do it. If you had a friend who would not do what you told him to do, would you waste your time giving your friend your advice or counsel? No! Neither does God show His will to His children who are unyielded. You cannot find God's will without yielding to His will.

Fourth, you find God's *perfect will* through the spiritual gifts that have been given to you. We all have spiritual gifts, special abilities to help us serve God. God's *perfect will* is for you to use the combination of spiritual gifts He has given you, in the best possible way, for the best possible results. You cannot be in the will of God if you ignore the spiritual gifts given to you or try to use gifts you don't have.

Fifth, you will find the will of God in talking with godly people (Prov. 11:14). While an individual Christian may lead you astray, look to the counsel of many mature Christian friends who love you, know the Word of God, and want the best for you. These are the ones who can help you find God's will. However, remember that all parties can agree but still be wrong. (The consensus at one time was that the world was flat!) Everyone but Paul wanted to abandon the ship, but Paul understood what the will of God was concerning the physical safety of those aboard the ship (Acts 27).

Finally, God's will is found through circumstances. To understand His will for you, look where God has placed you in life. If you are born to African parents in the heart of Africa, God's will for you is not to live in China, nor to be raised like a Russian. You should be raised like an African to live as best you can in Africa to glorify God. Therefore, in finding the future will of God for your life, look in the rearview mirror. What God has done for you in the past is predictive of how He wants you to live in the future.

Is it the will of God for everyone to go to Bible college?

No, those who go to Bible college usually are people with (1) an opportunity to attend, (2) a great desire to serve God, (3) a great hunger to learn the Bible, and (4) a desire to go into full-time Christian service. While it would be good for every Christian to attend Bible college because of what he would learn about the Bible, it is not God's will that all go to Bible college. God wants some people to go into secular fields; He has not called everyone into full-time Christian service. He wants some to begin early in life to perfect their secular vocations to which God has called them to be. God also wants certain young people to go to a university so they get a proper foundation to enter medical school or law school or some profession to which they are called.

Can we miss the will of God by following the examples of other Christians?

Sometimes Christians follow the example of another godly Christian, but what worked for *that* godly Christian does not work for the others. As an illustration, George Mueller built orphanages by faith and never asked for money. All he did was send out a magazine telling of great answers to prayer. Some people believe Mueller had more faith to raise money than almost any other Christian. Some have followed Mueller's example and never asked for money, and their work faltered or collapsed. Why? Because they didn't have adequate finances. God's plan is to ask the Lord through prayer and ask others: "Yet you do not have because you do not ask" (James 4:2).

There are some people who get up very early in the morning to pray. When other Christians try to follow their example, they may not be effective because they're not "morning people." Rather, they are most wide-awake late at night, and could easily spend their evening hours praying to God. Hence, they are most effective *not* following the "morning person." God's will for one person may be different for another. However, all people should pray: "Men always ought to pray and not lose heart" (Luke 18:1).

Can I be in the will of God when I do things contrary to Scripture?

Sometimes people *feel* that they know God's will because of an internal urge or certainty. However, when your *urge* or *certainty* is contrary to the Bible, make sure that you have correctly interpreted the Bible, and faithfully follow the Word of God. As an example, a young woman may pray about marrying an unsaved man simply because she loves him, is attracted to him, or for some other reason. However, God tells the Christian to be separate from the unsaved (2 Cor. 6:14–18). God clearly says, "Do not be unequally yoked together with unbelievers" (v. 14).

The same goes with bartending. Can a Christian pray about the will of God to be a bartender? Even if a Christian feels a desire for the job, and circumstances seem to be leading him to the job, the Bible says, "Woe to him who gives drink to his neighbor, pressing him to your bottle, even to make him drunk" (Hab. 2:15). This seems to say that a Christian can never be responsible for giving any alcoholic beverage to another person.

Should I enter a good "doorway" if I don't know the doorway is God's will?

Sometimes Christians have difficulty finding the will of God. Then a great opportunity opens up to them and they are not sure whether they should take that opportunity or not. Many opportunities come to every believer that are usually not decided by Scripture, prayer, or any other Christian resource. Simply ask and answer, "Is this a good opportunity?"

How can a Christian determine whether an act or attitude is acceptable or unacceptable?

The following principles will guide such a believer when facing decisions about acts or attitudes that he/she feels are questionable:

An act or attitude is against the revealed will of God if it is contrary to Scripture.

An act or attitude is wrong if it is against biblical principles.

An act or attitude is wrong if it will hurt my body or destroy the testimony of God through my body.

An act or attitude is wrong if it will harm other people or believers.

An act or attitude is wrong if it is fleshly motivated and not spiritually motivated.

An act or attitude is wrong if it will draw me away from fellowship with God.

Lot, Abraham's nephew, chose outwardly, making a bad choice. When the land was before Abraham and Lot, Lot chose the portion that was well watered. The best soil was in the valley. He chose the land with cities and civilization nearby. Lot chose with the outward eye, and it seems as though he made the best choice. However, when Lot isolated himself from believers (specifically Abraham), and associated with sinful people, he brought a rebellious attitude into his home, so that some of his children would not follow him when danger was lurking. Lot ended up destroying his present family and his future family influence (Genesis 19).

Is it possible to jump ahead of God's plan and miss the will of God?

It seems all of life is timing. Sometimes people are not willing to wait for God's timing, which may be natural timing or the laws of nature. As an illustration, if you plant your seeds too early, they might freeze in the snow. If you plant them too late, they might burn up in the hot summer sun. God promised Abraham a son, but Abraham and Sarah ran before the timing of God. Abraham and Hagar gave birth to Ishmael (literally, "wild horse"), and the seed of Ishmael has been a thorn in the side of Abraham to this day. When you seek the will of God, also seek to know the right time to implement His will.

Am I in the will of God if I have difficulties?

Some people enjoy the will of God when they're in church, when God is answering their prayers, or when they are fellowshipping with other Christians. But what about when they have difficulties? What about when there has been an accident, their house has burned down, or a serious disease or bankruptcy comes to call? Are they still in the will of God?

Job was a wealthy man who had everything going for him. He had material wealth: land, resources, servants, a wonderful family, and a wife. But then Satan asked God to remove the "hedge" that protected Job (Job 1:10). First, God allowed Satan to take away all of Job's physical assets and family. Next, God allowed Satan to take away his physical health. God's one restriction was, "He is in your hand, but spare his life" (2:6). Even Job's wife wanted him to "curse God and die" (2:9).

Notice Job's response: "'Shall we indeed accept good from God, and shall we not accept adversity?' In all this Job did not sin with his lips" (2:10). He remained in the will of God even in his trouble.

For reasons unknown to us, money, health, and other resources are sometimes taken away from God's children. That does not necessarily mean one is out of the will of God. And when God prospers His children, it is not always physical or financial prosperity. However, God's prosperity is always *spiritual*, whether we have money or not. God wants us to *walk with Him* and *fellowship with Him*. That is true prosperity!

What was Job's conclusion? "Though He slay me, yet will I trust Him" (13:15). Job was yielded to the will of God.

Think of all the sufferings of Paul. He was beaten, stoned, imprisoned, shipwrecked, robbed, and continually criticized and verbally attacked. Paul called it his "light affliction" (2 Cor. 4:17). But what did he see as its purpose? "A far more exceeding and eternal weight of glory" (2 Cor. 4:17 KJV). Paul could say, "For I have learned in whatever state I am, to be content" (Phil. 4:11). And why was he content? Because his heart, cry, and passion was "that I may know Him and the power of His resurrection, and the fellowship of His sufferings, being conformed to His death" (Phil. 3:10).

There have been a host of missionaries—David Livingstone, Hudson Taylor, and many others—who have gone into great difficulties; yet God took care of all their needs. God's spirit will never lead you where God's grace will not provide for you.

Should you pray for the will of God for others?

Because the will of God is good, perfect, and acceptable (Rom. 12:2), every person should be in the will of God. However, just because you pray for them to be in the will of God does not mean that every person is submissive to God, nor will all do the will of God. Nonetheless, you should pray for all people, as did Paul, "The will of the Lord be done" (Acts 21:14).

Should parents pray for the will of God in the lives of their children?

Yes! Every parent should want his or her children to do the will of God. No parent wants his/her children to suffer from disease, financial difficulties, or accidents, but it is much better to have a child prosper spiritually *in* the will of God than to have him prosper physically or financially *outside* the will of God. Jesus says, "And do not fear those who kill the body but cannot kill the soul. But rather fear Him who is able to destroy both soul and body in hell" (Matt. 10:28).

Is it God's will for every person to marry?

In certain cultures there are great societal pressures put on all young men and women to marry. At the same time, in other situations pressure is put on young men and women *not* to marry. This is the same question that was asked of Jesus by His disciples: "It is better not to marry?" (Matt. 19:10). Jesus went on to say that there were three answers why people did not marry: "For there are some unmarried people which were born from their mother's womb and there are some unmarried people which are physically made that way, and there are others who have made themselves unmarriageable, because of their commitment to the kingdom of heaven" (Matt. 19:12, author's translation). This verse seems to tell us that God has predetermined that it is God's will for some not to marry; they are born that way. Second, some people are not married because of circumstances (disease, poverty, incarceration, a particular vocation, or other situations). Finally, others have committed themselves to not marry for the kingdom of God. These have chosen to be single for Christian service, for instance, missionaries who have gone into extremely difficult situations where they would not take a family.

What does the Bible teach about marriage?

God intends for two people to marry who are committed to each other for life, "one man for one woman for one lifetime." No matter what the burdens and responsibilities, no matter what the tests and trials, no matter whether in youth, in middle age, or in old age, in sickness or health, God intends for a man and his wife to be faithful to each other till death parts them. Moreover, God's Word has sanctified the marriage relationship because

(1) marriage was instituted by God (Gen. 2:21–24).

(2) marriage was, and is to be, monogamous (God gave Adam only one wife—"one wife for one lifetime").

(3) the husband and wife are to be unified physically and spiritually (Matt. 19:6).

(4) the husband is to be the head of the wife (Eph. 5:23); marriage is to be heterosexual (a homosexual marriage does not fit God's standards in the light of biblical revelation).

God performed the first marriage; He sanctified and blessed the first home and the first family. "He brought her to the man . . . Therefore a man shall leave his father and mother and be joined to his wife, and they shall become one flesh" (Genesis 2:22, 24).

What does the Bible teach about Christians marrying non-Christians?

The first requirement for marriage for a Christian is that he or she marry a Christian. Paul tells us that a Christian has a right to marry "only in the Lord" (1 Cor. 7:39). Again Paul tells us, "Do not be unequally yoked together with unbelievers" (2 Cor. 6:14). A Christian should not marry someone who is not a Christian. It is dangerous for a Christian to even think about marrying someone who is not a Christian because it violates the Bible's clear commandment about marriage.

"A prudent wife is from the LORD" (Prov. 19:14). Christians should not only be determined to marry Christians, but should also earnestly seek the Lord's guidance as to *whom* to marry among those Christians. Genesis 24 gives the beautiful story of Abraham sending his spiritual and prayerful servant to search out a wife for his son Isaac who would be "of the Lord."

What authority does the husband have in the home?

God's plan for the family is that the husband be subject to Christ, the wife be in submission to the husband, and the children be in submission to the parents. The husband is not to rule over his wife as a dictator, but he does have the responsibility to make decisions on matters affecting the family. However, he should make those decisions with his wife.

Ephesians 5:25 tells us, "Husbands, love your wives, just as Christ also loved the church and gave Himself for her." In Ephesians 5:25, Colossians 3:19, and 1 Peter 3:7, we are told that the husband is to treat and love his wife as Christ loved the church and gave Himself for it. When this principle is violated, there is a tendency for the remainder of God's plan for the family to also break down. The wife will start to lose respect for her husband and rebel against his authority. The children will notice this attitude and will themselves become rebellious. Friction in the family is generated when the husband fails to genuinely love his wife and provide clear leadership in the family.

Colossians 3:18 tells us, "Wives, submit to your own husbands, as is fitting in the Lord." The wife should submit to the leadership of her husband as long as he does not violate God's will.

When God's principles are followed—the husband under the authority of Christ, the wife under the authority of the husband, and the children under the authority of the parents—and they are living their lives according to God's Word, we will always find a happy, strong, and stable family. Psalm 127:1 tells us, "Unless the LORD builds the house, they labor in vain who build it."

Does the Bible teach that a woman is equal to a man?

The equality of the sexes can be supported by examining the Scriptures: "There is neither Jew nor Greek, there is neither slave nor free, there is neither male nor female; for you are all one in Christ Jesus" (Gal. 3:28). Being "in Christ Jesus" removes all race or national distinction. Class differences vanish, and sex rivalry disappears. All are equal at the foot of the cross, and no one enjoys special privileges.

While the sexes are equal, they have different roles. There are many Scriptures that address the position of women with regard to their roles in the family and in the church (1 Cor. 14:34–35; 1 Tim. 2:11–15; 1 Peter 3:7). It should be recognized that God has placed the wife under the authority of her husband (Eph. 5:22; Col. 3:18; 1 Cor. 11:8–9). God's chain of authority within the family places the wife over the children.

A fulfilled man or woman is one who finds the will of God for his/her life and lives according to the Scriptural pattern given for him/her. Certainly, women are special. They are loved and valued by the God of the universe. The wife is to be the helper (helpmate) for her husband. It should be noted that the chain of authority exists because God instituted it, not because anyone thought it up.

QUESTIONS
ABOUT
THE CHURCH

What does the word *church* mean in the Bible?

The word *church* is used in the Scriptures in two senses: one, in a universal sense; and two, in a local sense.

In the universal sense the church consists of all those who, in this dispensation, have been born of the Spirit of God and have by that same Spirit been baptized into the body of Christ (1 Cor. 12:13). The gospel of Jesus Christ is simply His death, burial, and resurrection for the forgiveness of our sins and our justification before God (1 Cor. 15:3–4). The blood of Jesus Christ actually cleanses an individual from his sins (Eph. 1:7; Col. 1:14, 20–22; Rom. 3:25; Heb. 9:12–14; 1 John 1:7). When an individual believes the gospel and invites Jesus into his heart as his personal Savior by faith, that person automatically becomes a part of the universal church.

The second way the word *church* is used in the Bible is in the local sense. That is, a local church is a group of professed believers in any locality who have banded together to carry out the Great Commission. Thus, we read in the Bible about the church at Ephesus, the church at Corinth, the church at Galatia, the church of the Thessalonians, the church in Jerusalem, and others. In other words, once an individual accepts Jesus Christ into his heart as his personal Savior, it is God's plan for that individual to join a local church in his own area. Christians around the world are part of the universal church that the Bible describes as being the body of Christ, or the bride of Christ. Yet at the same time, the Lord wants each Christian to unite with a local church.

What is the root meaning of the word *church*?

The word *church* comes from the original word *ekklesia*, which means "assembly." The Greek *ek* means "out" and the Greek word *kaleo* means "to call." Thus, a church is an assembly of people who have been "called out" from sin and called to worship and serve God.

How is the word *church* used in the Bible?

The church is the *body of Christ* (Eph. 1:22–23; 5:23–29; Col. 1:24; 2:19), which means it is the universal, mystical, invisible, or triumphant body. The body is composed of all believers in this dispensation from Pentecost to the rapture. So the word *church* could be either singular (one local body) or plural (many churches referred to as "the church") (Acts 9:31).

The word *church* indicated an *unassembled assembly*, such as those Saul of Tarsus sought to arrest as he entered "every house" looking for Christians (Acts 8:3). It also indicated an *assembled assembly*, people who came together in one place in worship.

In Revelation 2 and 3, the "church" was *an assembly that did not belong to God*, those who practiced heresy and/or evil sins.

How is the word *church* defined?

A church is an assembly of born-again believers in whom Christ dwells by the Holy Spirit, an assembly that exists for the glory of God, under the discipline of the Word of God. It must be spiritually prepared to carry out the Great Commission. Its credibility is evident through the manifestation of spiritual gifts to nurture and reproduce itself. Hence, a local church is more than just a gathering of Christians. It must assemble for the right purpose and have the right organization and authority. It must have God's seal on its existence. When a group of Christians is characterized by these distinctives, it is a church in the biblical sense of the word.

What is the body of Christ?

The church is more than an organization; it is an organism. The life of the church is the very life of Christ Himself. Paul recognized the presence of Christ in the church when he called it "the body of Christ" on a number of occasions (1 Cor. 12:27; Eph. 1:23). Jesus observed the uniqueness of the church when He predicted, "For where two or three are gathered together in My name, I am there in the midst of them" (Matt. 18:20). Paul spoke also of Christ being the head of the Body (Eph. 4:15). While these truths are spoken of the universal body, what is true of the whole should be true of each individual part, each local church. In the same way, individuals are a part of the universal body by the Holy Spirit's work of joining us to the body of Christ: "For by one Spirit we were all baptized into one body—whether Jews or Greeks . . . and have all been made to drink into one Spirit. For in fact the body is not one member but many" (1 Cor. 12:13, 14).

Why does the Church worship on Sunday instead of Saturday?

For over fourteen hundred years the Old Testament Jews worshiped on the Sabbath (Saturday) because it was ordained in the fourth commandment (Ex. 20:8). But we observe Sunday. Why?

First of all, the greatest event in history happened on a Sunday—the Resurrection of Jesus Christ. "Now on the first day of the week, very early in the morning . . ." (Luke 24:1). We also observe Sunday because of the example of the early church, who worshiped on Sunday and were commanded to bring their tithes on Sunday (Acts 20:7; 1 Cor. 16:1–2). Jesus endorsed this practice; most of His postresurrection appearances occurred on Sundays (John 20:19–26), including His last recorded appearance: "I was in the Spirit on the Lord's Day, and I heard behind me a loud voice, as of a trumpet" (Rev. 1:10).

When the Colossians were struggling with how to observe Old Testament religious days, Paul instructed them, "So let no one judge you in food or in drink, or regarding a festival or a new moon or Sabbaths, which are a shadow of things to come, but the substance is of Christ" (Col. 2:16–17). By this Paul was telling Christians that they were under grace, not under the Law (Eph. 2:8–9; Rom 4:1–4; Gal. 3:1–5). They were no longer required to keep the Old Testament laws and dictates because the death of Christ "wiped out the handwriting of requirements that was against us, which was contrary to us" (Col. 2:14). The verse goes on to say, "And He has taken it out of the way, having nailed it to the cross." In His life Jesus perfectly kept the Law, and in His death He fulfilled the Law. When Jesus said, "It is finished," He set aside the judgment of the Law that was against us. So we no longer have to keep the Law, including the Law that relates to the Sabbath.

Sunday observance didn't catch the early church by surprise. In the Old Testament, Sunday was observed on many occasions as a *day of promise*. Three of the more important Old Testament feasts ended on Sunday: (1) The week of Passover ended on Sunday with the Feast of Firstfruits; (2) Pentecost was celebrated on Sunday, fifty days after Passover; (3) the Feast of Tabernacles ended on the eighth day, a Sunday (Leviticus 23:1–44). Finally, there is a rich stream of tradition that the Christian church has celebrated Sunday since the early-church fathers.

There has always been a group of Christian people who have celebrated the Sabbath rather than Sunday. But if they know Jesus Christ as Lord and Savior and if they accept the authority of the Bible as their standard of living, we should not judge them, but neither should we let their teaching on the Sabbath make us feel guilty or less Christian. We must not let their legalism destroy our freedom of serving Christ on the Lord's Day.

Should Christians tithe today?

Tithing was an Old Testament practice. Malachi 3:10 says, "'Bring all the tithes into the storehouse, that there may be food in My house, and try Me now in this,' says the LORD of hosts, 'if I will not open for you the windows of heaven and pour out for you such blessing that there will not be room enough to receive it.'"

First, what was established in the Old was to be carried out in the New Testament unless it was specifically prohibited. Giving to God 10 percent of one's earnings was specifically commanded in the Old Testament, and Christians are to give to God in the New Testament (Matt. 23:23; Heb. 7:8); so why not the 10 percent?

Tithing was not an issue during Bible times. Only in contemporary societies who misunderstand grace do we find people raising questions about it. Jesus described the scribes and Pharisees paying tithes (Matt. 23:23). Jesus said to not leave undone the tithe, but to observe love and mercy with the law. This proves they paid the tithe, as they were supposed to; they were just missing the weightier matters.

When we pay our tithes today, we give them to Jesus. Hebrews 7:8 says, "Here mortal men receive tithes; but there [Jesus in heaven] He receives them."

Does the Bible teach that Christians should give money to the Lord on earth?

Jesus said, "Do not lay up for yourselves treasures on earth, where moth and rust destroy and where thieves break in and steal; but lay up for yourselves treasures in heaven, where neither moth nor rust destroys and where thieves do not break in and steal. For where your treasure is, there your heart will be also" (Matt. 6:19–21). Believers have the privilege and opportunity to be a part of what God is doing in the world. Luke 6:38 says, "Give, and it will be given to you: good measure, pressed down, shaken together, and running over will be put into your bosom. For with the same measure that you use, it will be measured back to you."

When does the local church stop being a church in God's sight?

A church ceases being a New Testament church when it ceases carrying out its objective of the Great Commission, when it ceases teaching and believing biblical doctrines, when it ceases evangelizing and baptizing new converts, when it ceases serving the Lord's Table, and when a group of people allows the entrance of false teaching or sinful living. In so doing it ceases to recognize its Head, Jesus Christ; thus it stops being a New Testament church.

When did the Church begin?

Those of a reformed or covenant view say the church began with Adam or with Abraham. Other certain people believe the church began with the ministry of John the Baptist. These churches trace their baptism back to John the Baptist, teaching they are the only ones with valid baptism (hence, theirs is a valid church). Some people think the church began with the ministry of Jesus Christ when He *called* His twelve apostles together (the word *church* comes from the word "to call out"). A dispensational view accepted by another group teaches that the church began on Pentecost. Still others believe the church began somewhere in the book of Acts (these people make a separate dispensation from the Cross until an event in Acts when the gospel is taken to the Gentiles). But most people believe the church began at Calvary when the physical body of Jesus Christ was crucified for sins. Since the church is the body of Christ, it obviously began in identification with Jesus' death, burial, and resurrection.

Are denominations scriptural?

The word *denomination* does not occur in the Bible, neither is there an organizational attachment of one church to another in the Scriptures. However, there are "seeds" of the formation of denominations evident in Scripture (for instance, when the churches sent representation to the Council in Jerusalem to solve together a doctrinal problem in A.D. 15).

What is a denomination?

A denomination is a group of churches with similar doctrinal beliefs, traditions, and backgrounds, who share the same goals in ministry, desire fellowship to encourage one another, and have organically bound themselves to establish corporately in ministry what they feel they cannot bring together separately.

Are all denominations the same?

Most denominations are separated by their interpretations of doctrine. There are a few denominations that have separated over practice or methodology. A "tight" denomination exercises strong control over each local church. A "loose" denomination gives little centralized direction or control of the churches. These are sometimes called fellowships, conventions, or associations.

What is a deacon?

The Greek word *diakonia* means "a servant"; therefore, a deacon is one who serves the churches. The church at Philippi had bishops and deacons (Phil. 1:1). Paul gave instructions concerning the qualifications of deacons (1 Tim. 3:8–13).

What do deacons do?

Deacons apparently take responsibility for routine labors in the church. They smooth human relationships (Acts 6:1, 6) and they give Spirit-guided counsel. One was required to be spiritually mature to be a deacon. Deacons also cared for the widows in the early church.

What is a deaconess?

The word *deaconess* does not occur in the English Bible, but Phoebe was called a "servant," and her task was identified in the Greek text as *diakonies*, which is a feminine word for servant. Some churches feel that a deaconess is a woman married to a deacon. Other churches have a separate office for deaconesses, and they serve the church. These deaconesses are elected to their office apart from their husband. They are appointed based on their unique qualifications. Other churches do not treat *deaconess* as an office, but simply look at certain women who have the spiritual gift of serving the church.

Should deacons ever preach?

To be a deacon one had to be spiritually mature and faithful. When a deacon faithfully performed his responsibility, it led to the promotion to a larger Christian service. Philip was a faithful layman, hence, he became a deacon.

Then he became a preacher (Acts 8:5), and after successfully preaching, he became an evangelist (Acts 21:8–9). Anyone called of God to preach should preach.

What is a pastor?

The word pastor means *shepherd*, and comes from the word *poimen* used by Paul in Ephesians 4:11. Obviously, Jesus Christ is the chief Shepherd of the church, but He appoints "undershepherds" who lead, feed, and tend the church of God.

What is a bishop?

The church at Philippi had bishops (Phil. 1:1). The word comes from the Greek *episcopos*, which means "bishop," or "overseer." A bishop had the administrative responsibility of the local church and usually fulfilled that task as a pastor. Shepherds or pastors were also called bishops.

What is an elder?

The Greek word for elder, *presbyteros*, is used twenty times in the New Testament to describe a church leader. The word *Presbyterian,* as in the Presbyterian Church, comes from *presbyteri*. Elders were known for their wisdom and decision-making ability. They were called leaders in the church (1 Tim. 5:17). Those who were elders were also called bishops and shepherd/pastors.

What does the word *elder* mean?

The word *elder* is translated directly from the Greek *presbyteros*. Elders served as pastors of churches in Bible times. For instance, Timothy was the head elder (or pastor) at Ephesus. He had other elders who shared the load with him. In the churches founded by the apostles, "elder," "presbyter," and "bishop" were interchangeable designations (Acts 20:17), though not strictly synonymous. The terms *elder* or *presbyter* had primary reference to the dignity of the office and the term *bishop* had reference to its supervisory duties.

Elders already existed in the church at Jerusalem by A.D. 44 (Acts 11:30). Paul, on his first missionary journey, appointed elders in every church (Acts 14:23). The office of elder in the Christian church was evidently suggested by the office of elder among the Jews, and was invested with similar authority. Elders were associated with the apostles in the government of the church (Acts 15:2, 4, 6, 22, 23; 16:4; 21:18). They led the spiritual care of the congregation, exercising rule and giving instruction (1 Tim. 3:5,17; Titus 1:9; James 5:14; 1 Peter 5:1–4; Heb. 13:17), and were ordained to office (1 Tim. 4:14).

There were several elders in the early local church (Phil. 1:1 and Acts 11:30). As in the synagogue, so in the Christian church of apostolic times, preaching was not the peculiar function of the elders, nor was it restricted to them. They were, indeed, the regular pastors and teachers. Aptness to teach was an essential qualification for the office (1 Tim. 3:2; Titus 1:9).

In the government of many churches, the teaching elder is the minister, and the ruling elder is a layman. "Plurality of elders" means "multiple"; in other words, more than one "elder."

Who are priests?

A priest is an Old Testament term for one who ministered for God and was a mediator between God and man. A priest sacrificed to God for people. In the Old Testament, all priests came from the tribe of Levi. Now Jesus Christ is our High Priest (1 Tim. 2:5) and has fulfilled the functions for us of sacrifice, intercession, and worship to God. We come to God through Christ, not through a priest.

Does the Bible teach there should be priests today?

Many denominations use the word *priest* in reference to their pastors or ministers. While the term *priest* is an acceptable term in modern society, most evangelicals do not use the term.

Who were the apostles?

After Judas hung himself, the remaining eleven disciples felt the need to appoint someone to take Judas's place. First they established criteria for being an apostle: one who "accompanied us all the time that the Lord Jesus went in and out among us, beginning from the baptism of John" (Acts 1:21-22), which meant a candidate must have known and experienced the baptism of John. Second, an apostle had to be "a witness with us of His resurrection" (v. 22). Because of these two criteria, the majority of evangelical Christians do not believe there are apostles today.

Why do some think there are apostles today?

There is a group who believe the office of apostleship has been either continued or restored in modern days. They believe that when certain leaders have
"the signs of an apostle" (2 Cor. 12:12), which are miracles, tongues, healings,
and so forth, then those persons should be recognized as apostles. Next, they
believe that when a person comes preaching the authority of Christ with a
"word of prophecy" or "word of knowledge," he should be recognized as an
apostle because he speaks God's Word, just as the original apostles. Obviously,
their churches recognize the gift of prophecy in those who are called apostles.

What does the Bible say about prophets?

The last section of the Old Testament includes the Major Prophets (the
longer books) and the Minor Prophets (the shorter books). There are two
Hebrew words for *prophet*. The first is *roeh*, used twelve times, translated
seer. The prophet saw both the glory of God and coming judgment. He
then delivered a message from God. The second Hebrew word was *nabhi*,
meaning "announcer." This prophet heard God and announced to the
people the message of God ("Thus saith the Lord"). So a prophet was one
who gave God's message (*forthtell*), pronounced God's judgment (*foretell*),
and predicted the future (*fortell*).

The church was founded upon the "prophets and apostles" (Eph. 2:20).
A prophet was a New Testament spiritual gift: "And He Himself gave some
to be apostles, some prophets, some evangelists, and some pastors and teachers" (Eph. 4:11). Since prophets deal with the message, most conservatives
have believed that the gift of prophecy was given to those who brought and
wrote the revelation of the grace of God. They were responsible for writing
the New Testament Scriptures concerning the grace of God.

Are there prophets today?

Most conservatives believe that there are no prophets today. Since the canon
of the Scriptures has been completed and nothing is being added to the
Canon, this suggests that there is no new revelation being given today.
Therefore, there is no need for prophets who are called to announce and
write the Word of God. Conservative Christians have usually taught that
Ephesians 4:11 means apostles and prophets were given to the church only
for its foundation, to establish the original foundation of the church.

Other Christians believe that there are modern-day prophets, just as they believe there are modern-day apostles. They believe that prophets have a "word from the Lord," a "prophecy," or a "word of knowledge," which is the interpretation of biblical truth. Since they display the "signs of an apostle," they argue that there are apostles or prophets who exist today.

What is a false prophet?

The apostle John said, "Many false prophets have gone out into the world" (1 John 4:1). Who are these false prophets? "Every spirit that does not confess that Jesus Christ has come in the flesh is not of God" (1 John 4:3). At another place John says, "He is antichrist who denies the Father and the Son" (1 John 2:22). A false prophet is also a false teacher.

Most false prophets who come with false teaching usually put their positions in a positive light. They don't want people to know that their doctrines or teachings are contrary to conservative Christianity. However, when examined carefully and asked penetrating questions, you will find that at some point a false prophet has denied some essential of Christianity.

Does the Bible teach footwashing as a Church ordinance?

The majority of Protestant churches observe only two ordinances—baptism and the Lord's Supper. However, there are a few groups of churches that view footwashing as an ordinance of the church. Consequently, a highlight of their church calendar is the ceremony at which they wash each other's feet. This, to them, is a time of deep heart searching, confession of sin, and rededication to do the will of God. Those who do not recognize footwashing as a church ordinance should be careful not to condemn churches and individuals who do observe footwashing. Anything that draws an individual closer to Christ should be commended and not condemned.

The Bible passage describing the act of Jesus washing the feet of His disciples is found in John 13:1–15. This was a lesson in humility that Jesus taught His twelve disciples. Jesus taught them by example through the actions of a slave washing the feet of guests at a banquet. The occasion of the footwashing was because His disciples would not condescend (Luke 22:24–27).

Jesus Himself points out that His taking the place of a servant and washing the feet of the disciples was given as an example (John 13:14–15). He

was not initiating an ordinance of footwashing for the church, but was showing an example of humility in service. He did not command us—the
church—to perform this act, but to acquire the attitude that this activity displays (humility and service).

Those who do not wash feet as an ordinance base their belief on (1) the
lack of a commandment to the churches by Paul, (2) the lack of an example
of footwashing by churches in Scripture, (3) the true purpose of Jesus (to
teach humility), and (4) the "lesser" symbol of footwashing when compared
to the "higher" symbol of baptism and the Lord's Table. (Baptism is a symbol
of the death, burial, and resurrection of Jesus. The Lord's Table is a symbol of
His broken body and spilt blood, that is, the heart of the substitutionary
death of Christ). The symbolism of footwashing is humility, while a noble
trait is "lesser" when compared to the sacrificial death as symbolized by the
Lord's Table.

Can we call a human minister by the title "father"?

The Scripture seems to indicate we should not: "And call no man your father
upon the earth: for one is your Father, which is in heaven" (Matt. 23:9 KJV).
This passage should be taken in the context in which Jesus spoke. The first
verse of chapter 23 identifies Jesus addressing "the multitude and the disciples." Jesus was speaking about "the scribes and the Pharisees" (Matt. 23:2).
The entire twenty-third chapter gives Jesus' final condemnation of the
scribes and Pharisees as He exposed the true hostility and hypocrisy of these
religious leaders of Israel.

With this context in mind, Jesus says, "Call no man your father . . ." in
reference to human religious authority. This appears to condemn the use of
the word "father" in addressing the clergy.

You may refer to a priest as *Father* only to acknowledge the common
form of address for the office of the priest. This is an act of generic identification. But you should not reverence him or attribute to him special spiritual authority or spiritual control over your life.

What is the difference between the Roman Catholic Church and the Protestant Church?

There are many similarities between the Roman Catholic Church and the
Protestant Church: Both churches pray, use the same Bible (though Catholic

Bibles include a section known as the Apocrypha), sing some of the same hymns, and share some similar doctrines (the Trinity, inspiration of Scriptures, blood atonement, the Creation by God, and so forth). However, there are some major differences between the Roman Catholic and the Protestant Church.

First, Roman Catholics put great stock in tradition, the Church, and the Bible (making these three equal) as ultimate authority for faith and practice. Protestants disagree with tradition and the Church being ultimate authorities, believing instead in *sola scriptora*—in Scripture alone. Protestants believe that the Bible is their only rule of faith and practice.

Second, the Roman Catholics teach that salvation comes through grace, a person's cooperation with God (works), and through the sacraments. Protestants believe in salvation through Christ alone, without any addition of works, sacraments, etc.

What does the Bible teach about Communion or the Lord's Table?

God's Word teaches that only those who are saved should partake of the Lord's Supper. The Lord's Supper does not save anyone but is taken in obedience to the instructions of the Lord Jesus Christ in memory of His death until He comes again. The Lord's Table points backward to His suffering, death, and shed blood on Calvary's cross, and forward to his promised return to earth.

What is the purpose of the Lord's Supper?

On Jesus' final night with His disciples, He observed the Passover and ate the Passover meal. After dinner, He gathered His disciples around to initiate the second ordinance of the church. The church practices the Lord's Supper as a constant reminder of Christ's death on Calvary. "For as often as ye eat this bread, and drink this cup, ye do shew the Lord's death till he come" (1 Cor. 11:26 KJV). The observance of this ordinance also provides an opportunity for self-examination (1 Cor. 11:28). God provided this ordinance as one means whereby He could keep His church pure and separated from the world.

What elements are used in Communion?

God's Word teaches that the elements to be used in the Lord's Supper are unleavened bread and the fruit of the vine (grape juice). The bread symbolizes

His body and the grape juice symbolizes His shed blood. The juice does not turn into the blood of Christ, nor the bread to the body of Christ. These emblems only represent the body and blood of Christ in a symbolic and figurative sense (a memorial).

How often should one take Communion, or the Lord's Table?

The Bible does not tell us how often to partake of the Lord's Supper. The Lord Jesus simply reminded us that as often as we do partake, we remember His death on the cross for us and His promise to return to earth for us.

The Lord's Supper took the place of the Old Testament Passover. The Passover was instituted as an ordinance to commemorate the deliverance of the children of Israel from slavery in Egypt. Because the Passover was celebrated only once a year, some churches serve communion only once a year (usually at Easter).

Many churches observe the Lord's Supper weekly; others observe it once a month, or once every three months. It should be taken often enough to cause the believer to take seriously the call to reconsecrate one's life and renewed appreciation for Christ's death on the cross. Nevertheless, the Bible does not explicitly state how often we should observe the Lord's Supper.

Is it possible for Christians to celebrate Communion in a wrong manner?

The Corinthian church members were commended by Paul for their keeping of the ordinances (1 Cor. 11:2), but they were sharply criticized for their abuses in the Lord's Supper. They had been guilty of carnality (vv. 17–22). They needed to be corrected (vv. 23–26) as to the proper procedure and attitude of observing the Lord's Supper before they received chastisement from the Lord (vv. 27–34). "What! Do you not have houses to eat and drink in? Or do you despise the church of God and shame those who have nothing? What shall I say to you? Shall I praise you in this? I do not praise you" (v. 22).

"When you come together . . . it is not to eat the Lord's Supper" (1 Cor. 11:20). The church members were having a supper, but not the Lord's Supper. It was a disorderly gathering of people going through the motions. "For in eating . . . one is hungry and another is drunk" (v. 21). In the early church, the Lord's Supper was commonly preceded by a fellowship meal, later known as the "Agape Feast." Eventually these feasts were strictly forbidden at the Council of Carthage (A.D. 397). In their coming together, they were not eating together, so it could not be called "communion," and their behavior was so dishonoring to the Lord that it could hardly be called "the Lord's Supper." Some were actually getting drunk.

Is baptism taught in the Bible?

On the day of Pentecost, Peter and the other apostles preached to Jews from around the world. Each person heard the gospel in his own native tongue. Many were saved as they responded to the gospel preached that day. "Then those who gladly received his word were baptized; and that day about three thousand souls were added to them" (Acts 2:41). Baptism is the first step after salvation. Members of the New Testament church were baptized soon after conversion. The New Testament gives no illustration of an unbaptized Christian except the thief on the cross, and his yieldedness to Christ indicates he would have been baptized if given the opportunity. While baptism has no merit in securing salvation, this act of obedience is a "badge of discipleship" in which a believer publicly identifies with Christ and His church.

What is the purpose of baptism?

The first ordinance of the church is baptism. It was practiced by the church with every believer, as far as we know. As people were baptized, they were symbolically identifying with the church (Acts 2:41) and their Savior (Rom. 6:37; Gal. 2:20). Usually baptism was an evidence to their friends and neighbors that they were serious in their decision to follow Christ. It became known as a "badge of discipleship."

Should a local church exercise discipline over its members?

Whenever individuals (members of a church) cause offenses or divisions within their church, then it is the responsibility of that church to exercise church discipline.

The purpose of church discipline is to rebuke a brother or sister for causing an offense or trespass in hopes of causing them to seek repentance and to right the wrong they caused by their actions. The church has an obligation to show Christlike love and assist the individual toward cleansing, forgiveness, and restoration.

The correct procedure in church discipline is included in the following five steps:

First step: Note and mark those who are in need of discipline (2 Thess. 3:14; Rom. 16:17). Second step: Arrange a private meeting with the offender (Matt. 18:15). Third step: If this fails, set up a second meeting, this time with several other members of the church present (Matt. 18:16). During these preliminary private and semiprivate meetings, the individual should be admonished (Titus 3:10), rebuked (2 Tim. 4:2), and warned (1 Thess. 5:14). Fourth step: As a final resort, the unrepentant one is to be brought before the entire church (Matt. 18:17; 1 Tim. 5:20). Fifth step: Upon refusal to submit to church discipline, the guilty party is to be spiritually excommunicated. This constitutes two fearful things: a denial and a deliverance. When a person is disciplined, he is *denied* Christian fellowship: "Avoid" (Rom. 16:17); "Withdraw" (2 Thess. 3:6); "From such withdraw yourself" (1 Tim. 6:3, 5); "Reject" (Titus 3:10); "Do not keep company with him" (2 Thess. 3:14; 1 Cor. 5:9, 11). He is to be *delivered* over to Satan (1 Cor. 5:5; 1 Tim. 1:20).

Within the process of church discipline, all individuals are to maintain a proper heart attitude toward the individuals being disciplined. They are to avoid both vengeance and arrogance. "Brethren, if a man is overtaken in any trespass, you who are spiritual restore such a one in a spirit of gentleness, considering yourself lest you also be tempted" (Gal. 6:1).

What does the Bible say about women preachers/pastors?

Some teach that women are not to hold authority over men. "Let a woman learn in silence with all submission. And I do not permit a woman to teach or to have authority over a man, but to be in silence" (1 Tim. 2:11–12).

Those who reject "women preachers" say if a woman were to be a pastor, she would clearly be in a position of authority over the men in the church. "But I want you to know that the head of every man is Christ, the head of woman is man, and the head of Christ is God" (1 Cor. 11:3).

God gives here His divine order of the submission of woman to man, man to Christ, and Christ to God. In the matter of preaching and teaching then, the man should have the leadership role in bringing people into a better relationship and knowledge of God. This does not diminish the work of women in witnessing, teaching, counseling, and giving testimonies, etc.

Another indication of God's intention to have only men as pastors is found in the verses that describe a minister (elder, bishop). He should be the husband of only one wife (Titus 1:6 and 1 Tim. 3:2). Nothing is said about a minister having one husband. In 1 Timothy 3:5, Paul says a man should rule his house well in order to also rule the church; this supports the man as both head of home and the church.

There are others who teach women can be preachers/pastors. They point out that Philip's four virgin daughters had the God-given gift to prophesy (Acts 21:9). Deborah also was a prophetess (Judg. 4:4), as were Huldah (2 Kings 22:14) and Moses' sister, Miriam (Ex. 15:20).

Also, women were promised the gift of prophecy in the day of Pentecost (Acts 2:17) and were actually preaching on the day of Pentecost (Acts 2:18). Women preached to women and men to men.

Sarah, Ruth, and other great women of God were greatly honored and blessed by God and given mention in His Word for generations to come. Mary Magdalene, not some preacher or prophet or apostle, was chosen by Jesus as the first person to be allowed to see Him alive after His resurrection from the dead. Therefore, women have great positions of service, even the position of pastor, say those who hold this view.

Can a divorced man be a pastor of a church?

The first qualification for a pastor/bishop is, "A bishop then must be blameless, the husband of one wife, temperate, sober-minded, of good behavior, hospitable, able to teach" (1 Tim. 3:2). These verses teach that a "bishop" (an overseer of one of Christ's flocks) must be the husband of one wife. To many this verse means no divorced man shall pastor a church. Some other Christians teach these verses simply mean a pastor must be the husband of one wife at a time. They think this verse does not prohibit a man who has been divorced from serving as a pastor.

Ordained positions may be closed in some churches for those who have suffered divorce, but God can and does use divorced persons in these churches. Many are excellent witnesses for the Lord, lay evangelists, church workers, and missionaries (ordained positions are not the only tasks performed in the mission field—some mission boards use divorced persons in full-time Christian service in engineering; construction; program production for radio and television outreach; writing, printing, and distribution of literature; medical services; teaching; and administrative and clerical positions, and so forth).

However, there are other Christian churches that will take a divorced person as their pastor. When someone has truly repented of any sin or sins—

whether that person has been or is divorced or remarried—God will forgive and will use that person, within the boundaries of His Word. He wants to use each Christian to serve Him to his/her utmost. Although some doors are closed, God may open other doors of service, and it is important to remember that God's Word teaches forgiveness, acceptance, and blessings for all who turn to Him and are willing to serve Him. If you are divorced, do not spend your time looking at closed doors; find open doors and walk through them.

What is ministerial ordination?

According to the teaching of the New Testament, ordination is official recognition by a local church or Christian denomination of a member's call of God to the gospel ministry. The recognition consists of the candidate's conversion to Christ, his call to the ministry, and his conviction or beliefs. Ordination involves four aspects: First, ordination recognizes God's call to a full-time responsibility to serve the Lord. Second, ordination involves identification—the church publicly identifies itself with the man. Third, it further represents the church's judgment that the candidate has the ability to perform the duties of the gospel ministry. Fourth, ordination meets certain legal requirements in the performance of wedding ceremonies, serving as chaplain, and the like.

Should local churches be organized?

God is a God of order and organization. That is obvious as you consider the immense universe around us that was created by God. That is also obvious when you look closely at the church in the New Testament. While some may suggest there was no organization in the early church, the Bible tells us otherwise. Members were added (Acts 2:41), job descriptions were present (1 Tim. 3), votes were conducted to expel immoral members (1 Cor. 5:4), and votes were taken to elect church officers (Acts 6:5; 14:23). The church also organized a missionary team and sent them out (Acts 13:27). There may even have been some "order of service" in the early church. Paul advised, "Let all things be done decently and in order" (1 Cor. 14:40). To accomplish this task, the Holy Spirit endows certain ones with the gifts of government and leadership (Rom. 12:8; 1 Cor. 12:28). The church should be organized and equipped to carry out its purpose, which is the Great Commission.

QUESTIONS
ABOUT
CREATION

Which member of the Godhead created the earth?

All three members of the Godhead created the universe. First, the Father was involved because the Bible says, "The heavens declare the glory of God; and the firmament shows His handiwork" (Ps. 19:1). The Son was also involved: "All things were made through Him, and without Him nothing was made that was made" (John 1:3). The Holy Spirit was involved, as proved by Genesis 1:2: "The earth was without form, and void; and darkness was on the face of the deep. And the Spirit of God was hovering over the face of the waters."

What was God doing before He created the heavens and the earth?

The Trinity was fellowshipping among themselves throughout eternity past. The Bible says that Jesus was loved by the Father "before the foundation of the world" (John 17:24). Also, the Bible says, God was choosing from the foundations of the earth, "just as He chose us in Him before the foundation of the world, that we should be holy and without blame before Him in love" (Eph. 1:4). Finally, God was planning and decreeing what would come to pass: "He indeed was foreordained before the foundation of the world, but was manifest in these last times for you" (1 Peter 1:20).

What was included in the creation of the heavens?

The term *heaven* in the King James is actually plural, that is, *heavens* in other modern translations. The heavens include the whole of God's created universe— the atmosphere, stratosphere, and heaven, where the localized presence of God dwells—as well as the enumerable parts (the throne, angels, and so forth).

What is the "Big Bang Theory"?

Evolutionists have observed data that suggest that all the elements of the universe appeared simultaneously, or in their opinion, at least nearly simultaneously. Scientists also point out that the interrelatedness of the universe dictates that many elements cannot exist without the other, demanding that the universe was all created and/or appeared at the same time. The big bang theory is one argument against gradual evolutionary appearance of the earth, suggesting that the universe originated from an explosion from a single point of dense matter.

How are the apparent signs of longevity in the earth explained?

God created the world with apparent age. In other words, He created everything as it would later appear, as though the earth had been in continuous existence. Trees were not created as seeds in the ground to grow to full fruition, but each one was created with the appearance of maturity. God also created many trees at the same time, not just one tree from which all others came. And since each ring in a tree's trunk represents a year of growth, some trees were created that appeared one, ten, or more years old. The rock formations we know as stalactites and stalagmites in caves also give the appearance of age. Some of them appear to be millions of years old, because that is how they would have looked if water had seeped through the rock formations for multiple years. The burning stars of the universe were created instantaneously and the same light rays that travel at 186,000 miles per second were also created stretching from the star to the earth from millions of light miles away. God actually created the light of the stars we see each evening in process between the earth and that star.

Why do most Christians reject evolution?

Christians have taken the first chapter of Genesis at face value because it describes what God accomplished on each of the six days of Creation. To accept evolution, a Christian would have to reject the events of Creation described in the Bible.

What are the weaknesses of evolution?

First, while evolution is presented as fact, it is an unverified hypothesis, a suggested law that has not been proven, but is built on conflicting data, absence of data, and data that cannot be demonstrated. Second, scientists have never found the "missing link," the link between human and animal life. If man had evolved from a lower form, surely there would be some verifiable "link." Third, scientists claim evolution is the result of a *mutation* of the species, but mutations are the corruption of a superior to an inferior, while evolution suggests the evolving of lower forms to the human being, who is the highest of all living things. Finally, scientists have failed to identify the origin of life or matter; they cannot explain how something came from nothing.

How have some Christians tried to explain away the apparent longevity of the earth, yet still believe that God created everything?

First, there are *theistic evolutionists*, those believing that the universe was created by God, but that He used evolution to control the process.

Second, there is the *Day Age View* that the universe was created in six periods of time, each one called a "day." Supporters of this view say that each "day" could have actually been thousands or millions of years, because 2 Peter 3:8 says, "Beloved, do not forget this one thing, that with the Lord one day is as a thousand years, and a thousand years as one day."

Some believe in the *Revelatory–Pictorial Day* view, believing that God took six days to tell the story of Creation, but actually took millions of years of evolution to accomplish the process.

Others believe in *Progressive Creation*—that God created matter, but the world evolved by evolution.

Finally, some believe in the *Gap Theory:* that God created the universe millions of years ago, but when Lucifer fell, his sin destroyed everything, including the earth. They maintain that there is a gap between Genesis 1:1 and 1:2 so that "The earth was without form, and void; and darkness was on the face of the deep" (v. 2). The gap of time explains the apparent longevity of the earth.

Does the Bible teach a Gap Theory relating to Creation?

This theory teaches that in the dateless past God created a perfect heaven and a perfect earth. Lucifer (Satan) was ruler of the earth that was peopled by a race of "men." Eventually, he rebelled by desiring to become like God (Isa. 14). Because of Lucifer's fall, sin entered the universe and brought on the earth God's judgment in the form of a flood (indicated by the water of Genesis 1:2), and then a global ice age. All the plant, animal, and human fossils on the earth today date from this gap. If a gap is allowed between Genesis 1:1 and 1:2, there is ample time for the geological ages suggested by scientists in the eons of cosmic history.

The Gap Theory locates the fall of Satan between Genesis 1:1 and 1:2. In Genesis 1:1 God created a perfect and complete universe. Between Genesis 1:1 and 1:2 Lucifer's rebellion marred this perfect universe. From Genesis 1:2 on, God remolds or re-creates the earth.

What are the arguments against a Gap Theory of Creation?

The Gap Theory was (in part) a Christian attempt to reconcile the Creation account with the long periods of time suggested in the theory of evolution. But evolution itself as a theory is unscientific, defying the second law of thermodynamics.

If the Gap Theory was correct, Adam would have walked atop a gigantic fossilized graveyard. But Paul in Romans 5:12 and 8:20–22 states that Adam was the first man, so there were no humans before Adam, and that sin brought about death, even of animals.

The most natural interpretation of Genesis 1 and 2 is taking it at face value, without addition or subtraction. Isaiah 45:18 says, "[God] did not create it in vain [*tohu*], [He] formed it to be inhabited." Genesis 1:1 thus becomes a summary statement of Creation. In the first verse God tells us *what* He did. In the remaining verses He tells us *how* He did it.

What are the weaknesses of the Gap Theory?

Creation seems to be a singular act, not one divided by a long period of time. Exodus 20:11 teaches that Creation happened in six days, followed by a seventh day of rest (Sabbath). When the Bible says, "The earth was without form, and void" (Gen. 1:2), the word *was* is the Hebrew *hayeta,* which does not mean the earth *became* void, but that it was that way when created by God. The words for "form" and "void" are the Hebrew *tohu* and *bohu,* which do not mean devastation or something destroyed, but rather that nothing was there. These are empty words. Also, if there were some pre-Adamic race or civilization before the gap, it is not mentioned in Scripture. There is no redemption for those individuals. There is no support for a pre-Adamic race anywhere in Scripture. Facts seem to support a recent Creation that has apparent age.

What is the firmament?

"Then God said, 'Let there be a firmament in the midst of the waters, and let it divide the waters from the waters.' Thus God made the firmament, and divided the waters which were under the firmament from the waters which were above the firmament; and it was so. And God called the firmament Heaven. So the evening and the morning were the second day" (Gen. 1:6–8).

The word for *firmament* comes from a verb that means "to spread out." The noun in this instance is best rendered by "an expanse." *Firmament* as used in Genesis 1:6–7 refers to the atmospheric heavens immediately surrounding the earth.

Genesis 1:7 suggests a greater state of density in the original atmosphere than is the case today. Apparently a water vapor canopy encompassed the earth, creating a warmth and moisture on the earth's surface that sustained life. The explosive release of this water vapor was one of the sources of the Flood waters during Noah's time (Gen. 7:11).

"Firmament" as referred to in Genesis 1:8 must include the area above the canopy, because in verse 17 God set the sun and moon in "the firmament of the heavens to give light on the earth," seemingly the same as in verse 8 when it says, "And God called the firmament Heaven." Therefore, in a sense, you could say *firmament* refers to both water vapor (v. 6) and the atmosphere (v. 8ff).

Is the Creation story inconsistent (God created light on the first day, but He created the sun, moon, and stars on the fourth day)?

No, there is not an inconsistent report. On the first day God created "cosmic" light (Gen. 1:4); He created the existence of light. Before the first day there was neither light nor darkness, there was nothing but God. Technically, on this first day God also created darkness (Isa. 45:7).

On the fourth day God created the "light holders" (Gen. 1:14–16), the sun and moon. He also created the stars that shine in the universe, allowing them to give off light. However, light that they produce as they burn was created on the first day.

Why did God create stars?

Stars that shine in the sky are "for signs, and for seasons, and for days, and years" (Gen. 1:14 KJV). There was no time before God created anything (Gen. 1:1). Since time is the sequence of events, there were no earthly or human events before God created the world. Since time did not exist for God—no yesterday, today, and tomorrow—then there was no time in eternity past. Once God created time, He also set the earth spinning on its axis, and from human perspective people can observe the passing of time by comparing themselves to the apparent stationary positions of the moon and stars in the sky. Stars help us tell time and dates.

Why are there so many stars?

Today we are not sure how many stars there are, just as the number of stars observed a hundred years ago was nowhere near accurate. The Hubble Telescope has identified over fifty billion galaxies, each with over two hundred million stars, while the naked eye can only observe approximately three thousand stars. When God told Abraham that he would have more "seed" than the stars in the sky, Abraham could only number a few thousand. Abraham had no idea the vastness of the promise that God was making to him (Gen. 15:5–6).

What does the phrase "Let us" imply when God said, "Let us make man in Our image"? (Genesis 1:26)

This suggests the existence of the Trinity because God was speaking to Himself; there was more than one Person in the Godhead. It also suggests that God took counsel with Himself, not with angels, or anything else when He made man. But it also suggests that man is made in the mirror likeness of God. Man is not like animals, birds, fish, or vegetation. Finally, it suggests man's personality because he reflects God, who is Personhood, that is, intellect, emotion, will, self-perception, and self-direction.

What does it mean, man was made from "the dust of the ground"? (Genesis 2:7)

This suggests God used clay to form man. Man was made from the same *elements* (carbon, hydrogen, oxygen, etc.) from which both plants and animals were made. Modern science has recently determined the unity of man's physical composition, a fact originally taught in Scripture.

What did Adam know?

Adam was created without sin, and he knew everything he needed to carry out the commands of God: to multiply the race, replenish the food supply, subdue the earth, and have dominion over Creation. "And God blessed them, and God said unto them, Be fruitful, and multiply, and replenish the earth, and subdue it: and have dominion over the fish of the sea, and over the fowl of the air, and over every living thing that moveth upon the earth" (Gen. 1:28 KJV). Adam understood the physical world about him, plus social relationships, psychological reactions, and spiritual matters.

Did Adam have a navel?

Since the earth and man were created with *apparent age*, Adam had the physique and appearance of a man who was completely grown. He had hair on his head—not the hair of a baby—that gave the appearance of growth. Since a navel is a prerequisite to life, Adam had a navel.

Did God use a rib to create Eve?

While the King James Bible suggests that God used a rib to create Eve—"He took one of his ribs" (Gen. 2:21 KJV)—the Hebrew word suggests it was *bone* or *flesh,* and that God took part of Adam's side to create Eve.

Did Adam have a scar in his side?

Adam did not have a scar because God "closed up the flesh in its place" (Gen. 2:21), suggesting that in this miracle Adam was made whole.

Do modern men have one less rib than women?

The myth has been suggested that men have one less rib because God took one of Adam's ribs to create woman. However, that is a myth; both men and women have the same number of ribs. It could be possible that Adam had one less rib than others who were born into the world after him. However, when Cain, the first male child, was born, he was born with the normal number of ribs.

QUESTIONS ABOUT DEMONS

What is a demon?

A demon is a fallen angel with the power of intellect, emotion, and will. Demons are incorporeal beings who are invisible to humans. They carry out the work of the devil on this earth.

What is a demon like?

The word for demons in the Greek language is *daimon* and is found more than seventy-five times in the Greek New Testament. While it is translated *devil* in the King James Version, it refers to demons, Satan's evil angels. We know from certain Scriptures that Satan fell from heaven, and that other angelic beings shared in his fall and became evil (Ezek. 28:18; Matt. 25:41; Rev. 12:4). Demons are those fallen angels. The Bible calls them "unclean" (Matt. 10:1).

How many demons are there?

Some believe that Satan took one-third of the angels of heaven with him when he fell (Rev. 12:4). There are many, but they are not limitless.

What do demons do to Christians?

"For we do not wrestle against flesh and blood, but against principalities, against powers, against the rulers of the darkness of this age, against spiritual hosts of wickedness in the heavenly places" (Eph. 6:12). Christians are engaged in spiritual warfare with demons, who carry out the work of the devil against their lives. Demons tempt Christians to sin. They corrupt morals, prompt doubt and unbelief, and blind the minds of unbelievers (2 Cor. 4:3–4). They can also "possess" individuals to do the work of the devil.

Why are demons sometimes called "devils?"

The word *daimon* is usually translated "devils" in the King James Bible but should be better translated demons.

Where do people say demons come from?

There are a number of theories concerning the origin of demons. Among these are the following:

(1) They are spirits of deceased wicked men. This is the underlying assumption of much popular occult literature. However, this cannot be, for the Bible declares the unsaved dead are in Hades, not roaming the earth (Ps. 9:17; Luke 16:23; Rev. 20:13).

(2) They are spirits of a pre-Adamic race. Those who embrace this view believe that before the creation of Adam and Eve, there was a perfect world in which Lucifer lived. For some reason, God destroyed that world, and the spirits of those who lived in that world now inhabit the earth as demons. This is called the Gap Theory, because there was a "gap" of time after Genesis 1:1, before God re-created the world as we know it. There is no scriptural support whatsoever for this view. The Bible declares that Adam was the first man (1 Cor. 15:45).

(3) They are the children of angels from the unnatural union between angels and women. Believers in this theory base their belief on Genesis 6:4: "There were giants on the earth in those days, and also afterward, when the sons of God came in to the daughters of men and they bore children to them. Those were the mighty men who were of old, men of renown."

(4) They are fallen angels who were created when Lucifer was created and fell when he fell. This is the correct view, as seen in Matthew 25:41: "the devil and his angels."

What is the nature of demons?

Demons have a spirit nature. "They brought to Him many who were demon-possessed. And He cast out the spirits with a word" (Matt. 8:16). Demons have the same type of nature as angels, only demons are fallen angels, or evil spirits.

How are demons directed?

They are a loyal and organized kingdom under Satan. "If Satan casts out Satan, he is divided against himself. How then will his kingdom stand?" (Matt. 12:26).

How strong are demons?

In Scripture angels are called mighty (Rev. 10:1), and demons are described as having tremendous strength (Mark 5:3–4). They are powerful, but they are not omnipotent.

How smart are demons?

They have been observing and retaining knowledge since their creation. They obviously have enough intellectual ability to design and propagate various false doctrines (1 Tim. 4:1–3). They have great knowledge, but they are not omniscient.

Can demons read our thoughts or hear the prayers we pray silently?

Only the Holy Spirit is able to read our thoughts and hearts. Demons are limited in their knowledge and ability to acquire knowledge. The very nature of demons does not allow them to know our thoughts.

What freedom do demons have today?

Apparently some demons have limited freedom to operate within the permissive will of God, but others are confined in some type of restraint until the Tribulation and/or judgment seat of God. These angels God has "reserved in everlasting chains under darkness for the judgment of the great day" (Jude 6).

Why do some believe the "sons of God" in Genesis 6:2 and 4 are demons?

They are fallen angels because God's people are never called the "sons of God" in the Old Testament. The phrase "sons of God" refers to angels (Job 1:6; 2:1). The rabbis in the Old Testament and believers of the early church held that these sons of God were fallen angels who were tempting men to sexual sins with a view of corrupting the human race. The progeny of the cohabitation between the sons of God and the daughters of man had such a character to imply a supernatural-superhuman union. To say that the daughters of men were all evil and the sons of God all good doesn't quite fit the picture. There were no other "good" sons of Seth, because Noah and his family were saved in the ark. There were other Semites who were lost in the judgmental flood.

How do demons carry out their work?

The book *The Screwtape Letters* by C. S. Lewis describes the effort of one demon to hinder a person in his walk with God. On occasion in the Bible, physical afflictions are attributed to demons. For example, Jesus cast a demon out of a dumb man who immediately began to speak (Matt. 9:32–33). However, a *very small* percentage of physical problems (disease, sickness, or other physical ailments) are related to demon activity. While demons are capable of causing physical pain and suffering, do not fall into the error of attributing all physical sufferings to demons.

Some manifestations of mental diseases seem to be related to demons. We read in Luke 9:37–42 of a young boy who was possessed with a demon. The child involuntarily fell into an apparent convulsion. He was called a "lunatic" (Matt. 17:15 KJV). But after the demon was cast out, the apparent mental problem disappeared. Again, not all mental diseases are caused by demonic influences; only a small percentage is demon inspired. Mental illness is caused by a variety of other sources (relational problems, psychological problems, physical problems, and so forth).

What role do demons have in false doctrine?

Apparently many people are led astray by demonic activity, or "doctrines of demons" (1 Tim. 4:1).

What is demon possession?

There is no word for *demon possession* in the original Greek language. The phrase *demon possession* suggests a noun form, but the Greek uses a verb form, which should be translated *demonized.* Demon possession or a demonized person is demon influenced or demon controlled, or the demon directs the life of the one who is demonized.

How is a person demonized?

When a demon enters a person, it is similar in process yet opposite to the filling of the Holy Spirit. To be filled with the Holy Spirit, a person must be yielded to God, and must pray and ask for the filling. One must also have faith to believe the Spirit will fill him and act upon the filling of the Holy Spirit. In a similar yet opposite way, when a person is demonized, he desires to be controlled by demons, reads about it, seeks it, then yields himself to demonic power. Then when he has received a demon or the power of a demon, he acts upon it and expresses his demonization in various ways.

Why does there seem to be growing evidence of demonic activity in the United States that was not evident in the past?

Just as darkness fills a room when light is removed or turned off, so the darkness of demonic activity is filling the United States as the light and influence of Christianity is being removed from public places (no prayer or Bible reading in schools, no posting of the Ten Commandments, zoning, laws against churches, and so forth).

Why do some say a true child of God cannot be demon-possessed?

Because God dwells in the Christian: Jesus (Gal. 2:22), the Father (John 14:23), and the Holy Spirit (Rom. 8:11). God and demons cannot possess the same person.

Why do some people teach that a Christian *can* be demon-possessed?

Because it seems that there are illustrations in the Bible of believers who are externally harassed or influenced by demons, like King Saul. Even Paul said, "Satan hindered us" (1 Thess. 2:18).

What are transitional experiences a person has when being demonized?

Sometimes the person being demon-possessed is severely depressed, melancholy, or is given to idiocy. At other times he is thrown into paroxysms and may foam at the mouth, all the while appearing in every other respect healthy and normal. Sometimes there is no outward or physical change in the person because demonization is only inward and spiritually related.

What happens to the person who is demonized?

Usually one's physical health eventually suffers, his moral life deteriorates, and he reacts violently to any expression of true Christianity about him.

What characterizes demon possession?

Sometimes the person is entirely ignorant of everything that goes on around him while manifesting demon possession. At other times he or she displays traits of character that are utterly different from previous personality. Usually there is a complete change of moral character, and sometimes the person gives evidence of knowledge that cannot be accounted for in ordinary ways.

How does one become possessed by demons?

First of all, a person becomes *obsessed* with a demon and demonic power; second, there is a struggle for *possession* between the person and the demon; the third stage is designated *subjection* and *subservience* and the person serves the demon, developing capacities for using the demon; and finally the person is used by the demon.

What is divination?

This is the practice of killing a chicken or some small animal and perhaps observing the liver of the animal to determine the state of affairs or the direction of the immediate future. It is an illegitimate means of trying to determine the will of God.

What is necromancy?

It is an illegitimate effort to communicate and interrogate the dead. The Bible teaches that the dead are unable to communicate with the living (Luke 18:27–31). God calls the necromancer an "abomination" (Deut. 18:11–12).

What is black magic?

Black magic is used by a demon-possessed person, witch, psychic, or sorcerer to employ evil spirits to bring calamity and sorrow upon another.

What is white magic?

A demon-possessed person, sorcerer, psychic, or witch employs demonic power to do "good things" for people, usually for a small price.

Should Christians go to magic shows?

Do not confuse white magic with illusion, tricks that are done by people called "magicians." An illusionist (better termed than magician) simply entertains people, usually for a price, and does not have any power or supernatural force.

What is sorcery?

Sorcery relates to calling upon demons to create situations around people. This may include mood changing. Sometimes this is done with psychedelic drugs and is sometimes advocated in certain rock or antisocial music.

What is witchcraft?

A witch is one who makes use of magic and sorcery to accomplish the will of demons. The work of a witch is called *witchcraft,* which is directly opposed to God (Deut. 18:10).

What is an exorcist?

An exorcist is one who casts a demon(s) out of people. This person must be spiritual, having dedicated his life to God, and familiar with demonic activities. He must allow the Holy Spirit to control his life and practice when casting out demons.

What are the general steps to casting out demons?

First, there must be a choice by the demonized person for the demon to come out. Next, the possessed must decide whether he or she is going to follow God and be free of possession. The role of the exorcist is to share faith to strengthen the "choice" of the possessed person, and use his wisdom in casting out the demon. The exorcist must follow God's principles to cast out the demon, and must recognize that he has no power of his own to exorcise a demon. The blood of Jesus Christ is the only power that cleanses from sin (the possessed person's *and* the exorcist's sin).

Some feel that the demon must be exposed as a demon before he can be cast out. Others feel the demon must not be given any recognition. Whatever the case, the ultimate exorcism is not in the power of either the possessed or the exorcist, but in the power of God. The demon is cast out by the blood of Jesus Christ.

What is meant by the term "death angel?" Does the Bible actually teach that there is a "death angel?"

The actual term "death angel" is not found in the Scriptures. In reference to the meaning of the term "death angel," the Bible uses the term "destroyer," as in Exodus 12:23: "For the LORD will pass through to strike the Egyptians; and when He sees the blood on the lintel and on the two doorposts, the LORD will pass over the door and not allow the destroyer to come into your houses to strike you." The "destroyer" was the agent used in judging the first-born of the Egyptians. In the *Moffatt Version* of the Scriptures, the term "destroying angel" is used in Exodus 12:23. In 1 Corinthians 10:10, the term "the destroyer" is used: "Nor complain, as some of them also complained, and were destroyed by the destroyer."

Angels are considered executors of God's judgment. They were used by God in the destruction of Sodom and Gomorrah (Gen. 19:1; 12–13). God also used angels to deliver the plagues on Egypt (Ps. 78:43, 49). Therefore, the popular term *death angel* is used.

Can living people talk to the dead?

There are Christians who would like to talk to a deceased loved one, perhaps a child talking to a parent or a spouse talking to a dead mate. There are even television personalities who imply that they can talk to the dead. However, God condemns this practice.

"When you come into the land which the LORD your God is giving you, you shall not learn to follow the abominations of those nations. There shall not be found among you anyone who makes his son or his daughter pass through the fire, or one who practices witchcraft, or a soothsayer, or one who interprets omens, or a sorcerer, or one who conjures spells, or a medium, or a spiritist, or one who calls up the dead. For all who do these things are an abomination to the LORD, and because of these abominations the LORD your God drives them out from before you" (Deut. 18:9–12).

The dead cannot talk to those who are alive. Remember, the rich man died and wanted to warn his family about hell but was prohibited. Abraham answered the rich man's request: "'And besides all this, between us and you there is a great gulf fixed, so that those who want to pass from here to you cannot, nor can those from there pass to us.' Then he said, 'I beg you therefore, father, that you would send him to my father's house, for I have five brothers, that he may testify to them, lest they also come to this place of torment.' Abraham said to him, 'They have Moses and the prophets; let them hear them'" (Luke 16:26–29).

God has given the Scriptures to tell people all they need to know of life after death. No one needs to hear from those who have died.

Did the witch of Endor conjure up dead Samuel for King Saul?

Many Christians teach that Samuel was not brought back from the dead, but that it was just the image, spirit, or illusion of Samuel that came back from the dead, because no one can come back from the dead apart from the power of God. Apparently the witch of Endor had certain demonic powers, but demons cannot bring people back from the dead. However, Saul knew Samuel; they had a long relationship before Samuel died, and Saul should have known the "one" who appeared to him. Saul spoke to the one who appeared as though he were alive.

God can do anything He wants to do. One time He spoke through a donkey. So why couldn't God allow Samuel to return from the dead to speak to Saul through "Samuel"?

So what is the answer? Was Samuel alive or was he spirit? The answer is, it doesn't make any difference. God condemns necromancy: "When you come into the land which the LORD your God is giving you, you shall not learn to follow the abominations of those nations. There shall not be found among you anyone who makes his son or his daughter pass through the fire, or one who practices witchcraft, or a soothsayer, or one who interprets omens, or a sorcerer, or one who conjures spells, or a medium, or a spiritist, or one who calls up the dead. For all who do these things are an abomination to the LORD, and because of these abominations the LORD your God drives them out from before you" (Deut. 18:9–12).

Can the devil or demons read your mind or thoughts?

Most Christians say "no" because the devil is not omniscient (he does not know everything). Since the devil is a person, he can only know what he perceives; he receives through means of communication.

Sometimes Satan may put a thought in your mind concerning a sin, and because of your response to that thought it may appear that the devil knows your mind and how you are thinking. Because of this, some people do not pray out loud because they do not want Satan to know the projects they are attempting for God. They feel if Satan knows the things for which they are praying, he will use extra energy or manipulations to thwart their prayers from being answered.

Can a child be demon-possessed?

Some Christians believe that children cannot be demon-possessed because they are innocent—they do not know good or evil. The assumption is that a child must choose evil to be demon-possessed. However, when a father brought his son to Jesus, Jesus asked the question, "How long has this been happening to him?" (Mark 9:21). Jesus didn't need to ask that question for self-knowledge. He knew all things. He asked that question for the sake of the father and to include it in Scripture so we would know the answer. The father answered, "From a child." This implies that this boy was demon-possessed as a small child. So when a child sits before a television set and is exposed to movies, rock music, or video clips that express demonism, that child can open himself to possession.

Can a child become demon-possessed from a mother who was demon-possessed?

Technically, the process of the filling of the Holy Spirit is the same as the process of being possessed of a demon but with opposite results. This means that when a person desires to be filled, seeks the filling, reads the Scriptures about the filling, and places himself so that he can receive the filling, that person is filled with the Spirit. In the same way, for a person to be demon-possessed, the person must desire demon possession, seek demon possession, study various aspects of demon possession, and allow himself to be possessed by the demon.

If that is true, then a demon could not possess a child without the child opening himself up to the demon. However, many missionaries have testified of casting out demons that have entered a child from birth. These missionaries feel that a demon that was in the mother transferred to the child. This fulfills the Old Testament prophecy, "Visiting the iniquity of the fathers upon the children to the third and fourth generations of those who hate Me" (Ex. 20:5). But normally, most Christians feel that the person who is demon-possessed must open *himself* up to possession.

Does my godliness make the devil angry?

No, you can't "make" Satan angry. He is already angry. Because of his rebellion against God, he has suppressed anger, as well as suppressed jealousy, bitterness, and revenge. The devil has all of the negative feelings that any rebel against God would have. He is the source of the "works of the flesh" (Gal. 5:19–21) and he wants to produce these results in every person: "Now the works of the flesh are evident, which are: adultery, fornication, uncleanness, lewdness, idolatry, sorcery, hatred, contentions, jealousies, outbursts of wrath, selfish ambitions, dissensions, heresies, envy, murders, drunkenness, revelries, and the like; of which I tell you beforehand, just as I also told you in time past, that those who practice such things will not inherit the kingdom of God" (Gal. 5:19–21).

Should Christians fear the devil?

No, they should not fear the devil, because fear is part of worship. Throughout the Scriptures the believers are told to "fear God." In fact, almost every time an angel appeared, humans were fearful of the supernatural manifestation of the angelic being. They were fearful because they didn't know what it was, or perhaps they feared God, or anything that comes from God.

Christians should not be fearful of Satan; however they must respect the evil power. A person picking up a poisonous snake is not afraid of the snake if he knows how to handle it, but he still respects the danger of the snake. The same illustration holds true with electricity: Respect a wire with ten thousand volts of electricity. but don't be afraid of it. In like manner, the Christian should respect the danger of Satan and "flee [evil] things" (1 Tim. 6:11) but should also heed Christ's warning in Matthew 10:28: "Do not fear those who kill the body but cannot kill the soul. But rather fear Him who is able to destroy both soul and body in hell." Fear God only, and rely on the power of the Holy Spirit, for "He who is in you is greater than he who is in the world" (1 John 4:4).

How can a Christian overcome the fear of the devil or demons?

There are many Christians who are fearful of Satan because they have heard, "The devil will get you if you don't behave," or, "The devil will get you if you don't watch out." However, *knowing* is the first step to overcoming fear.

If a person has a serious physical problem, he might avoid going to the doctor, fearing the worst. However, when he learns the truth from the doctor and properly treats the problem, the truth casts out fear. Remember, "perfect love casts out fear" (1 John 4:18).

Fear is a controlling spirit, and "God has not given us a spirit of fear, but of power and of love and of a sound mind" (2 Tim. 1:7). So the Christian should say, "The LORD is my helper; I will not fear. What can man do to me?" (Heb. 13:6).

Has the devil stolen the fear of God?

There was a time when people feared the Lord. Unsaved people were actually fearful of what God would do to them. People were afraid to take God's name in vain, work on the Lord's Day, or commit any other vile sin for fear that God would judge them. Because fear is the first step in worship, God wants people to fear Him. He wants the worship of people.

However, the young people of today attend horror movies, play "extreme" computer-generated games, and enter into all types of activities that generate fear. Even though being "scared" is a disquieting experience, young people seek after "fear" for excitement and to fulfill sexual fantasies. People enjoy the "fear" they get from evil, black magic, demons, and other diabolical activities. Because the devil said, "I will be like the Most High" (Isa. 14:14), he wants and has stolen the fear from men that has been naturally reserved for God.

Can people be addicted to fear?

Yes, when they continually watch the scariest movies or ride the scariest roller coasters to get a "rush." Each experience is so overwhelming that they want to repeat it again and again. And like a drug, it takes a greater dose of fear to satisfy the desire for excitement each time. "Fear" can be addictive.

Why does it seem that modern people struggle with the question "Who am I?"

In the past, people in the United States had a God consciousness, and when people know who God is, they know who they are. Remember, man was made in the image of God (Gen. 1:26–27), and since we are mirror images of God, when we know God we know ourselves. But when people reject the presence and knowledge of God in their lives, as is the case today, they also lose consciousness of who they are.

What are some of the reasons people are turning to a female god?

Many women turn to a female deity because they have been hurt by men. They may have been abused, raped, abandoned, or in some way violated by the males in their lives. As a result, they may blame the heavenly Father, who is male. Notice, when people ask why God would allow starvation, cancer, or other problems in the world, they never ask why "Mother Earth" or a female deity has caused the problems. It's always a male deity that they blame. People are starving all over the earth, but they never say, "If Mother Earth is a gracious goddess, why doesn't she feed everyone?"

A Christian father must be an example to his children of the heavenly Father. He must be the "priest" in the family and pray for the family, guide the family, and lead the family to salvation. A godly Christian father gives his family a view of what the heavenly Father is like.

Can psychics or demons tell the future?

No, they cannot tell the future. Only God knows the future (Dan. 2:28), and no human or angelic created being has the power of omniscience to know all things possible or all things future. However, at times it seems as though psychics or demons can predict the future. If they know the future, or seem to predict the future, it is because of demonic influence. Remember, there was a demon-possessed girl in Philippi (Acts 16:16) that made money for her owners by telling fortunes (predicting the future). When Paul cast the demon out of the girl, she could no longer tell the future, and the owners threw Paul into prison. The point is that it appeared that the girl could predict the future.

There are two reasons why a demon appears to be able to tell the future. First, they have access to knowledge concerning things that are about to happen. For instance, they may know evil people not related to the immediate surroundings who have some association with the events that are being prophesied. As an illustration, a psychic may help find a dead body. The demon who was in that body or associated with that body (for example, the person's murderer) knows where the body is; therefore, the psychic seems to know how to find dead bodies.

Demons also have access to other demons, and through that knowledge may even know what is about to happen, perhaps evil acts planned by another demon. They also know of activities that will be caused by people controlled by demons. Therefore, demons seem to know the future. But remember, their predictions of the future are never exact; they only have inferences concerning the future.

But there's a second thing. Demons are able to manipulate the future through their supernatural power. Without having any true foreknowledge, they can predict that you are going to have an accident. But what really happens is that demons may cause another person to crash into you. You thought they knew the future accident, but they were only manipulating circumstances that influenced your future. If demons (or psychics) really knew the future, we'd never have a rollover on lotto (the state lottery). They would know the right number and win the lotto every time.

Psychics often "fish" for information to give them a "hunch" or insight into what might happen in the future. When Nebuchadnezzar had a supernatural dream from God, the magicians (psychics of his day) began to "fish" for information from Nebuchadnezzar so they might interpret his dream. They knew they couldn't interpret the dream without a little bit of data. Then they said, "There is not a man on earth who can tell the king's matter; therefore no king, lord, or ruler has ever asked such things of any magician, astrologer, or Chaldean" (Dan. 2:10). They went on to say that no one could do this, "except the gods, whose dwelling is not with flesh" (Dan. 2:11).

What is the spirit of Jezebel?

There seems to be two teachings about the *spirit of Jezebel.* Just as evil Queen Jezebel persecuted the people of God and tempted them to give up their godliness, so women shall come into the church to seduce men who are following God to make them think that illicit sex is acceptable. For example, the church at Thyatira had "symbolic" women who used sexual temptation to destroy God's work in the church: "Nevertheless I have a few things against you, because you allow that woman Jezebel, who calls herself a prophetess, to teach and seduce My servants to commit sexual immorality and eat things sacrificed to idols" (Rev. 2:20). Thus, the *spirit of Jezebel* can be any woman in any church who tempts men sexually, and justifies her temptation with her teachings.

There are some who feel that the *spirit of Jezebel* is found in certain demons who will destroy the work of God through sexual adultery and fornication. Just as some demons are given over to destroying Bible doctrine (1 Tim. 4:1), other demons are given over to destroying sexual purity (2 Tim 3:5, 6). When this demon appears, the *spirit of Jezebel* must be driven out (see questions regarding demon possession).

Do Satanists believe in God?

Yes, the Bible says, "Even the demons believe—and tremble!" (James 2:19). Many people who minister to the occult say, "I've never met a Satanist or a witch who doesn't know there is a God." The problem is their anger toward God and their rebellion against God has driven them to their evil practices. You can't rebel against something you don't know, and "rebellion is as the sin of witchcraft" (1 Sam. 15:23).

Who is more susceptible to devil worship or heathenism, a person who has never heard of God or a person who is angry at God?

Obviously, the answer is the person who is angry at God. In driving God out of one's life, one opens himself up to the only alternative to God, which is Satan.

Is there such a thing as a "good witch"?

No. Sometimes witches claim to be "good" because they can use supernatural power to heal, bless, and bring "good" things into the lives of people. Technically, this is called "white magic," which supposedly helps people, whereas "black magic" harms people. However, when a "good" witch is asked, "Can you curse me?" The answer is always, "Of course." Therefore, her "goodness" is not in her nature, but in her relationship to the person, so she can be either good or bad depending on the circumstances or whether she likes or dislike a person.

Can a witch doctor or witch do good things?

Yes, there is *white magic* and *black magic*. White magic is when a witch or witch doctor will do good things for a person, for example, heal, prosper, or bless them. A witch doctor or witch usually does "white magic" for a fee. Black magic is when a witch or witch doctor curses a person, with intent to harm or persecute that person. When a witch doctor or witch releases the power of demons or Satan upon another person, that is an illustration of "black magic."

Is *yin-yang* Christian?

No. The ancient Chinese were the originators of the "yin" and "yang." *Yin* was the feminine passive principle in nature that combined with *yang,* the masculine active principle in nature, to produce all that comes to be. Today, the idea of yin-yang is related to black magic and white magic. *Yin* is the blessing; *yang* is the curse. There is white magic through which Satan or his agent (a witch doctor or a witch) can bless a person physically, financially, or in other ways. The *yang,* or black magic, is when the agent of Satan curses, harms, or releases torments upon the person.

Can Christians believe in the "force" taught about in *Star Wars?*

No, the "force" is an extension of *Paoism,* which is an Eastern religion that teaches good versus evil, and that good always overcomes evil. However, a Christian believes in a God who has the power of personality, that is, intellect, emotion, and will. God is not an impersonal "force" that only does good or only judges evil. God loves people, and God relates to people based on His nature. God blesses people with eternal life, based on their responses to Him in repentance and faith.

While many Christians read God into the statement, "The force be with you," those words actually represent the *opposite* of Christianity. Christians using those words simply fill them with Christian meaning. Additionally, those who used the force in *Star Wars* were told, "Trust your feelings," but the child of God walks by faith, not by sight.

What should Christians understand when they see *Harry Potter* movies?

Harry Potter and other "horror" films teach that good will overcome evil, and that *good magic* will ultimately overcome *bad magic.* Notice, the issue always comes back to *magic.* However, being good has never gotten rid of demonism, and a person cannot buy his own goodness or make any choices to exorcise a demon from his or her life. Exorcism does not come from goodness; only Jesus Christ can get rid of evil, and only Jesus Christ has the power to cast a demon out of a person or an environment. Exorcism happens when Christ comes to dwell in that person or space. It is the power of God that overcomes bad magic.

Is reincarnation taught in the Bible?

One of the verses used to teach reincarnation in the Bible is John 9:1–2: "[Jesus] saw a man who was blind from birth. And His disciples asked Him, saying, 'Rabbi, who sinned, this man or his parents, that he was born blind?'" Those who believe in reincarnation point out that this man's sin caused him to be blind, that he was being punished for a sin in his or his parent's previous existence.

Reincarnation teaches that you return to pay for the sins of past lives. Judaism taught that the sins of the father influence the children (Ex. 20:5), which is implied here in John. However, each person is responsible for his or her own sins before God.

The miracle that Jesus did to give sight to the blind man had nothing to do with the sin of the father, but everything to do with the mercy and forgiveness of God. Jesus answered, "Neither this man nor his parents sinned, but that the works of God should be revealed in him" (John 9:3).

Those who believe in reincarnation say that John the Baptist is actually Elijah reincarnated because Malachi said that Elijah would return: "Behold, I will send you Elijah the prophet before the coming of the great and dreadful day of the LORD. And he will turn the hearts of the fathers to the children, and the hearts of the children to their fathers, lest I come and strike the earth with a curse" (Mal. 4:5–6). They further attest that the angel promised Zacharias that his son (John the Baptist) would embody the spirit of Elijah (Luke 1:17). But notice, this is not a reincarnation of Elijah, but the spirit of Elijah.

There are certain answers to the claim of those who believe in reincarnation. When John the Baptist was asked, "Are you Elijah?" (John 1:21), John answered, "No." This was a direct denial that he was Elijah. When they asked the direct question, "Who art thou?" he answered them, "I am 'the voice of one crying in the wilderness: "Make straight the way of the LORD,"' as the prophet Isaiah said" (John 1:23).

Before a person is reincarnated, that person must die. Elijah never died. The Scriptures said, "Elijah went up by a whirlwind into heaven" (2 Kings 2:11).

When Jesus went into the Mount of Transfiguration, notice Elijah appeared with Jesus: "Moses and Elijah appeared to them, talking with Him" (Matt. 17:3). Elijah is a distinct personality; he is not John the Baptist, which means John the Baptist was not a reincarnation of Elijah.

In addition, Hebrews 9:27 points out that "it is appointed for men to die once," negating the reincarnationist's view that you could die multiple times at the end of various lives.

Is astrology Christian?
First of all, astrology is not scientific. It is based on the belief that the sun circles the earth, when in fact the opposite is true. The earth circles the sun.

Astrology is practiced by most pagan cultures, and "Thus says the LORD: 'Do not learn the way of the Gentiles; do not be dismayed at the signs of heaven, for the Gentiles are dismayed at them'" (Jer. 10:2). We are not to look at the stars to follow them. Rather God has given us the Son, and we are to follow Him. Only Jesus knows the future, and only as we are connected to the Son do we have any confidence about the future.

Do the stars determine our destiny as claimed by the astrologers?
Throughout Scriptures when you find the word *astrologers,* they are always associated with those who deny God, who work contrary to God, and in whom there is no truth (Dan. 2:27–28).

Can we find our future by studying astrology?
When you follow astrology, you are allowing unsaved people and the spirit of this world (Satan) to have control over your life. "You are wearied in the multitude of your counsels; let now the astrologers, the stargazers, and the monthly prognosticators stand up and save you from what shall come upon you" (Isa. 47:13).

Actually, to find your future other than by God and His Word is a form of idolatry; you are replacing God with something tangible. God tells us throughout Scripture that we are to turn from idols (Lev. 19:4).

Many of the astrologists say that God used the wise men to worship Jesus, and God uses astrology today to lead "wise men" to Jesus. They quote the following: "Wise men from the East came to Jerusalem, saying, 'Where is He who has been born King of the Jews? For we have seen His star in the East and have come to worship Him'" (Matt. 2:1–2).

The star did not lead them directly to Jesus; apparently the star led them first to Jerusalem and to Herod. If the star had not led them to Herod, many children would not have been killed. But when Herod heard that there was a new babe born "King of the Jews," he sent and killed the babies in Bethlehem.

Herod and the Jews knew the Scriptures and where the Messiah was to be born. They looked at Micah 5:2, which said the child would be born in Bethlehem of Judah. Thus Herod sent them to Bethlehem.

When they left Herod, they saw the star in the sky again. This was not a natural star, for it led them to the actual home where Jesus was (Luke 2:9). The star and the wise men are not examples of astrology, but rather an example of a supernatural sign, a miracle God used in connection with the birth of His Son. They do not give us an excuse or example to use astrology today.

Can you sell your soul to the devil?

No, you can't sell what doesn't belong to you. You were born in sin, and you were a child of the devil, so you belonged to him from the beginning (John 8:44). But God has the title deed to your soul, and you can't bargain with Satan if the title deed belongs to God. "You are not your own . . . you were bought at a price" (1 Cor. 6:19–20). That price was the blood of Jesus Christ. Some people have mistakenly thought they have "sold" their souls to the devil and can't be saved today, but that is obviously not true in light of Scripture.

QUESTIONS ABOUT THE DEVIL

Who is the devil?

Originally the devil was named Lucifer, one of the angels that worshiped God. He fell because of pride. The devil is the origin of evil, the force behind evil today, and the personification of evil.

How does the devil carry out his work?

First, the devil opposes the will and work of God. Second, he tries to destroy all that is good. And third, the devil imitates the work of God. His desire is to be like the Most High (Isa. 14:14), and some of his work is to counterfeit righteousness and the work of God.

How does the devil imitate God?

First, there is a satanic Bible, and there is a church of Satan. There are also satanic ministers who do the work of Satan (2 Cor. 11:15). During the future Tribulation, it is the devil who will send the Antichrist, who will be a "substitute Christ," to perform miracles just as Jesus did.

What is the primary source for correct information about Satan?

We learn about Satan from the Scriptures, because the truth of the Bible is accurate. Because the very nature of Satan/the devil is to deceive, he will mislead people about his identity and purpose.

Does the devil have a tail and horns and wear a red suit?

No! In the Middle Ages, an actor in a play acted out the role of Satan, or the devil, with a red suit, horns, and a pitchfork. Since secrecy is one of the characteristics of Satan, it is understandable why so many believe the caricature of Satan. Satan is very happy for you to have a wrong or humorous view of his nature.

What is the nature of the devil?

He is a real person with a personality; he has intellect, emotion, and will. He doesn't have a body but has manifested himself physically. The devil has great power, but he is not omnipotent. He has great wisdom, but he is not omniscient. He is seemingly everywhere present to tempt believers, but he is not omnipresent.

Since God could not create anything evil, where did the devil come from?

God originally created Lucifer with the power of "free will" so that he could voluntarily worship and exalt God. But Lucifer used his power of choice to exalt himself. First it was pride ("lest being puffed up with pride he fall into the same condemnation as the devil" [1 Tim. 3:6]). Second, in unbelief, he rebelled against God. Lucifer did not believe that God could know what he was doing or judge him. Third, in self-deception, Lucifer actually believed he could wrestle the throne away from the Almighty. Finally, there was an unwillingness on the part of Lucifer to abide in the stead where he had been placed by the Creator. After the fall Lucifer is also called "great dragon . . . that serpent of old . . . the Devil and Satan" (Rev. 12:9).

What are some names or titles of the devil?

His original name before the fall was Lucifer (Isa. 14:12). He is also called Satan (Job 1:6), Apollyon (Rev. 9:11), Beelzebub (Matt. 12:27), the old serpent (Rev. 20:2), the evil one (John 17:15), the god of this age (2 Cor. 4:4), the accuser of the brethren (Rev. 12:10), and father of lies (John 8:44).

If Satan is the "god of this world," who is in his kingdom?

First, Satan directs the angels who fell during rebellion against God. Second, he controls the hearts of unregenerate men (Luke 8:44) and the world system that is in association with the lust of the flesh, the lust of the eyes, and the pride of life (1 John 2:15–18). The kingdom of Satan denies the supernatural (Eph. 2:2) and opposes all that God is and does.

Why does God tolerate the devil?

Many would think that an all-powerful God would go ahead and destroy or kill Satan, or at least get him out of the way. But if there were no devil to resist us, we could not show God our love for Him by resisting the devil (James 4:7). By resisting temptation from Satan, we demonstrate our love for God and build up our Christian character.

If there were no devil, we would not see the mighty power of God or how He can demonstrate Himself in the face of evil and temptation.

If there were no devil, we would not receive crowns, or rewards, for resisting Satan and overcoming temptation. And if God destroyed Satan before the end of the world, then God would not be faithful to the timetable that is written in Scripture. God has promised to bruise Satan's head (Gen. 3:15), but He will not do it before His appointed time. God has a "fullness of time" when He will do what He plans to do (Gal. 4:4).

Does the devil have wings? Can he fly?

Many pictures show the devil as a demonic character with wings. This is because originally the devil and his demons were angels. Because of the misconception that angels fly, the devil is depicted as also having wings and flying. But remember that many times when angels appeared to individuals in the Old and New Testaments, they were often mistaken for normal people. They did not appear to be superhuman, nor did they have wings. Therefore, most evangelicals teach that neither angels nor the devil have wings. However, both cherubim and seraphim are pictured as having wings (Isa. 6:3), and they fly (Ezek. 1).

No one knows for sure if the devil has wings, but he probably does not. He does not need to fly; apparently he can travel at "the speed of thought."

What is your favorite name for the devil?

The devil has many names. He is called Satan, the devil, Beelzebub, Lucifer, the evil one, murderer, a liar, the prince of the power of the air, and the god of this age. However, one favorite name is one that is not found in Scripture. It is *counterfeiter*. Lucifer fell because his ultimate desire was "to be like the Most High God." He wanted to be Jehovah El Elyon, the possessor of heaven and earth. Since the devil wants to be like God and rule a kingdom like God, he has created false religions, false Bibles, and false salvation (2 Cor. 11:13–15). He wants to have a religion, but it is a counterfeit religion. As counterfeit money is a replica of real money, the devil is a counterfeit of the real God, and offers counterfeit supernatural experiences. Remember, no one makes counterfeits of play money or worthless money. They make counterfeits of the real thing.

Has anyone actually seen the devil?

While many people think the devil will manifest himself, in polls taken of audiences, very few claim to have seen the devil. But at the same time, many have claimed to see angels (Heb. 13:2). The one person who saw the devil physically on the earth was Jesus (Matt. 4:1–11). The devil manifested himself to Jesus in the wilderness and tempted him with the well-known temptation to make stones into bread, to jump off the temple mount, and to worship him so he (the devil) could give Jesus the kingdoms of the world.

Can the devil know our minds?

The devil is not omniscient; he does not know all things present, nor does he know anything future. He does not know what you are thinking; therefore, there are times when you pray that you might not want to pray out loud lest the devil knows what you are asking. However, the devil is brilliant, and he can "read our minds" like a wife can "read" her husband's mind. He has past knowledge of us, and he knows our inclinations, so he quite often knows what we are thinking. This ability helps him "guess" what will happen in the future.

Is it true, "The devil made me do it"?

That statement was made famous by the comedian Flip Wilson, and many repeat it as gospel fact. Actually if you think, *The devil made me do it,* you make your accountability for your sin the responsibility of the devil. That way, it's very easy for people to not take responsibility for their actions.

We are tempted to sin by (1) the lust of the flesh, (2) the lust of the eyes, and (3) the pride of life. These all come from the devil, which he uses in tempting us. However, our sin comes from within; everyone has a sinful nature. *We* want to satisfy our physical needs contrary to God's law (lust of the flesh). *We* have been guilty of seeking possessions apart from God's law (lust of the eyes). And *we* often take credit for ourselves, contrary to God's law (the pride of life). So rather than saying, "The devil made me do it," we should take responsibility by confessing our sins, asking God to forgive us by the blood of Jesus Christ, and repenting, turning from sin to God.

What did Jesus do to the devil on the cross?

God predicated that "the seed of the woman" would crush "the seed of the serpent." On the cross, Jesus received a "heel bite" which was the equivalent of physical death. As painful as this was, Jesus rose again on the third day; the heel bite was not permanent. However, Satan received a "head blow," which means permanent destruction.

As Jesus was facing the Cross, He said, "Now is the judgment of this world; now the ruler of this world will be cast out" (John 12:31). In the context of the Cross, Jesus was describing Satan being cast out from God's presence. Also on the night before He died, Jesus said, "The ruler of this world is judged" (John 16:11). In essence, the death of Jesus on the cross was a "judgment" of Satan. The Cross was Satan's judgment, and eventually he will be cast into the lake of fire.

If Satan is judged, why does he still have "bite and poison" to destroy lives?

Even though Satan was judged by the Cross, that judgment will not be carried out until the future coming of Christ in judgment. Just as a sentence is handed down to a criminal in a court of law, so Satan received the death sentence at God's court of law, the Cross judgment. Just as a criminal is told, "Ye shall hang by the neck until dead," the punishment of Satan was announced. However, just as in the American legal system there is a period of time between judgment and execution, so in God's legal system is there a period of time between Satan's judgment by the Cross and God's carrying out Satan's "execution" in the lake of fire (Rev. 20).

Where will I most likely confront Satan today?

Most people think that the devil will be found in places of moral debauchery where rampant alcohol, drugs, and sex abound. However, remember that Satan already has these people under his control. He does not have to display himself in these evil settings to capture more followers. He has these addicts captured.

You're more likely to confront Satan in a liberal theological seminary where the professors and students deny the blood atonement of Jesus Christ, the authority of Scriptures, the existence of God, and even the existence of the devil himself (2 Cor. 11:13–15).

Is Lucifer the brother of Jesus?

Certain people have taught that Lucifer is the brother of Jesus because angels are called sons of God (Job 1:6), and Lucifer is an angel. Therefore, Lucifer being originally an angel of God was a son of God. Those who believe that Lucifer is the brother of Jesus base their opinion on the Scripture that Jesus is called "the Son of God" (John 1:49). However, Jesus is not just another son of God like the angels. Jesus is *the Son of God*, also known as the only begotten Son (John 1:14, 18; 3:16). Jesus is also called *the Beloved Son* by the Father at the baptism. Conservative Christians have always taught *eternal generation*, in other words, that Jesus Christ is the Son of God, being eternally generated in relationship to the Father. Jesus was not a created being. Angels, like Lucifer, are called "sons of God" because God created them. Satan is not Jesus' brother. Satan is a created being.

What should my response be when I am attacked by the devil?

First, you should always *respect* Satan because of his immense power. But remember, "He who is in you is greater than he who is in the world" (1 John 4:4). While the Holy Spirit is much greater, Satan has great power. Jesus said, "Do not fear those who kill the body but cannot kill the soul. But rather fear Him who is able to destroy both soul and body in hell" (Matt. 10:28). Just as one would *respect* a deadly rattlesnake and stay far from his bite, you should have the same respect for Satan. That means do not joke about him, trivialize him, or flirt with him.

Second, is the principle of *removal.* Paul tells Timothy, "Flee" (1 Tim. 6:11). This means stay completely away from anything having to do with Satan.

Third, Paul gives us the principle of *resisting:* "Resist the devil and he will flee from you" (James 4:7). Just because Satan tempts does not mean we should give in. And when he appeals to our weaknesses, we should be strong. Scripture reminds us that "you have not yet resisted to bloodshed, striving against sin" (Heb. 12:4).

Finally, Paul gives us the principle of *readiness.* He tells us, "For we do not wrestle against flesh and blood, but against principalities, against powers, against the rulers of the darkness of this age, against spiritual hosts of wickedness in the heavenly places" (Eph. 6:12). You should always be ready and expect Satan's attack. Like the soldier on sentry duty, be alert and expect an attack at any moment. When you do, Satan will not catch you with your defenses down and will not overcome you spiritually.

How can a Christian overcome Satan?

First, by the principle of *respect,* knowing his power. Second, by the principle of *removal,* leaving the presence of sin, "abstain[ing] from every form of evil" (1 Thess. 5:22). Third, by the principle of *resistance* to sin: "Resist the devil and he will flee from you" (James 4:7). And fourth, the principle of *readiness:* "Watch and pray, lest you enter into temptation" (Mark 14:38).

Should I rebuke Satan?

There are those who rebuke Satan when he comes to attack them. In light of the principle of *respect,* you should never rebuke Satan in your own strength or even in your own faith. Notice that the Scripture teaches that the archangel Michael "dared not bring against him a reviling accusation, but said, 'The Lord rebuke you!'" (Jude 9). You should let the Lord rebuke Satan; you should not rebuke him.

What should my response be when I feel the "presence" of Satan or "evil"?

Satan cannot stand in the presence of the Word of God, so when you feel the presence of "evil," begin quoting Scripture. This was Jesus' response (Matt.

4:4) when He was confronted by Satan. Next, Satan cannot stand the blood of Jesus Christ and cannot remain in the presence of the power of Jesus Christ. Therefore, when you feel the presence of evil, begin quoting Scriptures about the blood: "But if we walk in the light as He is in the light, we have fellowship with one another, and the blood of Jesus Christ His Son cleanses us from all sin" (1 John 1:7). Also, when you feel the presence of the evil one, begin singing hymns out loud about the blood. As an illustration, sing the hymns, "There Is Power in the Blood," "The Blood Will Never Lose Its Power," or "Nothing but the Blood."

Can the devil be saved?

No, the devil cannot be saved. He was given an opportunity to serve God at the beginning of time but fell to evil because of his pride (Isa. 14; Ezek. 28). Once a "window of opportunity" is past, a person doesn't get a second opportunity to be converted. The opportunity that was given to Satan is also given to people who die outside Jesus Christ. There is no second chance after death.

Apparently hell was created after the fall of Satan. It is his place of punishment along with all who deny God and side with Satan. Jesus said, "Depart from Me, you cursed, into the everlasting fire prepared for the devil and his angels" (Matt. 25:41).

If Satan knows that God will judge him in the future (he knows Scripture that says "hell is prepared for him"), then why does He still fight God and keep up his activity?

Actually, Satan has no other choice but to keep up his activity. He has an evil nature and will continue to do evil because he *is* evil. But also, Satan is blinded to the perfect will of God. Perhaps in his evil desires Satan believes he can somehow thwart the will of God and escape from hell, because he is driven by pride and arrogance. Perhaps he believes that somewhere, somehow, under some conditions, he can win the victory over God. But Satan cannot win that victory because God has indicated the victory belongs to Him.

QUESTIONS

ABOUT

HEAVEN AND HELL

What does the Bible teach about *sheol*?

The common word for "hell" in the Old Testament is *sheol,* which means "the grave," where people go when they die. In the King James Version, *sheol* is translated "hell" thirty-one times and "pit" three times. When both saved and unsaved died, they were said to go to sheol, the place of the departed dead. The Hebrew word *sheol* was translated into Greek as *hadees* (Hades). Hades, or sheol, is the place the Old Testament unsaved went. Jesus, in the parable of the rich man and Lazarus, said that Lazarus had gone to a place called "paradise" (Luke 23:43), and "Abraham's bosom" (Luke 16:22). Two people died, the rich man and Lazarus (Luke 16:19–31), but in their after-lives they were treated differently.

What does the Bible teach about *hades?*

The rich man went to hades at death and was tormented in flames (Luke 16:24). The punishment of hades is (1) burning, (2) separation/loneliness, (3) conviction by memory, (4) thirst, (5) falling, and (6) stench. The rich man could look across "a great gulf fixed" (Luke 16:26) and see where the saved were located. However, the Scripture is silent on whether the saved could see the torment of the unsaved. The one thing the rich man could not do was escape his torment. He could not even send a warning to his family.

What does the Bible teach about *Gehenna?*

This word appears only twelve times in the New Testament and is translated "hell and "lake of fire." The Lord Jesus used this term eleven times. The name is probably related to the Valley of Hinnom, a dumping ground for the city of Jerusalem. During the time of Jesus, it was used to burn garbage. Hence, the Lord used the word *Gehenna* to describe the place of eternal punishment because it was a place of filth and stench, of smoke and pain, and of fire and death (Matt. 5:22; 18:8–9; 23:33; John 3:36).

What does the Bible teach about the "lake of fire"?

John refers to hell in terms of a "lake of fire" (Rev. 20:15). Some have suggested this is nothing more than a metaphor to describe a place of suffering, but since the Bible uses flames to describe its torment, there is no reason to think the cause of suffering will be otherwise. Human language limits a perfect identification of the horrors of hell, as it also does when we seek to describe the glories of heaven. Only in this aspect can the "lake of fire" be considered a metaphor. It is as if John were saying, "Hell is so horrible I cannot completely describe it. Hell is like a vast sea covered in flames, and that is only the beginning of the pain and suffering I saw there."

Does hell have literal fire?

The first torment a person encounters in reaching hell is the torment of burning. Jesus said His angels "will cast them into the furnace of fire. There will be wailing and gnashing of teeth" (Matt. 13:42). John the Baptist identified hell in terms of an "unquenchable fire" (Matt. 3:12). The rich man in hell acknowledged, "I am tormented in this flame" (Luke 16:24). While it is wrong to say all the torture in hell comes from the flame, it would also be wrong to explain away the literal flames of hell.

What will hell be like?

Hell is a place of unquenchable fire: "He will burn up the chaff with unquenchable fire" (Matt. 3:12). It is also a place of memory and remorse. In Luke 16:19–31 the unsaved rich man experienced memory and remorse over his lost condition. Hell is also a place of thirst: "Then he cried and said, 'Father Abraham, have mercy on me, and send Lazarus that he may dip the tip of his finger in water and cool my tongue; for I am tormented in this flame'" (Luke 16:24). Those in hell suffer misery: "And being in torments in Hades, he lifted up his eyes" (v. 23). "And these will go away into everlasting punishment" (Matt. 25:46). Hell is described as a place of "wailing and gnashing of teeth" (Matthew 13:42) and "weeping and gnashing of teeth" (Matt. 24:51). Those in hell are not begging to get out, nor do they sorrow; rather, they express anger and hatred to God. Their rejection of God is greater in death than in life.

Often the unsaved man jokes about hell saying, "If I do go to hell, I won't be lonely, for all my friends will be there too." But the opposite is true! Hell is called the "second death" (Rev. 2:11; 20:6, 14; 21:8). Death in the Bible does not mean cessation of existence but refers to separation. Sinners will be forever separated from God, and from others. Finally, hell is a place of darkness, which will doubtless isolate the sinner from the companionship of unsaved friends as well.

Will all the millions of people who have not heard the name of Jesus, who have been ignorant of God, go to hell when they die?

Would a God of love throw them into eternal torture without giving them an opportunity to be saved?

The premise of the question is wrong. Every person who has ever lived has had a chance to be saved. The Bible says,

"For the wrath of God is revealed from heaven against all ungodliness and unrighteousness of men . . . because what may be known of God is manifest in them, for God has shown it to them. For since the creation of the world His invisible attributes are clearly seen, being understood by the things that are made, even His eternal power and Godhead, so that they are without excuse." (Rom. 1:18–20)

The Bible is very clear that the heathen who have never accepted Jesus Christ are lost and going to hell. While they do not have as much "light" as those who sit in a gospel-preaching church, they know of God from creation and realize there must be a Creator. And what do they know about the Creator? That He is all-powerful to have created the world, and that He has the power of choice; He had knowledge to create the world, and chose to do so. The heathen know the Creator exists, but refuse to believe in Him.

Again, Paul tells us about the lost: "For when Gentiles, who do not have the law, by nature do the things in the law, these, although not having the law, are a law to themselves, who show the work of the law written in their hearts, their conscience also bearing witness, and between themselves their thoughts accusing . . . in the day when God will judge the secrets of men by Jesus Christ, according to my gospel" (Rom. 2:14–16).

This verse says that the unsaved will be judged by their consciences. In their hearts they know what is right, but they have refused to do what is right. They are judged by their knowledge of "right."

In a final way Paul says, "Therefore you are inexcusable, O man, whoever you are who judge, for in whatever you judge another you condemn yourself; for you who judge practice the same things. But we know that the judgment of God is according to truth against those who practice such things" (Rom. 2:1–2). Paul says that every person who judges other people will be judged. Therefore, when they judge another, they must realize that they, too, will be judged. Because there was a law, they must recognize the lawgiver and how far they fall short in light of the law.

Every person who has lived has had the chance to be saved. Jesus "was the true Light which gives light to every man coming into the world" (John 1:9).

This light is their understanding of God, and their obligation to Him. A man who has never heard the gospel, yet has done wrong, knows he has broken the law and that he is condemned. It is contrary to the Bible to say that some men did not have an opportunity to seek God. Every man has had that opportunity—granted, some more than others, but all have had a knowledge of God. No man can say in hell, "I didn't know there was a God; I didn't know what was right to do. I didn't have an opportunity."

After Creation, people knew about God, but eventually most turned against God. How did that happen? Romans 1:18–32 explains how the heathen became godless and rebellious against the truth. Rebellion against God results in idolatry and sexual immorality. People would rather please themselves than please God. When people turn from God in unbelief, they give themselves over to lust and self-satisfaction. Their knowledge of God and their knowledge that what they do is wrong become the basis of their condemnation.

Will people in the presence of Jesus be able to see what is happening on Earth?

There are some who believe that the dead can look back to see what is happening on earth. "Therefore we also, since we are surrounded by so great a cloud of witnesses, let us lay aside every weight, and the sin which so easily ensnares us, and let us run with endurance the race that is set before us" (Heb. 12:1). The witnesses referred to are believers in heaven who observe what is happening on earth. Therefore, the writer of Hebrews exhorts living people to "run with endurance the race" because they are observed by those who have gone before.

Many other Bible teachers believe that those in heaven *cannot* see what is happening on earth. Because those in heaven have no sadness and disappointment (Rev. 21:4), they must not be able to see the sins and mistakes of loved ones who are still living. Those who teach this view state the "witnesses" in Hebrews 12:1 are not those in heaven, but are those mentioned in the previous chapter. (Hebrews 11 lists great people of faith in the "Christian Hall of Fame" who have died and have become a testimony to those who are still alive.)

Perhaps the answer is halfway between these two positions. Those in heaven don't see all that happens on earth. However, God allows those in heaven to see only what He wants them to see: joys, victories, and those things that glorify God. People in heaven don't see the failures, sins, and defeats of their loved ones on earth. That would not glorify God. They only know what God wants them to know.

How can we be happy in heaven if some of our loved ones are lost?

The problem with this question is that we are judging our lives in heaven by our earthly-minded existence here on earth. Here, we are burdened for our loved ones; and they disappoint us in many ways. We project our earthly disappointment onto our existence in heaven.

So we have to ask the question, "How can Jesus be happy in heaven, knowing people are lost in hell?" Obviously, the joy and peace of God is greater than ours. The Bible says, "Who for the joy that was set before Him endured the cross, despising the shame, and has sat down at the right hand of the throne of God" (Heb. 12:2). Jesus apparently has joy in heaven. He has joy knowing that all things were done right, and that everything possible was done for the salvation of every soul on earth.

After the last judgment, every person will experience the joy and peace of God. Although every wife or husband whose spouse died unsaved will apparently know what happened to that mate (Rev. 20:11–21:3), they will turn away with the peace of God, for the Holy Spirit will comfort them. "God Himself will be with them and be their God. And God will wipe away every tear from their eyes; there shall be no more death, nor sorrow, nor crying. There shall be no more pain, for the former things have passed away" (Rev. 21:3–4).

What happens to me at death?

According to Genesis 35:18, your soul and body separate: "as her soul was departing (for she died)." Angels take/escort you to heaven (Luke 16:22), and you immediately enter the presence of God: " . . .to be absent from the body and to be present with the Lord" (2 Cor. 5:8). Your earthly body decays.

What will I be like in heaven until the resurrection?

You will be a "spirit being," with active personality (intellect, emotion, and will). You will be incorporeal (without a body).

What happens to me at the resurrection?

You will come back bodily with Jesus. "Even so God will bring with Him those who sleep in Jesus" (1 Thess. 4:14). Your physical and immaterial will be joined: " . . . shall be caught up together with them in the clouds to meet the Lord in the air" (1 Thess. 4:17). You will be transformed, having a converted body-soul that will not be subject to the laws of nature and death. "Who will transform our lowly body that it may be conformed to His glorious body" (Phil. 3:21).

Will we have physical bodies in heaven?

"[Jesus] shall change our vile body, that it may be fashioned like unto his glorious body, according to the working whereby he is able even to subdue all things unto himself" (Phil. 3:21 KJV).

"Beloved, now we are children of God; and it has not yet been revealed what we shall be, but we know that when He is revealed, we shall be like Him, for we shall see Him as He is" (1 John 3:2).

These verses tell us that those of us who die, having trusted Christ as our personal Savior, will be given bodies like that of the Lord Jesus Christ. They will no longer be subject to disease and death.

It should be noted that the Christian will not receive a body until the time of the rapture. Those Christians who die before the rapture must wait until the Lord comes in the clouds to call His church. At that point, those who have died in Christ will have their bodies resurrected and will be changed and united with their souls once again, receiving glorified bodies.

Will we remember our sins and failures in heaven?

Though we cannot be dogmatic concerning our memory of the affairs of this life when we get to heaven, it is our belief that once we enter into eternity with the Lord, which is at the conclusion of the millennial reign, the sins and struggles of this life, with all the tragedies and sorrows and sufferings, will be permanently erased from our minds. Therefore, we simply will not have any remembrance of the affairs, the struggles, the sufferings, and heartaches of this life. "God will wipe away every tear" (Rev. 21:4).

What will I look like in heaven?

"Then shall I know even as also I am known" (1 Cor. 13:12 KJV). Not only will you be known by Jesus, but you will also be recognized by those who knew you on earth. You will have those features in heaven that characterized you on earth. If two people looked similar on earth (twins, for example), they will look similar in heaven.

How old will I be in heaven?

There are many answers to this question. Some say you will be the age at which you were converted (1 Cor. 13:12); others say you will be the age at which you died. Still others say you will be the age of Jesus when He died, or the age Adam and Eve appeared to be when they were created. Perhaps we'll be an unknown mystical age. Probably the correct answer is, "No one knows."

Will I recognize my friends in heaven?

Yes, we will know as we are known (1 Cor. 13:12). Perhaps our experience in heaven will be similar to those in Scripture when, "the graves were opened; and many bodies of the saints who had fallen asleep were raised" (Matt. 27:52–53). We will know many people in heaven, but not everyone.

Will I be perfect, or can I displease God in heaven?

At death we lose our sin nature, for "the former things have passed away" (Rev. 21:4). We will be like the angels, we will only be able to do right things, and please God. Some theologians teach that in heaven some will do more to serve God, learn and know more about God than ever before, and grow in grace and maturity more than ever before.

Will I be married in heaven?

No one is married in heaven. "'In the resurrection, whose wife of the seven will she be?' . . . Jesus answered and said to them, 'You are mistaken, not knowing the Scriptures nor the power of God. For in the resurrection they neither marry nor are given in marriage, but are like angels of God in heaven'" (Matt. 22:28–30). Just as the woman in this passage is no man's wife in the resurrection, you will not be married in heaven, though you will have a special relationship with your spouse. Since heaven is an amplification of the joys of life on earth, you will progress from the point at which the relationship was broken. Young couples taken in death will grow from their initial relationships, while older couples will continue maturing.

What will the relationship in heaven be between two believers who were divorced?

They will remember the positive things about one another. They will not consider themselves in a relationship with one another in heaven. Any animosity will be gone. Jesus said, "I make all things new" (Rev. 21:5).

Will I know everything in heaven?

You will not know all things. Things will happen in heaven of which you will not be aware nor know about. Only God knows all things. Your awareness will not be negatively influenced by sin, so you will be aware of more and know more than you knew on earth. Since aging toward death is a product of sin (Gen. 2:17; Rom. 5:12), you will not suffer the corruption and decline of memory; hence, you will remember more. There is "no more curse" (Rev. 22:3). You will grow in knowledge, but you will never reach all knowledge or perfect knowledge.

Will I be able to do everything in heaven?

The curse and limitation of the Fall will be removed. Heaven is likened unto a garden (Rev. 21:23– 22:6), so you will not be unlike Adam and Eve in the garden. You will be able to do "exceedingly, abundantly, above" what you are now able to do. You will not be limited by the laws of gravity and time (angels travel at the speed of thought).

What will I wear in heaven?

Because the Bible speaks of the "robes of righteousness," some think we'll wear robes, but no one really knows.

Will I eat in heaven? Drink?

In His resurrected body Jesus ate. "So they gave Him a piece of a broiled fish and some honeycomb. And He took it and ate in their presence" (Luke 24:42–43). You will probably be a vegetarian, as were Adam and Eve before the Fall. Heaven will have "a pure river" (Rev. 22:1) and "fruit trees" (Rev. 22:2). Just as angels have incorporeal bodies, yet manifested themselves physically and have eaten in that state (Gen. 18:3), so will you. You will eat in heaven for enjoyment, but not of necessity for physical growth or sustenance.

Will I work in heaven?

Yes, you will work in heaven, but the curse that was associated with work will be removed (Gen. 3:17–19). You will work and be productive, grow because of it, and glorify God through it. The Bible says of the Lord, "His servants shall serve Him" (Rev. 22:3). Your main work will be the "service of worship" or praise. God has "made us kings and priests to our God; and we shall reign on the earth" (Rev. 5:10).

Will I get money for work in heaven?

Money is barter or a medium of exchange. Money places value on work, products, and time. Money is our objective standard whereby sinful, selfish people can relate one to another. Where there is no standard, people steal, lie, fight, and kill because of their selfish desires.

Money will not be the motivation of work in heaven because there will be no sinful selfishness. People will readily do the work that they have to do. They will also have what they want and need because heaven is perfect. There will be no need to stockpile money, and no gates for protection from theft will be necessary (Rev. 21:25). What's more, the negative attitudes that some have concerning money will no longer exist. "But there shall by no means enter it anything that defiles, or causes an abomination or a lie" (Rev. 21:27).

Will I grow in heaven?

Not physically. And there will be no physical problems associated with the growth of disease, tumors, rotten teeth, failing eyesight, and so on.

You will grow spiritually. You will constantly become more like Jesus, but no one will ever be exactly like Him, because He is God.

You will also grow mentally and emotionally (your personality of intellect, emotions, and will). The reference to the "healing of the nations" (Rev. 22:2) means "growth."

Will I retain my ethnic characteristics in heaven?

Yes, you will be known as you are known. Heaven has "the nations of those who are saved" (Rev. 21:24). "And they sang a new song, saying: 'You are worthy to take the scroll, and to open its seals; for You were slain, and have redeemed us to God by Your blood out of every tribe and tongue and people and nation'" (Rev. 5:9).

What language will I speak in heaven?

"And every creature which is in heaven and on the earth and under the earth and such as are in the sea, and all that are in them, I heard saying: 'Blessing and honor and glory and power be to Him who sits on the throne, and to the Lamb, forever and ever!'" (Rev. 5:13). What language will we use when we praise God in this way?

Some think you will speak an unknown language in heaven, or Greek, the language of the New Testament. Others think you will speak the heavenly language of Hebrew, or the language that angels now speak. Still others think you will speak what you spoke on this earth, but you will be able to understand and be understood by those who speak a different language. The Bible does not say for sure.

Will I sleep in heaven?

The Bible says there will be "no night there" (Rev. 21:25). You need sleep here on earth because of the curse. Your toil and hard work wears down the body, and sleep replenishes strength and renews stamina. You won't need to sleep in heaven because you will always have all the energy you need. But that doesn't mean you won't be allowed to sleep and enjoy it.

Will heaven be fun?

We think of fun as (1) physical stimulation, (2) diversion from work, (3) dream fulfillment, (4) self-fulfillment. Heaven will not be "fun" as defined above because (1) you will not need stimulation, (2) you will enjoy work, (3) all aspirations will have been fulfilled, and (4) you will be complete in Jesus, and need nothing. The sensation we seek on earth called "fun" will be automatically fulfilled in heaven.

Where will I live in heaven?

You will actually live on earth. "I saw a new heaven and a new earth, for the first heaven and the first earth had passed away" (Rev. 21:1). Earth will not be new in substance, but new in kind and sequence. You will live in a city.

"Then I, John, saw the holy city, New Jerusalem, coming down out of heaven from God" (Rev. 21:2). You will live in an apartment/condominium. "In My Father's house are many mansions; if it were not so, I would have told you. I go to prepare a place for you" (John 14:2).

What will my body be like in heaven?

You will have a perfect body, no more results of sin and aging (false teeth, hairpieces, and so forth). We will appear to others with our same unique personalities and physical characteristics.

What is not in heaven?

According to Scripture, there will be no sea, no more death, no sorrow, no crying, no pain, no abomination, no murderers, no whoremongers, no sorcerers, no idolaters, no temple, no sun, no moon, no shut gate, no night, no cures, no need for candles (Rev. 21).

What *is* in heaven?

Jesus, God, the Holy Spirit, a throne, a tree of life, a pure river, God as the sun, different ethnic groups, twenty-four elders, angels (Michael, Gabriel), the Lamb's bride, choir, lightning, thunders, the Lamb's Book of Life, and golden streets are all found in heaven.

QUESTIONS ABOUT THE DOCTRINE OF GOD

Why should we study God?

Because God has demanded, "Be still, and know that I am God" (Ps. 46:10). Also, we are made in the image of God, and the more we understand Him, the better we understand ourselves. When people have a wrong view of God, it causes a multitude of problems in their daily lives as Christians. There is only one true God, the God of the Bible. We all have an inner desire to know Him, and by studying about Him in Scripture and nature, we better understand the true God.

Can we really know God by studying Him?

Zophar, a friend of Job's, asked, "Can you search out the deep things of God?" (Job 11:7). The answer is "No!" God is the wholly other One, and we cannot *know* Him by our study. We know what God is like from what He has revealed about Himself in the Scriptures. We can never know everything about God, even as we will spend all eternity learning more about God. But we should learn as much about God on this earth as we can.

What is a definition of God that most Christians would accept?

Many people think the best definition of God is found in the Westminster Catechism: "God is a spirit, infinite, eternal and unchangeable in His being, wisdom, power, holiness, justice, goodness and truth."

What is meant by the phrase "God is spirit"?

When we call God "spirit," we mean He has an immaterial nature, that is, incorporeal, nonphysical, and invisible.

Why is God described as having ears, hands, and feet?

These are *anthropomorphisms,* which means we have projected onto God man's characteristics for the sake of understanding God and knowing Him better. Actually, God does not have ears, hands, feet, etc., but he can perform the functions that are necessary in a human being that are reflected in these physical instruments. This means God hears, can perform things that we do with our hands, and can go places for which we use our feet.

Since man is made in the image of God, what does that say about God?

Since man is a person, having personality, then God is not just an impersonal being or a "force." God is a person, who has intellect, emotions, and will. As a person, God has both self-awareness (He knows Himself) and self-determination (He can direct Himself).

What is *atheism?*

Atheism is the disbelief in and negation of deity, so an atheist is one who does not believe in God. Usually a *practical atheist* is one who has been disappointed because of Christianity and does not believe in God. A *dogmatic atheist* is one who teaches the principles of the nonexistence of deity. A *virtual atheist* feels that belief in God is inconsistent with the principles of truth.

What is an *agnostic?*

An *agnostic* believes it is impossible to know anything for certain because all knowledge is relative. Since you cannot know anything, one cannot know the existence of God.

What is *polytheism?*

Polytheism is the belief in the multiplicity of many gods.

What is *henotheism?*

Henotheism recognizes one god is supreme among many gods.

What is *tritheism?*

Tritheism is the belief in the existence of three gods, coequal in every respect, yet distinct deities, each with its own personality.

What is *dualism?*

Dualism is the view that there are two distinct and irreducible substances or principles that have always existed. Some explain this as "good and evil have always existed." Some explain it as "God and Satan have always existed." Some say, "Mind and matter have always existed."

What is *pantheism?*

Pantheism says everything in the world is part of one eternal self-existent being, which is god. A pantheist views all material objects, including mind, as a part of the infinite single substance that is god.

What is *deism?*

Deism teaches that God created the world by His power and endowed the world with laws that govern the oversight of nature. God has also created people and left them to work out their destinies by their own power within the laws of the universe.

What are *attributes* of God?

Attributes are those qualities of God whereby He manifests His nature and character.

What are some of the attributes of God that we know?

God is holy, loving, good, merciful, gracious, benevolent, and longsuffering. God is *omniscient*, knowing all things; *omnipresent*, meaning He is everywhere present at the same time; and *omnipotent*, able to do everything that is in harmony with His nature.

What does "God is holy" mean?

By *holiness* we mean that God is absolutely pure. He is separate from all of His created world, as well as equally separate from moral evil and sin. The word *holiness* means "to separate or to cut off."

Can God know things that are possible but didn't happen?

Yes, God has knowledge of all things that could have existed. "[He] calls those things which do not exist as though they did" (Rom. 4:17). All potential knowledge is bound up in the omniscience of God.

Does God have a hard time remembering?

No, there is no past to God, just as there is no future. Therefore, God never needs to recall or to remember. He knows all things equally well, including Himself.

Is there anything that God doesn't know?

If we were to say that God doesn't know anything, we would be saying that God does not have perfect knowledge, and that God is not the Supreme Being.

What is an illustration of God's knowledge?

The Hubble telescope has suggested that there are over 50 billion galaxies, and each galaxy has over 200 million stars. Yet, "He counts the number of the stars; He calls them all by name. Great is our Lord, and mighty in power; His understanding is infinite" (Ps. 147:4–5).

What is the *omnipresence* of God?

God is everywhere present at the same time. That means God is not limited by space or time.

How big is God?

Because God is omnipresent, He is everywhere present. But "omnipresence" also implies immensity. God is beyond space; He extends beyond the last star. (Stars are not limitless; only God is limitless, so there must be a last star). God exists where there is no space. There is no such place where God does not exist (Psalm 139:7–10).

If God is omnipresent, how close is He to me?

Because God is everywhere present, He is very intimate to every person.

> Where can I go from Your Spirit?
> Or where can I flee from Your presence?
> If I ascend into heaven, You are there;
> If I make my bed in hell, behold, You are there.
> If I take the wings of the morning, and dwell in the uttermost
>   parts of the sea,
> Even there Your hand shall lead me,
> And Your right hand shall hold me. (Ps. 139:7–10)

What is the *transcendence* of God?

Transcendence means God is up and over above all of His Creation. God is both close to His Creation, as well as high above His Creation.

What is the *omnipotence* of God?

The *omnipotence* of God means He can do everything that is in harmony with His nature and perfection.

Are there some things that God can't do?

Yes, God cannot create sin, nor can He sin. God cannot change Himself, nor can He change His decrees. God cannot do impossible things, such as creating a rock bigger than He can lift or making yesterday not happen.

How has God limited Himself?

Because God lives by His nature, He has limited His omnipotence (power) by His will and character. God has submitted His nature to carry out His plan.

What can God do?

God can do whatever He wants to do, but He has not necessarily willed to do everything.

Does God have to do anything?

God only does what His nature and power tell Him to do. If God had to do anything out of necessity, He would cease being a free being, and He would cease being sovereign. If God had to do anything to satisfy any person other than Himself, God would cease being God.

Does God have to work hard to get big things done?

No, God's power is comprehensive; He can do anything without effort.

How can I see God's power?

One can see the power of God by observing nature and its forces: "For since the creation of the world His invisible attributes are clearly seen, being understood by the things that are made, even His eternal power and Godhead, so that they are without excuse" (Rom. 1:20).

Do Christians believe in three gods?

No, that is *tritheism*. Christians are *monotheists* (see "What are *Monotheists?*" later in this Chapter), meaning they believe in one God. "Hear, O Israel: The LORD our God, the LORD is one!" (Deut. 6:4).

What is the *Trinity?*

The word *trinity* is not found in the Bible, but is used by Christians to define and describe the threefold nature of God. "We worship one God in trinity, and trinity in unity, neither confounding the persons, nor dividing the substance" (Athanasian Creed). This creed explains that there is one God, but He is three persons: Father, Son, and Holy Spirit. There are not three gods, but one God.

What does the Bible teach about God as a Trinity?

The Bible teaches that God is three persons in one nature. The three persons are equal in nature, separate in person, and submissive in duties. This is difficult for our finite minds to understand. Nevertheless, God is three persons in one nature. Jesus is a person. The Holy Spirit is a person. First John 5:7 says, "For there are three that bear witness in heaven: the Father, the Word, and the Holy Spirit; and these three are one." Bible scholars point out that this verse may not be in some of the oldest manuscripts of the New Testament. However, there are many other passages where there is no textual problem that teach God is three persons, yet one God.

The apostolic church taught that the best place to see the Trinity was to visit the Jordan River where Jesus was baptized. The Father spoke from heaven audibly, the Holy Spirit came down visibly, and Jesus the Son was being baptized: "When He had been baptized, Jesus came up immediately from the water; and behold, the heavens were opened to Him, and He saw the Spirit of God descending like a dove and alighting upon Him. And suddenly a voice came from heaven, saying, 'This is My beloved Son, in whom I am well pleased'" (Matt. 3:16–17).

Two separate persons are seen in Luke 23:34. While Jesus the Son was on the cross, He prayed to God the Father: "Then said Jesus, Father, forgive them; for they know not what they do" (KJV). In Psalm 2:7, God the Father said to God the Son, "You are My Son, today I have begotten You." In John 10:30, Jesus said, "I and my Father are one" (KJV). Then Jesus told Philip, "He who has seen Me has seen the Father" (John 14:9). And in Colossians 2:9, we are told of Jesus, "For in Him dwells all the fullness of the Godhead bodily."

Jesus, Himself, spoke of the Holy Spirit as a person: "And I will pray the Father, and He will give you another Helper, that He may abide with you forever—the Spirit of truth, whom the world cannot receive, because it neither sees Him nor knows Him; but you know Him, for He dwells with you and will be in you . . . But the Helper, the Holy Spirit, whom the Father will send in My name, He will teach you all things, and bring to your remembrance all things that I said to you" (John 14:16–17, 26).

God the Father, God the Son, and God the Holy Spirit are seen as three distinct persons. Jesus teaches that He and the Father will dwell in Christians by means of the presence of the Holy Spirit: "Jesus answered and said to him, 'If anyone loves Me, he will keep My word; and My Father will love him, and We will come to him and make Our home with him'" (John 14:23).

It should be noted that the Godhead is both a Trinity and a Unity, three yet one, God of very God. The unity of God means that there is but one God, and that the divine nature is undivided and indivisible. There can be, therefore, only one infinite and perfect being. That the divine nature is undivided and indivisible is presented in Scripture: "Hear, O Israel: The LORD our God, the LORD is one!" (Deut. 6:4; see also Mark 12:29 and James 2:19). God does not consist of parts, nor can He be divided into parts. His being is simple, numerically one, free from the composition of man's composition, which has both a material and an immaterial part. But God is Spirit and is not susceptible to any such division.

How can one God be three persons?

Both the Old and New Testaments teach that God is Unity as well as Trinity. The Trinity means that the Father, Son, and Holy Spirit are each equal Persons and eternally One. The Persons of the Godhead are equal in nature, separate in person, but submissive in the duties that They perform.

In the Old Testament, the Trinity is implied when the Godhead is seen talking among Itself: "Let Us make man in Our image" (Gen. 1:26), "Let Us go down" (Gen. 11:7), and "Who will go for Us?" (Isaiah 6:8). The three-fold Trinity is implied from the three-fold reference to deity who act in Creation: "For thus says the LORD, who created the heavens, who is God, who formed the earth and made it, who has established it, who did not cre-ate it in vain, who formed it to be inhabited: 'I am the LORD, and there is no other'" (Isa. 45:18). Again the three-fold nature of God is seen in Isaiah 48:16. "I have not spoken in secret from the beginning; from the time that it was, I was there. And now the LORD God and His Spirit have sent Me." The speaker is obviously God the Father, the "Me" is a reference to Jesus Christ, the Messiah, who is speaking, and the "Spirit" is the Holy Spirit.

The New Testament teaches the Trinity when Jesus said, "But when the Helper comes, whom I shall send to you from the Father . . . He will testify of Me" (John 15:26). This is the Holy Spirit, who is the Comforter, being sent from the Father by Jesus Christ. And the baptismal formula teaches the Trinity: ". . . baptizing them in the name of the Father and of the Son and of the Holy Spirit" (Matt. 28:19).

Jesus, the only begotten Son of the Father (John 3:16) also claimed to be God when He said, "'I am the Alpha and the Omega, the Beginning and the End,' says the Lord, 'who is and who was and who is to come, the Almighty'" (Rev. 1:8).

What have Christian leaders in history said about the Trinity?

The oldest existing identification of the Trinity is the Athanasian Creed: "We worship one God, in trinity, and trinity is unity, neither confounding the persons, nor dividing the substance." About a hundred years ago, Baptist theologian Robert Dick put the same truth this way: "While there is only one divine nature of God, there are three persons called the Father, Son, and Holy Spirit who possess, not a similar, but the same numerical essence, and the distinction between them is not merely nominal, but real."

What are *monotheists*?

Christians are *monotheists*, meaning they believe in one God. "Hear, O Israel: The LORD our God, the LORD is one" (Deut. 6:4). When we acknowledge that the Father, Son, and Holy Spirit are each part of the triune God, we still hold to the unity of God.

Why is the Trinity not three manifestations of God?

One of the early heretical groups in the early church taught what was known as Sabellianism or Modalism. They held that the Trinity was three different manifestations of the same God, as water can be seen as ice, liquid, and vapor. They explain "Person" to mean a representation of God, just as man could be father, husband, and brother at one time. According to Modalism, there was only one God who revealed himself as the Father and the Creator in the Old Testament, but as Redeemer in the New Testament. In this manifestation he is called Jesus. The Holy Spirit, they say, is the third manifestation of the same God who relates to people today. The basic error of Modalism is that it denies the eternity and distinctiveness of the three Persons of the Trinity.

Do Christians believe that the Father created the Son or Holy Spirit?

No! One of the hottest doctrinal controversies of the early church was Arianism. Arius taught that only the Father was eternally God from the beginning. He taught that both the Son and the Holy Spirit were created out of nothing by God before anything else. Because they were created Beings, they could not be considered divine or possessing the attributes of divinity.

The Bible, of course, does not teach the creation of the Son and the Holy Spirit, but recognizes the work of both in the creation of all things (John 1:3; Gen. 1:2). Historically, Christians have recognized the error of Arianism and taught the biblical doctrines of the deity of Christ and of the Holy Spirit. Even today, however, there are cults who twist the Scriptures to deny the Trinity.

Do Christians believe that Christ or the Holy Spirit was just a power or attribute of God?

A wrong view of the Trinity called *Monarchianism* teaches that Jesus was a mere man who was energized by God at the baptism but sacrificed His essential deity at His death. This error misunderstands the truth that Jesus is God. The Bible teaches, "And the Word became flesh and dwelt among us, and we beheld His glory, the glory as of the only begotten of the Father" (John 1:14). John described the return of Christ when He saw "heaven opened, and behold, a white horse. And He who sat on him was called . . . The Word of God" (Rev. 19:11, 13).

How do the members of the Trinity relate to one another?

The members of the Trinity are equal in nature (they all have the same nature), yet distinct in person (three distinct personalities) and submissive in duties. The Father sent the Son to the world to die for the sins of the world, and the Father and Son sent the Holy Spirit to carry out the work of salvation.

What are some Old Testament signposts that teach the Trinity?

First, the word for God, *Elohim*, is plural; the "im" at the end of the word is plural, and teaches that even though there was one God, there is a plural unity. Next, God said, "Let Us . . ." (Gen. 1:26; 3:22; Isa. 6:8), implying one talking to another. God is even worshiped with a Trinitarian formula: "Holy, holy, holy" (Isa. 6:3). All three persons of the Trinity are designated as God in the judgment of the Lord on Sodom and Gomorrah (Gen. 19:24); Jehovah has a Son (Ps. 2:7); and there was a child king who is called "God" (Isa. 9:6).

What are the New Testament teachings of the Trinity?

The Trinity was revealed at the baptism of Jesus Christ. The early church fathers said the Trinity is seen in the wilderness beyond Jordan when God the Son was raised from the water, God the Holy Spirit descended like a dove, and the voice of God the Father was heard breaking the silence of heaven to acknowledge His delight in His Son.

Next, the truth of the Trinity was taught when Jesus said, "But when the Helper [God the Holy Spirit] comes, whom I [God the Son] shall send to you from [God] the Father . . ." (John 15:26). Later, the Trinitarian baptismal formula was, "in the name of the Father and of the Son and of the Holy Spirit"

(Matt. 28:19). And the New Testament church recognized the Trinity in its benediction: "The grace of the Lord Jesus Christ, and the love of God, and the communion of the Holy Spirit be with you all" (2 Cor. 13:14).

Finally, the distinct work of each person of the Trinity points out their differences: The Son offered His blood, through the Holy Spirit, to God the Father for the atonement of our sins.

Did God create darkness?

Some have a question about the Scripture where God says He creates darkness: "I form the light and create darkness, I make peace and create calamity; I, the LORD, do all these things" (Isa. 45:7). In eternity past there was no throne and no heaven. There was nothing but God. Since God is light, there was no darkness. When God created the burning star we call the sun, both light *and* darkness appeared (darkness is the absence of light). When God created light, the opposite result was darkness because there was no darkness in eternity past.

Did God create evil?

When God created Lucifer, He created him with the power of choice. God wanted worship, and authentic worship only comes from the free-choice worshiper. God did not make Lucifer sin. Sin came from Lucifer's free will. When he chose to rebel against God, evil was conceived. God *allowed* Lucifer to sin, but God was not the direct creator of evil.

Is the Bible inconsistent because some claimed to see God, yet God said no one could see His face?

In Genesis 32:30, Jacob said, "I have seen God face to face," and yet John 1:18 says, "No one has seen God at any time." But Jesus said in John 14:7, 9, "If you had known Me, you would have known My Father also; and from now on you know Him and have seen Him . . . He who has seen Me has seen the Father." How then do we reconcile "see[ing] God face to face"?

Certainly, no man has seen the face of God. God told Moses in Exodus 33:20, "You cannot see My face; for no man shall see Me, and live." God actually hid Moses in the cleft of the rock so that Moses only saw the backside of God.

When Jacob said, "I have seen God face to face," he was seeing the face of a physical *manifestation* of God, but not God Himself (a *theophany*).

Moses certainly was in God's presence when he saw the bush burning. Although he did not see the face of God, he saw the effects (the burning bush) and knew the relationship of God, as God said, "Take your sandals off your feet, for the place where you stand is holy ground" (Ex. 3:5). So, here is an instance of God supposedly meeting someone "face to face."

Some argue that because Exodus 33:11 says, "And the LORD spoke to Moses face to face, as a man speaks to his friend," it means that Moses saw the face of God. But this verse is correctly interpreted to mean that they spoke "voice to voice," not face to physical face. You cannot see God because there's nothing to see.

If God can do anything, can I see a miracle today?

God always does a miracle for a purpose. Obviously, every conversion of an individual is a demonstration of the power of God. Obviously, every answer to prayer is a demonstration of God's ability to interact in the laws of nature.

So the question really is not, "Can God do miracles?" but "Does God perform signs today?" Probably not. God has revealed Himself through Christ, so why would He give a miracle today to accomplish what He has already done?

Some people ask for a miracle to build their faith. But God warned those who saw miracles yet hardened their hearts against God that they would be judged more severely because they did not believe. "How shall we escape if we neglect so great a salvation, which at the first began to be spoken by the Lord . . . God also bearing witness both with signs and wonders, with various miracles" (Heb. 2:3–4). Those who say they would have a stronger faith if they could see a miracle do not understand the nature of unbelief. The multitude not only *saw* Jesus feed five thousand people with five loaves and two fishes, but they *participated* in the miracle because they ate the loaves and fishes. Yet the very next day these same people asked Jesus, "What sign will You perform then, that we may see it and believe You? What work will You do?" (John 6:30). The reason God does not do miracles today is because of the nature of unbelief among people. People would not believe in Him even if they saw the supernatural. Saving faith is a belief of the human heart when the person sees God's plan in the Bible and sees Jesus Christ as the Savior for their sins.

How do miracles occur?

There are several different ways that miracles occurred in Scripture. First, a miracle can supersede or transcend all known laws of nature. The act of Creation was that miracle that transcended any laws of nature that we have ever seen. Second, a miracle supercedes or transcends natural laws, such as when Elijah went to heaven in a chariot, defying the law of gravity. Third, miracles suspend the laws of nature, as when Christ walked on the water. Fourth, miracles occur when the laws of nature are intensified to produce a miraculous result, as when Jesus changed water into wine. Fifth, a miracle can redirect the laws of nature, as when the Red Sea was parted. And finally, a miracle transpires when the consequences of the disease of sin are neutralized, that is, by a miraculous physical healing.

Is the work of God consistent with His nature?

There is nothing and no one capable of motivating God to work apart from His nature. There was no one to advise and counsel God or influence any of His decisions (Isa. 40:13–14). The nature of God demands the sovereignty of God in all areas of His work.

Some have misunderstood the sovereignty of God by denying it or misapplying it. Those who deny it fail to recognize that "salvation is of the LORD" (Jonah 2:9).

Does everything glorify God?

God has "created all things, and by [His] will they exist and were created" (Rev. 4:11). The psalmist wrote, "The heavens declare the glory of God" (Ps. 19:1). Paul told the Ephesians that their conversions were performed "to the praise of the glory of His grace" (Eph. 1:6). The purpose of God's work is to bring glory to Himself. The responsibility of all creation is to glorify God. If in our lives and conversation we bring dishonor to God, we have failed to do the will of God. When we do what God desires, we will naturally glorify God and direct honor to Him.

How is the work of God both passive and active?

Sometimes the work of God is active. This occurs when God causes things to happen to us according to His plan for our lives. Understanding what we need and what is best for us, God will sometimes direct the circumstances around us to provide experiences, opportunities, and provisions to aid us in our lives.

At other times, the work of God is passive. The classic example of this is found in the life of Job. God allowed the devil to afflict the life of Job but not the purpose of God. When the devil was permitted on two occasions to test Job, on both occasions divine limits were set on the testings. God used the devil to accomplish something in the life of Job while God remained passive. Today, when God allows the same to be accomplished in our lives, we have the promise of divine limits set by a God who knows us better than we know ourselves. "God is faithful, who will not allow you to be tempted beyond what you are able, but with the temptation will also make the way of escape, that you may be able to bear it" (1 Cor. 10:13).

How has God spoken in the past to people?

God has spoken through the natural world that surrounds us: "The heavens declare the glory of God; and the firmament shows His handiwork. Day unto day utters speech, and night unto night reveals knowledge" (Ps. 19:1–2).

Next, God speaks to us through the Scriptures, which are called the Word of God.

In a third way, God speaks through conviction of sin. Jesus sent the Holy Spirit to convict or convince us, which means the Holy Spirit causes people to be aware of sin, righteousness, and judgment (John 16:9–11).

Another way God has communicated to mankind is through miracles. Sometimes miracles are called "signs." Just as a road sign gives a special message, God has spoken to us through His miracles.

God has also spoken with an audible voice to people such as Adam, Cain, Noah, Abraham, Moses, and the children of Israel. At still other times God has communicated without using words but has communicated through inner urges. This is seen when Paul was going through Asia Minor: "They were forbidden by the Holy Spirit to preach the word in Asia . . . They tried to go into Bithynia, but the Spirit did not permit them" (Acts 16:6–7).

God can communicate through circumstances too, which has historically been called "the Providence of God." When Joseph was sent to Egypt, he told his brothers that they did it for evil, "but God meant it for good, in order to bring it about as it is this day, to save many people alive" (Gen. 50:20).

But the ultimate revelation of God is in Jesus Christ, "God . . . has in these last days spoken to us by His Son" (Heb. 1:1–2).

Can God speak today in an audible voice?

The answer to that is both yes and no. God could speak to us in an audible voice because God can do anything. And to say God could not speak is to say He is less than God. The very nature of God is to reveal Himself to His people (Deut. 29:29).

However, God has chosen not to speak audibly today, first, because He has said everything we need to know in the Word of God. Why should He say again what He has already said? If God did speak today, His message would be consistent with what He has already said. If people say that God has spoken to them in an audible message to do something contrary to Scripture, we rightly question whether they have heard from God (1 John 4:1 says to test a spirit).

If God would speak, what would He say?

If we could have an intimate discussion with God, He would not tell us doctrine, for that content is already included in the Bible. He would not tell us how to live, because that is also in the Bible. Nor would He tell us about salvation, because that too is included in Scripture. Would He warn us about danger? Again, He has done that in the writings of the prophets. Would God help us solve our problems? Our deepest struggles? He has done that in the Psalms and other books on spirituality. Everything God would say, He has already said. So rather than waiting for God to speak, we should study what He has already said, so we can understand what He wants us to know.

Why is God silent?

God is silent because He has already spoken in the Scriptures. Sometimes Christians don't feel His presence because He is testing them. Sometimes God doesn't communicate because He has already talked to them in the Scriptures. At other times God knows a person won't listen or has forgotten, or won't do what God said when He did speak to him.

Why does God seem far away when we call to Him in prayer?

Too often Christians rely on their feelings, and not on the facts of God's Word. While there are feelings associated with being a Christian, we should not base our relationship to God on them. After we have prayed about a problem, God may want us to talk to another Christian, or He may want us to work out the problem ourselves. Sometimes God wants us to learn patience or another Christian attribute.

God may also be distant because He wants us to learn to trust His Word. The hymn writer said it best: "When darkness veils His lovely face, I rest on His unchanging grace." Times of "lostness" when God doesn't speak make us unsure and take away our confidence. Perhaps God wants us to stop trusting in some physical thing and learn to trust Him. David asked the question, "Why are you cast down, O my soul?" (Ps. 42:5). In these times of "lostness," David was forced to remember the previous days when he had communion with God. "My soul longs, yes, even faints for the courts of the LORD; my heart and my flesh cry out for the living God" (Ps. 84:2).

Why can't people see God?

That's an easy answer: because most people are not looking for Him. Most people are sinners, and they don't look for God, just as a robber doesn't look for a policeman. But the real answer is that people can't see God because He is not seeable. "God is Spirit" (John 4:24). He doesn't have a physical body that can be seen.

Why do people want to see God?

First, some people want to see God out of curiosity; others want to see Him to worship Him. A third group of people wants to see God for personal fulfillment. "For in Him we live and move and have our being" (Acts 17:28). A fourth group wants to see God because they are naturally inquisitive. God placed in every person a natural longing for God, but sin has thwarted that desire.

What did Moses see when He saw God?

Moses prayed, "Please, show me Your glory" (Ex. 33:18). In response, Moses was permitted to see the back of God (Ex. 33:23). The Bible says, "No one has seen God at any time" (John 1:18), and Moses "endured as seeing Him who is invisible" (Heb. 11:27). Moses saw a manifestation of God, His glory (Ex. 33:22–23). While God is spoken of as having bodily parts—arms, legs, etc.—these are anthropomorphisms. These physical manifestations are attributed to God because they represent the functions that He does. But God doesn't have a physical body.

Why does God hide Himself?

First of all we have to remind ourselves of what Job said: "When He hides His face, who then can see Him?" (Job 34:29). So when God hides, no one can see Him. But God asked concerning Abraham, "Shall I hide from Abraham what I am doing?" (Gen. 18:17). God hides Himself or His plan because He has chosen not to reveal Himself to people because of their spiritual conditions.

Why can't I see God physically?

A famous prospector went looking for gold in the Northern Ontario bush country. He came back to say that there was no gold there. Later, a second prospector not only discovered gold, but also found the first prospector's boot print cast in the soft metal. The first prospector did not see gold because he failed to recognize gold when he stepped on it.

Because people can't see God does not mean that there is no God. We know that God has no physical presence. "God is Spirit" (John 4:24). Paul described "the image of the invisible God" (Col. 1:15).

There have been artists and sculptors who have rendered an image of God. But any portrayal of God is a picture of something less than God.

A Russian cosmonaut once announced from outer space that God did not exist because he looked out of his window and did not see God. Later, an American astronaut read from space the Genesis account of the creation of the world by God. God may not have a physical presence, but the physical earth that He created bears His fingerprints, proving He exists.

How can I know God if I can't see Him?

To see God, we should look to Jesus. John declared, "No one has seen God at any time. The only begotten Son, who is in the bosom of the Father, He has declared Him" (John 1:18). Jesus has shown us what the Father is like. "He who has seen Me has seen the Father," is what Jesus told Philip (John 14:9).

The inability to see God physically should not hinder us from trusting and obeying Him. We should be like the patriarchs, who "died in faith, not having received the promises, but having seen them afar off were assured of them, embraced them and confessed that they were strangers and pilgrims on the earth" (Heb. 11:13). They responded to God without depending upon physical sight, and so should we. Actually, not seeing God may aid us in knowing Him, because we are not distracted by the physical eye. Faith is demonstrated by the spiritual eye of the heart.

What can we learn from not seeing God?

A good scientist learns not only from what he or she sees, but from what cannot be seen. Our inability to see God physically may open up great areas of faith and trust. How big is God? Isaiah says the span of God's hand is as large as the entire universe (40:12). Since a man's span tends to be about one-eighth of his physical height, Isaiah's description of God makes Him eight times the size of the universe that He created.

We can't see a God that large, and we can't understand a God who is without limit, because we are finite. God is so large we can't comprehend it. By not being able to see a physical God, we realize He is bigger than our comprehension, and even bigger than that.

By not seeing God we realize how great He is, and what great things He can do, and what great potential He can be to our lives. "Now to Him who is able to do exceedingly abundantly above all that we ask or think . . ." (Eph. 3:20).

Why doesn't God do miracles today?

Maybe God is doing many miracles, but the person asking that question can't see what God is doing. After Jesus miraculously fed the five thousand, the following day the same crowd asked Him, "What sign will You perform then, that we may see it and believe You? What work will You do?" (John 6:30). They ate the food produced by a miracle, then complained that they hadn't seen one. People tend to make miracles a condition of their faith. Perhaps God doesn't allow us to see miracles today because we would base our faith on a miracle, rather than placing our faith in God.

Should I expect miracles in my life?

In one sense, look at all of the people in the Bible who did not experience an outward miracle: Adam, Jacob, Joseph, David, Isaiah, Jeremiah, and John the Baptist. We don't have to experience miracles to be spiritual men or women of God. Concerning John the Baptist, Jesus said, "Assuredly, I say to you, among those born of women there has not risen one greater than John the Baptist" (Matthew 11:11). Here's a man who was the greatest ever born, greater than Moses the miracle worker or Abraham, who had experienced miracles. Yet the Bible says of John the Baptist, "John performed no sign" (John 10:41). If he didn't do miracles or need miracles to serve God, neither do you.

However, when you seek miracles, make sure you properly define miracles. C.S. Lewis defines miracles as "an interference with nature by supernatural power." When most people think miracles, they think "sign-miracles." They think of God's interference in the laws of nature. However, every Christian has experienced the miraculous: conversion, answers to prayer, divine indwelling, divine insight into Scripture, divine leading, and divine protection.

Why does God keep secrets?

Have you ever thought that God doesn't tell you everything about your life? He knows what will happen to you in the future, but doesn't tell you. There are a lot of things God doesn't tell. Why does He keep secrets?

Sometimes God keeps secrets because He loves you. If you knew an illness was coming, it would take away your present joy.

Sometimes God keeps secrets to protect you. As an illustration, a travel agent may not give you a deep discount airline ticket because He knows it has safety violations that may put you in danger.

Sometimes God wants you to live a normal life. A mother won't tell her children about her serious illness so they can have a normal childhood. Just as humans keep secrets because they are concerned about the other person, God keeps secrets because He's concerned about us.

"The secret things belong to the LORD our God, but those things which are revealed belong to us and to our children forever, that we may do all the words of this law" (Deut. 29:29).

God may keep secrets from you because you haven't done what He's already told you to do. Why should God tell you something about the future when you haven't obeyed Him in the past?

And then there are reasons why God keeps secrets that we will never understand. Why? Because we don't understand the mind of God. "'For My thoughts are not your thoughts, nor are your ways My ways,' says the LORD. 'For as the heavens are higher than the earth, so are My ways higher than your ways, and My thoughts than your thoughts'" (Isa. 55:8–9). This tells us two things: Not only do we not know all of the content of God's thoughts, but we also don't know the way He thinks.

How can I live with the secrets of God?

First remember that God is committed to revealing His secrets under certain conditions. If you worship Him, He will tell you His secrets. "The secret of the LORD is with those who fear Him" (Ps. 25:14). Second, God reveals His secrets to those who live a holy life. "For the perverse person is an abomination to the LORD, but His secret counsel is with the upright" (Prov. 3:32).

Where is God when accidents happen?

When a truck plowed into a crowd of school children, killing many and injuring others, some people asked, "Where was God?"

They ask additional questions: "Is God not good to children?" "Did He not know what would happen?" "Doesn't He care enough about children to protect them?" "Couldn't God have prevented the disaster?"

An orderly God runs the world by laws, which are an extension of His nature. If a person falls out of an airplane without a parachute, God knows, loves, and is concerned for the person. But God cannot go contrary to His laws to cause a person to float to the ground. It's not that God can't save the person who's falling, but that God has chosen to run the world by His laws, and "He cannot deny Himself" (2 Tim. 2:13) or contradict Himself. The laws of gravity will cause that person to fall to the ground.

The questions about the school children are not asked properly. Yes, God is good because He gives us life and an opportunity to go to heaven. Yes, God knew that the children would be harmed. And obviously God cares about each one of them. God could have prevented the disaster, but sometimes God allows laws to work themselves out for a greater purpose. Perhaps some other children might be converted out of this disaster, and other people may be brought closer to the Lord. Sometimes a missionary becomes a martyr and is killed, and ten more people are called to pick up his work. What is the result? The work prospers tenfold.

Why do some people suffer?

Sometimes God allows a person to suffer to prepare that person for a special service. At other times God brings that person into a closer relationship to Himself. Disease is a result of sin in the world, and sometimes disease, like sin, is taking its course. Some people suffer because they don't pray and trust God for healing. Perhaps some people suffer because they don't get the proper medical care and medicine.

Sometimes suffering is a punishment for sin in the person's life and God wants to purify that person to bring him closer to the Lord. At other times, suffering is entirely circumstantial; it has nothing to do with God's punishment or the work of God in a person's life. A person may suffer sickness because of exposure to bacteria. Another may suffer physically because of an accident, or psychologically because of home conditions while growing up.

Why do good people suffer?

Sometimes God allows your suffering to manifest strength in other areas of your life. At other times suffering, like Paul's thorn in the flesh, manifests God's grace in your life. Sometimes suffering is to refine your life from impurities, and God wants you to be more holy. At other times suffering helps you find the perfect will of God. This is especially true when someone is not following the Lord. At other times suffering is from Satan. Job suffered because Satan took away his family, wealth, and finally his health.

Why doesn't God run to our rescue when we suffer?

God uses problems in our lives to test us and help us learn from our mistakes. "Now no chastening seems to be joyful for the present, but painful; nevertheless, afterward it yields the peaceable fruit of righteousness to those who have been trained by it" (Heb. 12:11). C. S. Lewis describes suffering as a "gift of God," so that when we suffer we become more godly. "My brothers, think well of all the various sources of your sufferings, knowing they mature you" (James 1:4, author's translation).

Sometimes God doesn't run to our rescue because He's told us in the Bible what we should be doing about our suffering or affliction. Instead of crying out to God, sometimes we should be studying the Scriptures to find God's will for our lives. When we are tempted, we should study 1 Corinthians 10:13 to find God's "way of escape." Finally, God does not expect us to live from "miracle to miracle," but from "faith to faith" (Romans 1:17). When people were following Jesus looking for a miracle, He rebuked them (John 6:26). We should look daily to Jesus, and not look for daily miraculous deliverance from suffering.

God doesn't run to our rescue each time we fall down, just like a wise parent will allow a child to struggle to get back up because that is the way the child will grow and become stronger.

When God intervenes in my problems, how does He do it?

Actually there are several ways that God intervenes in our lives, many times without our knowing it. Sometimes God uses friends to tell us what to do, as Mordecai told Esther how she could make a difference in the problem facing Israel (Esther 4:1, 8).

Sometimes God intervenes by giving us a special burden or desire. When Nehemiah heard Jerusalem had no walls, "[he] sat down and wept, and mourned for many days; [he] was fasting and praying before the God of heaven" (Neh. 1:4). God intervened in response to Nehemiah's prayer and fasting.

A third way God intervenes is through Scripture, because in the Bible we see how we should act and respond to a problem.

On other occasions, God uses angels to intervene, such as the angel of the Lord who released Peter from prison (Acts 5:19). The Lord may use an angel in your life (Heb. 13:2).

At times God intervenes by providence; that is, He works His perfect will through details and circumstances. When Joseph was in prison, it was God's working (providence) that brought him to power in Egypt. Joseph said to his brothers, "You meant evil against me; but God meant it for good" (Gen. 50:20). Sometimes a flat tire is used by God to keep you from an intersection where you might have been in a terrible accident.

QUESTIONS
ABOUT
THE HOLY SPIRIT

Who is the Holy Spirit?

The Holy Spirit is the third Person of the Trinity, equal with God the Father and God the Son in nature, but separate in personality from them.

Is the Holy Spirit a person?

The Holy Spirit is the third Person of the Trinity, and as such, He has personality. The Holy Spirit has intellectual ability to know things (1 Cor.

2:11), emotional capacity to feel things (Rom. 15:30), and volitional power to make choices (1 Cor. 12:11).

Why is there so much more attention given to the Holy Spirit today than in the past?

Some have called the Holy Spirit the forgotten Member of the Trinity. However, with the publication and distribution of millions of copies of the *Scofield Bible* in the last century, those who read the *Scofield Bible* have talked about the amplified ministry of the Holy Spirit in this present dispensation. Also, many dispensational teachers have pointed out that we are living in the dispensation of the Holy Spirit, that is, the church age. With the arrival of the gift of tongues at Azusa Street in 1907, and the subsequent planting and growth of many pentecostal denominations, there has been a growing emphasis on the ministry of the Holy Spirit. Then in the late 1950s when Roman Catholics and non-pentecostals began speaking in tongues, there arose a second wave, the charismatic movement, again giving attention to the Holy Spirit. In the past twenty years, the growing attention to practical service in the church connected to spiritual giftedness again has brought attention to the Holy Spirit.

In recent days other manifestations of the Spirit, such as being "slain in the Spirit," the apostolic church movement, and others have brought more attention to the ministry of the Holy Spirit.

Why is the Holy Spirit referred to as "It" several times in Scripture?

The Greek word for "spirit," which is *pneuma,* is neuter in the Greek language (All Greek words are classified as either male, female, or neuter); therefore, a neuter pronoun would normally be used for "spirit." Yet in other places in Scripture, masculine pronouns *he* or *him* are used for the Holy Spirit and are properly translated *He.* Also, the masculine pronoun *ekeinos* is used in the same passage where we find the neuter *pneuma,* as in John 14:17 and 16:13. While the Holy Spirit is referred to as "it" in some translations, "it" should have been rendered "He," because of the context.

How is the Holy Spirit treated as a person?

The Holy Spirit can be obeyed (Acts 10:19), lied to (Acts 5:3), resisted (Acts

7:51), grieved (Eph. 4:30), reverenced (Ps. 51:11), blasphemed (Matt. 12:31), and spited (Heb. 10:29).

What proofs are there that the Holy Spirit is God?

First, the Holy Spirit does the work of God (Gen. 1:2; John 3:5). Second, He receives the honor only due to God. Third, He has the title of deity. Fourth, in the baptismal formula, He is identified with God (Matt. 28:19). And the words He speaks are ascribed to God (Ex. 16:4; Ps. 95:6–7; Heb. 3:7; Isa. 6:8; Acts 28:25).

How can Jesus give direction to the Holy Spirit, yet Jesus and the Holy Spirit remain equal?

"When the Helper comes, whom I shall send to you from the Father, the Spirit of truth who proceeds from the Father . . ." (John 15:26). In this passage Jesus sends or directs the activities of the Holy Spirit. Jesus and the Holy Spirit are equal in nature, but the Holy Spirit is submissive in duties to Jesus, just as Jesus is submissive to the Father. The Father sent the Son to the world, so the Father and the Son sent the Holy Spirit. The Father, Son, and Holy Spirit are equal in nature, separate in person, and submissive in duties.

What are some representations of the Holy Spirit?

The Holy Spirit is called or likened to a dove (Matt. 3:16), a seal (Eph. 1:13), anointed oil (2 Cor. 1:21; 1 John 2:27), fire (Matt. 3:11), wind (John 3:8), river (John 7:38), dew (Ps.133:3), water (John 3:5), and a down payment or earnest money (2 Cor. 1:22).

What is the *conviction* of the Holy Spirit?

The word to *convict* comes from Latin, and its root means "to cause to see, or to know the truth." John 16:8 says, "When He [the Holy Spirit] has come, He will convict the world of sin, and of righteousness, and of judgment." When the Holy Spirit convicts, He will take away the blindness of Satan and cause people to see the nature and work of God.

What does the conviction of the Holy Spirit do?

Concerning the Holy Spirit, Jesus taught, "And when He has come, He will convict the world of sin, and of righteousness, and of judgment" (John 16:8).

The Holy Spirit today is actively reproving, or convicting, in the world. The terms *reprove, convict,* and *illuminate* all have similar meanings. These terms speak of the work of the Holy Spirit in setting forth the truth and causing a person to see it as such. This does not necessarily mean a person will respond positively to the gospel and accept the truth, but that the Holy Spirit will cause a person to see the truth.

What is the Holy Spirit's "ministry of restraint"?

In this world of sin, darkness, and corruption, the Holy Spirit prevents the complete corruption of the world. He does this by restraining sin, or striving against sin. "My Spirit shall not strive with man forever" (Gen. 6:3). The Holy Spirit will restrain sin until he is "taken out of the way" (2 Thess. 2:7). In this role the Holy Spirit is called the Restrainer.

How does the Holy Spirit restrain sin?

The Holy Spirit uses the institutions of society, such as the church, government, schools, family, and business, to enforce "laws" so society won't be lawless. Next, the Holy Spirit works directly in the human heart to stop sin. Finally, the Holy Spirit works providentially to enforce the laws of God in the world.

What is the Holy Spirit's "work of regeneration"?

Regeneration is the work of the Spirit of God whereby people are given eternal life (God's life and nature) and become part of God's family. They receive a new nature and have new spiritual desires. In regeneration a person becomes the child of God.

How is the word *regeneration* used in the Bible?

The Greek word translated "regeneration" is used only once in the Bible as it relates to this ministry of the Holy Spirit: "Not by works of righteousness which we have done, but according to His mercy He saved us, through the washing of regeneration and renewing of the Holy Spirit" (Titus 3:5). Jesus told Nicodemus, "Unless one is born of water and the Spirit, he cannot enter the kingdom of God" (John 3:5). Regeneration is that work of the Spirit of God whereby men are given God's life and nature and made a part of the family of God. Occurring at the moment of conversion, it lasts a lifetime and eternity to follow. Jesus said, "He who hears My word and believes in Him who sent Me has everlasting life, and shall not come into judgment, but has passed from death into life" (John 5:24). This passing "from death into life" is perhaps the chief feature of regeneration.

How does regeneration work in the individual?

When a person believes in Jesus Christ (Acts 16:31) or accepts Christ as his Savior (John 1:12), he becomes a child of God. He was dead in trespasses and sins (Eph. 2:1), but in a divine experience, the Holy Spirit gives new life to the individual, a new nature to serve God, new desires to do God's will, and appetites for righteousness. God creates a new nature in him and makes him His child.

What does the Bible teach about the *indwelling* of the Holy Spirit?

In Christ's prayer to the Father on the believer's behalf, John 17:23 says, "I in them, and You in Me; that they may be made perfect in one." Jesus promised in John 14:16 that the Holy Spirit would come to abide in the Christian: "And I will pray the Father, and He will give you another Helper, that He may abide with you forever." The words *abide* and *dwell* come from the same root meaning, "to stay [live] in a given place." This is a promise to *every* believer. The Holy Spirit comes to live in us at conversion (see John 7:37–39; Rom. 8:9; 1 Cor. 2:12; 6:19; 1 John 3:24). First Corinthians 3:16 says, "Do you not know that you are the temple of God and that the Spirit of God dwells in you?"

The purpose of the indwelling Holy Spirit is to control the believer (2 Cor. 5:17; Gal. 5:16–18; Eph. 3:16), guide the believer (John 16:13; Rom. 8:14), teach the believer (1 John 2:27), empower the believer (Acts 1:8), impart the love of God to him and through him (Rom. 5:5; Gal. 5:22), strengthen the believer (Eph. 3:16), and give assurance of salvation (1 Cor. 2:10; 1 John 3:24).

What is the *filling* of the Holy Spirit?

The filling is a wonderful experience when the Holy Spirit controls or influences a person to accomplish the purpose and glory of God. "Do not be drunk with wine, in which is dissipation; but be filled with the Spirit" (Eph. 5:18).

What happens to one who is filled with the Spirit?

Paul commanded the Ephesian Christians, "And do not be drunk with wine, in which is dissipation; but be filled with the Spirit" (Eph. 5:18). God has given men and women the opportunity to be continually filled with the Holy Spirit for effective service. Rather than allowing alcohol to control the mind of the Christian, it is God's desire that His Holy Spirit be in control. As we establish our fellowship with God through confession of sins (1 John 1:9) and yield to Him (Rom. 6:13), we can be filled with the Holy Spirit as commanded in Scriptures.

Some sincere Christians today seek spectacular signs to accompany the fullness of the Holy Spirit in their lives. Actually, the Bible does not teach these should be expected today. The Holy Spirit's fullness within us is primarily to produce the fruit of the Spirit (Gal. 5:22–23). The evidence in the book of Acts of the fullness of the Holy Spirit promised by Jesus was power to witness (Acts 1:8). On some occasions (but not every occasion) when Christians were filled with the Holy Spirit, the building shook (Acts 4:31). Sometimes they spoke in tongues (Acts 10:44–46). But always the gospel was preached and people were saved. These occasional outward occurrences were often tools God used at that time to accomplish the main objective of witnessing. These outward signs were similar to the purpose that miracles had in the early church: They were an objective authority for the message of God. But when God provided the full revelation of the Word of God as the authoritative message, the outward signs or authorities passed off the scene.

What is the *sanctification* of the Holy Spirit?

Various denominations interpret the word *sanctification* differently. The root meaning is "to be set apart." When the Holy Spirit sanctifies a person, he or she is set apart to God and should reflect the character of God. Because the Holy Spirit is *holy*, He makes the person desire holiness. Because the Holy Spirit is *spiritual*, He makes the person desire spirituality.

What is the *sealing* of the Holy Spirit?

The Bible teaches that Christians are sealed by the Holy Spirit: "You were sealed with the Holy Spirit of promise, who is the guarantee of our inheritance until the redemption of the purchased possession, to the praise of His glory" (Eph. 1:13–14).

When a man and woman agree to marry, it is customary in our culture for the man to give the woman an engagement ring as a symbol of his commitment to her. Paul was drawing on a similar custom of the first century to explain this aspect of the ministry of the Holy Spirit in salvation. When we are born again, we immediately become heirs to all God has promised us. God gives us the Holy Spirit as a down payment for His commitment to someday give us all the other things He has promised. By way of application, it is important that we "do not grieve the Holy Spirit of God, by whom you were sealed for the day of redemption" (Eph. 4:30).

What is the *illumination* of the Holy Spirit?

Illumination is the ministry of the Holy Spirit that causes the believer to understand the spiritual things or message of God. The god of this world (the devil) blinds the mind (2 Cor. 4:4), but the Holy Spirit takes away spiritual blindness so one is able to see more clearly God's will and purpose for his or her life.

What is the *fruit* of the Spirit?

The fruit of the Spirit is a result of the work of the Holy Spirit that occurs after conversion whereby the believer reflects the character of God in his life. The fruit of the Spirit is referred to in the singular because it is what He does in us. There are many reflections of this fruit: "But the fruit of the Spirit is love, joy, peace, longsuffering, kindness, goodness, faithfulness, gentleness, self-control. Against such there is no law" (Gal. 5:22–23). The fruit of the Spirit produces godly character and works inwardly with outer manifestations.

What is a *spiritual gift?*

A spiritual gift is an ability given by the Holy Spirit to the believer for serving the Lord in a spiritual way. One's spiritual gift should be exercised to the glory of God.

How many spiritual gifts may a person have?

There are many gifts in the local body of Christ (1 Cor. 12:4). Some people seem to be less gifted, and some even may appear to have no gifts (maybe they had spiritual gifts, but didn't use them and lost them), but every believer has been given a gift (1 Cor. 7:7). All people are expected to use their gifts for the glory of God. If you don't have specific gifts, you can desire or seek them (1 Cor. 12:31).

What is the relationship between a spiritual gift and natural ability?

A spiritual gift relates to building up the saints of God or doing something spiritual or supernatural in the ministry of God. Natural talents or abilities instruct, inspire, or entertain on a natural level. Nothing supernatural happens when a talent is displayed. However, people can yield themselves to God so that their natural abilities are used by God to become the expression of their spiritual gifts.

When does a person receive his spiritual gift?

Historically, spiritual gifts were given at the Ascension of Jesus Christ into heaven (Eph. 4:8,11). *Embryonically*, spiritual gifts were placed in a person at their conversions (Rom. 8:9; 1 Cor. 7:7). But *actually*, spiritual gifts come to light later in experience as a person grows in spiritual maturity (Rom. 1:11; 1 Cor. 12:31).

Can a spiritual gift in one believer be greater than in other believers?

Sometimes this is difficult to tell, because some who are less gifted are more faithful in their service to God than those who are more gifted. God would use the less gifted because of their faithfulness, and it would be difficult to compare their spiritual gifts to those God didn't use whose giftedness may be greater. All are exhorted to "earnestly desire the best gifts" (1 Cor. 12:31). The parable of the men with five talents, three talents, and one talent (Matt. 25:14–30) implies that people have varying degrees of giftedness.

Can a person seek a spiritual gift that he or she apparently doesn't have?

It appears that gifts are sovereignly given by the Holy Spirit (1 Cor. 12:4), but Paul wanted to give spiritual gifts to the Christians in Rome (Rom. 1:11), and people were told to earnestly desire spiritual gifts (1 Cor. 12:31).

Does a person have a prominent spiritual gift?

It appears that every person has a prominent or dominant gift in his or her life. First Corinthians 7:7 says, "Each one has his own gift from God." The Greek word *proper* suggests something that is unique to the person. This means a person can have a spiritual ability that best characterizes his or her service.

QUESTIONS

ABOUT

JESUS

Does the Bible teach that Jesus was God?

The Bible records many statements concerning the deity of Christ (Heb. 1:8). John says "the Word was God" (John 1:1). Writing hundreds of years before his birth, Isaiah called him "the Mighty God" (Isa. 9:6). Paul was "looking for the blessed hope and glorious appearing of our great God and

Savior Jesus Christ" (Titus 2:13). Paul quotes an early church doctrinal statement:

> God was manifested in the flesh,
> Justified in the Spirit,
> Seen by angels,
> Preached among the Gentiles,
> Believed on in the world,
> Received up in glory. (1 Tim. 3:16)

The teaching of both Old and New Testaments is clearly that Jesus is God.

Did Jesus live before He was born of a virgin?

Christ is eternal. The writer of Hebrews compared Melchizedek to Christ: "Without father, without mother, without genealogy, having neither beginning of days nor end of life, but made like the Son of God" (Heb. 7:3). When we think of the earthly life of Christ, however, we recognize that He came from heaven. John the Baptist said, "He who comes from above is above all; he who is of the earth is earthly and speaks of the earth. He who comes from heaven is above all" (John 3:31). Because of this, John could accept the growing popularity of Jesus at his expense. Jesus told the people of his home region, "For I have come down from heaven, not to do My own will, but the will of Him who sent Me" (John 6:38).

When did Jesus become the Son of God?

Some teach that Jesus became the Son of God at the Incarnation. To prove this they use the angel's prediction to Mary, "[He] will be called the Son of God" (Luke 1:35). Others say Jesus became a Son of God at His baptism. It *was* there that God broke the silence of heaven to announce, "This is My beloved Son, in whom I am well pleased" (Matt. 3:17).

A third view is that Jesus became the Son of God at His Resurrection, because Paul said, "Declared to be the Son of God with power, according to the Spirit of holiness, by the resurrection from the dead" (Rom. 1:4). And yet another group cites Hebrews 1:1–4, arguing that Jesus became the Son of God by "appointment" at His Ascension. All of these fail to recognize the teaching of one of the Bible's best-known verses: "For God so loved the world that He gave His only begotten Son, that whoever believes in Him should not perish but have everlasting life" (John 3:16). Jesus was recognized as the Son of God before He came to earth to provide eternal salvation. Jesus was the Son of God even before the first presentation of the gospel in Genesis 3:15: "And I will put enmity between you and the woman, and between your seed and her Seed; He shall bruise your head, and you shall bruise His heel." This verse recognized the coming of the Seed of the woman to bruise the head of the serpent.

The key to understanding when Jesus became the Son of God is to understand the meaning of the word *day* in Psalm 2:7: "I will declare the decree: the LORD hath said unto me, Thou art my Son; this day have I begotten thee" (KJV). The word *day* does not refer to a twenty-four hour period in time. God lives beyond time. This word means an eternal day. Technically this is called *eternal generation*. Jesus did not become the Son of God at a point in time. He has always been in the process of becoming the Son of God in God's eternal day. The conclusion is that there never was a time that Christ was not the Son of God.

What does the phrase "the only begotten Son of God" mean?

The term "only begotten" is used to describe the unique relationship between the Father and Jesus (John 1:14, 18; 3:16; 1 John 4:9). Though any individual who trusts Christ personally for salvation will become a child of God (John 1:12), there is only one "only begotten Son of God." In this phrase Christ possesses the nature of God, just as a son possesses the nature of his father. The only begotten Son of God is just like His heavenly Father, for He is God.

Was the virgin birth of Jesus the same as artificial insemination?

In our day artificial insemination creates the possibility of a woman experiencing birth without knowing a man in a sexual way. However, this is not true of the virgin birth in the biblical sense, which involved a virgin giving birth to a child *without* the seed of a man. The virgin birth is the supernatural method God used to send Jesus Christ to earth to become a man.

Is the virgin birth important or necessary?

The virgin birth of Christ is not an independent doctrine that we can receive or reject without affecting our Christianity. It is one of the foundation stones of Christianity; our faith will crumble if it is removed. This doctrine is tied to biblical inerrancy, Christ's sinless character, the Atonement, and other key doctrines of the Bible. If Jesus was not born of a virgin, then He would be unable to save Himself because He would not be a sinless Savior. If we cannot accept the virgin birth of Christ, very little credibility remains in the Bible. Therefore, we must understand the virgin birth if we are going to understand our faith.

What does the word *virgin* mean?

Some argue that Isaiah did not mean a "virgin" but rather a "young maid" when he wrote this verse: "Behold, the virgin shall conceive and bear a Son, and shall call His name Immanuel" (Isa. 7:14). Actually, the Hebrew word *almah* translated "virgin" could be translated either way, "virgin" or "young maid." But the context suggests Isaiah was talking about a virgin. A nonvirgin having a child would not be an extraordinary miracle but would be expected. The introduction of a miraculous sign implies the use of "virgin" rather than "young woman." Under Mosaic Law a young woman could be stoned if she was found pregnant out of wedlock. So even if Isaiah was referring to a young woman ready for marriage, it is reasonable to assume she had not known a man. When the *Septuagint*, the Greek-language version of the Old Testament, was translated, a Greek word was used that could mean only "virgin." Until recent times, it was generally assumed by translators that Isaiah here referred to a woman who had not known a man.

Not only is there a cultural and traditional reason for accepting the translation of the word *virgin*, but there is also a biblical mandate. When Matthew wrote under the inspiration of the Holy Spirit, he cited Isaiah 7:14 to demonstrate that Christ's birth was fulfilling Bible prophecy. In doing so, he followed the Septuagint translation and used the Greek word *parthenos*, which could only be translated "virgin." Matthew noted, "Now all this was done that it might be fulfilled which was spoken by the Lord through the prophet, saying: 'Behold, a virgin shall be with child, and bear a Son, and they shall call His name Immanuel,' which is translated, 'God with us'" (Matt. 1:22, 23).

Why is the doctrine of the virgin birth necessary?

At stake in the controversy surrounding the doctrine of the virgin birth of Christ are a number of other doctrines. If Jesus had a human father, He would have inherited a sin nature. In that case He would be unable to save

Himself, let alone be the sinless substitute for the sins of the world. With human parents, it would be impossible for Him to be the Son of God.

What does the Bible teach about Christ "emptying" Himself?

The term *kenosis* is a Greek word used in Philippians 2:7 to describe what happened when Christ became a man. The term is translated from "made Himself of no reputation," which appears in the King James Version of the Bible. It is translated "He emptied himself" in the *New American Standard Version.* One theologian described it, "He stripped himself of the insignia of mystery."

For Christ, who was God before time began, to take on "the form of a servant" was indeed a humiliating experience. For ages theologians have faced the dilemma of interpreting this one word, *kenosis.* They cannot deny that Christ "emptied" Himself, but "What was poured out?" is the question. Can Christ give away part of His deity and remain God? Can God be less than God? The answer is found in a threefold explanation. "Christ emptied Himself" by (1) veiling His glory, (2) accepting the limitations of being human, and (3) voluntarily giving up the independent use of His relative attributes.

How can Christ be both God and man at the same time?

When we think of the dual nature of Christ, we must somehow not divide Him into two parts as though He were a schizophrenic, or two persons in one body. Rather we must think of Him as a Unity; He is the God-man. His nature has been described a number of ways. At the Council of Chalcedon, an ecumenical gathering in A.D. 451 called in to settle some of the eastern church divisions, Jesus was described as having been "made known in two natures without confusion, without change, without division, without separation, the distinction of natures being by no means taken away by the union." In essence, when we examine the two natures of Christ, orthodox doctrine forbids us either to divide the Person or to confound the natures.

When the council said it could not divide the Person, it meant that Christ did not have two personalities (persons), but one. He did not have a perfect divine mind and a limited human mind—Christ had one mind. As humans we cannot understand it, but we can see it in the Gospels. As a person Christ had one mind, one set of emotions, and one will.

Did Jesus father any children?

There are some religions that teach that Jesus fathered children. First, there is no record or implication in Scripture that He did so. Second, if He did, that would mean that His children would have a divine nature or the nature of God, because Jesus Christ is God (John 1:1). It would also imply that those children were not conceived in sin (Ps. 51:5) and/or that they were born without a sin nature. The usual view among Christians is that the sin nature is passed on from parent to child through the father. Because of this, a virgin birth was necessary so that Jesus would be born from the human body of the mother, but without a sin nature because His divine nature came from God. In light of all of the above, no, Jesus did not father any children.

Did Jesus have physical brothers and sisters?

The Bible teaches that Jesus did have brothers and sisters. "Is this not the carpenter's son? Is not His mother called Mary? And His brothers James, Joses, Simon, and Judas?" (Matt. 13:55). Matthew 12:46–47 and Mark 3:31–32 tell of a time when Jesus was teaching the people, and Mary and His physical brothers stood outside the crowd, desiring to talk with Him.

The Bible tells in John 7:5 that even Jesus' brothers rejected Him at the beginning of His ministry: "For even His brothers did not believe in Him." The word *brothers* here must refer to His physical brothers. God's Word tells us later that His brothers did finally accept Jesus as their Savior. Acts 1:14 states that as the disciples waited in the Upper Room in Jerusalem, they were joined by Mary and Jesus' brothers: "These all continued with one accord in prayer and supplication, with the women and Mary the mother of Jesus, and with His brothers." One of Jesus' brothers' even became an apostle: "But I saw none of the other apostles except James, the Lord's brother" (Gal. 1:19).

Did Jesus ever claim to be God?

There are many who say that Jesus never claimed to be God. They say He was a son of God, or He was a son of the Father, but that did not make Him equal with God in nature. Yet He said that He was identical with the Father: "I and My Father are one" (John 10:30). Jesus also said that He was omnipresent (John 3:13), omniscient (John 11:14), and omnipotent (Matt. 28:18). Since only God can receive worship, Jesus demonstrated Himself as God when He received worship (Matt. 14:33). Also, when Jesus forgave sins,

He did something only God can do, because only God can forgive sins (Mark 2:5–7). When Jesus made the Jehovahistic statements ("I am bread . . . light . . . shepherd . . . and so forth), He was suggesting His deity.

What happened at the Last Supper?

The night began with the celebration of the Passover and the eating of the Passover meal. As the disciples gathered with Jesus, He took it upon Himself to wash His disciples' feet and teach them humility (John 13:1–20). As they ate, He announced His betrayal and made His last appeal to Judas Iscariot, the financial secretary of the group, who would betray Him (John 13:21–29). That night Jesus introduced the ordinance of the Lord's Supper (Luke 22:17–20) and gave His disciples the Upper Room discourse, which contained the embryonic teachings of the church age, including a life of love and fruitfulness, yet persecution. Right up to the end, Jesus was involved in the training of the Twelve.

How did Jesus actually die?

Crucifixion usually began with a beating. A man would be lashed with a whip that had bits of metal, bone, or stone at the end of each thong. The whip, as it cut the back of the convicted man, would wrap around him. When it was raised to be lowered again, it would tear the flesh. Often a condemned man would faint from the pain.

The second aspect of the crucifixion was the custom known as "bearing one's cross." The written-out accusation would be tied about his neck and he would be paraded to the place of execution. The shingle he wore would then be nailed above him on his cross so that those who witnessed the event knew his horrendous crime. Jesus' crime was published in three languages and read, "This is Jesus of Nazareth, the King of the Jews" (Matt. 27:37; Mark 15:26; Luke 23:38; John 19:19).

The third aspect of crucifixion was agony leading to death. A man was crucified in such a way that he could not easily breathe. His arms and feet were fastened to the cross so that he had to push his body up to breathe. Every time Jesus breathed, He had to raise His body to gasp for air. As He reached for air, He would scrape the open wounds on His back up and down the rough wood of the cross. The Romans knew their craft. They could execute a man and let him suffer for as long as nine days until he died.

When the soldiers came by to break Jesus' legs to speed up His death, they found a lifeless body. A spear thrust into His side produced blood and water. A friend of Jesus was granted permission to bury the body in His tomb. Jesus was anointed with spices and placed in the borrowed tomb. There He stayed for three days.

Where is the original spot where Jesus was crucified and buried?

There are two sites where Christians believe the tomb of Jesus is found: (1) Gordon's Calvary and the Garden Tomb favored by many Protestants; and (2) the Church of the Holy Sepulcher (this is the view held by Roman Catholics and other Orthodox churches).

In 1842, General Gordon discovered the tomb he believed was the tomb of Jesus. Nearby on a hill are two cavities that give the appearance of a skull. These two "eye sockets" give Gordon's Calvary credibility.

The nearby garden, although re-created during the nineteenth century, gives travelers the confidence that they are at the place where Jesus arose from the dead. However, sockets for bolts and hinges in the jambs indicate the tomb was closed by a door and not a rolling stone. The so-called "window" is the top of the doorway of the originally independent chamber, now partially blocked up with masonry.

On the other hand, the traditional site of the Church of the Holy Sepulcher as the location both of Calvary and of the Lord's tomb also has support for its authenticity. This site of Golgotha goes back to A.D. 327 when the emperor Constantine built the original Church of the Holy Sepulcher over the spot (he first had a temple of Venus torn down from that same spot). The crucifixion took place outside the second wall of Jerusalem (Heb.13:12). Archaeological excavations in Jerusalem conducted by Kathleen M. Kenyon in 1963 indicate that the Church of the Holy Sepulcher lay outside the second wall, so it could mark the site of Christ's death and burial.

We have difficulty knowing the exact site of Calvary and other areas sacred to Christians because they were deliberately desecrated by the emperor Hadrian in A.D. 135.

What does the Bible teach about Christ's substitution for Christians?

On the cross of Calvary, God placed our sin upon Christ and accepted Him in our place as He provided for our atonement. "For He made Him who knew no sin to be sin for us, that we might become the righteousness of God in Him" (2 Cor. 5:21). Paul reminded the Romans that "while we were still sinners, Christ died for us" (Rom. 5:8). The Bible teaches that Christ was the Christian's substitute at Calvary.

What does the Bible teach about *redemption*?

The word *redemption* means "to purchase." When Jesus died for our sins, He paid the price that satisfied the demands of God's holiness. The price of this redemption was the blood of Jesus (1 Peter 1:18–19).

What does the Bible teach about *propitiation*?

The work of Christ satisfied the necessary judgment on sin. When Jesus died on the cross, He satisfied the justice and holiness of God. A biblical term meaning "satisfaction" is the word *propitiation* (Rom. 3:25; 1 John 2:2; 4:10), from *hilasterion,* "a place of propitiation," or the mercy seat. In the Holy of Holies in the tabernacle, the mercy seat was the covering on the ark of the covenant. The priest sprinkled blood on the mercy seat on the Day of Atonement; hence it was symbolically the judgment seat. This was the place where the justice of God was satisfied.

What does the Bible teach about *reconciliation*?

In the act of reconciliation, Christ brought humanity into a favorable light of God's mercy. On the cross, Christ was bringing together two enemies and making them friends. "That is, that God was in Christ reconciling the world to Himself, not imputing their trespasses to them, and has committed to us the word of reconciliation" (2 Cor. 5:19). This work of reconciliation was accomplished by destroying the enmity between God and man and changing man himself.

Jesus came and died "that He might reconcile them both to God in one body through the cross, thereby putting to death the enmity" (Eph. 2:16). That enmity that formed "the middle wall of division" (Eph. 2:14) was the Law (Eph. 2:15). Christ abolished this in His flesh when He died.

The second step was for Christ to become our Mediator (1 Tim. 2:5). He presented two enemies to each other in a positive light. Because of the Cross, the unsaved man can meet God, not as a judge, but as a Savior. God looks at Christians as having been "crucified with Christ" (Gal. 2:20). When God saves a man, He saves him "in Christ." Essentially, Christ presents us to God as "savable sinners."

What does the phrase "water and blood" mean? (1 John 5:6)

"This is He who came by water and blood—Jesus Christ; not only by water, but by water and blood. And it is the Spirit who bears witness, because the Spirit is truth" (1 John 5:6).

The early church father Tertullian said the *water* is a reference to the baptism of Jesus when the Voice from heaven declared, "This is my beloved Son," and established that Jesus was the Christ. The *blood* was a common symbol for His death; hence, the emphasis on salvation.

A second interpretation calls attention to "blood and water" that came from the side of Jesus on the cross (John 19:34). These were important symbols to the deity of Christ. John also adds a third witness, the indwelling *Spirit.* Thus, according to John's count here, "there are three that bear record" (1 John 5:7).

Did Jesus go into hell during His death experience?

The Apostle's Creed does say, "He descended into hell." Paul seems to teach this in Ephesians 4:10–11: "He who descended is also the One who ascended far above all the heavens, that He might fill all things. And He Himself gave some to be apostles, some prophets, some evangelists, and some pastors and teachers." Also, the Bible teaches in prophecy, "For You will not leave my soul in Hades, nor will You allow Your Holy One to see corruption" (Acts 2:27). This passage is part of the apostle Peter's message preached on the day of Pentecost. Peter is quoting the Old Testament passage found in Psalm 16:8–11. These prophetic words, so Peter argues, were fulfilled in Jesus of Nazareth. Therefore, the Messiah whom David promised went into hell.

In the prophecy the statement is made, "For thou wilt not leave my soul in hell." Jesus declared His confidence that God the Father would not allow His soul to remain in hell (Hebrew *sheol,* the grave). The verb in this clause (Hebrew *azab*) means to forsake, abandon, or surrender. The Lord Jesus did not expect God the Father to just deliver Him from the *ordeal* of death and the grave, but from the *dominion* of death and the grave. He actually died and was placed in the grave, but the grave could not hold Him.

What does the Bible mean when it says, "Christ preached to the spirits in prison"?

"For Christ also suffered once for sins, the just for the unjust, that He might bring us to God, being put to death in the flesh but made alive by the Spirit, by whom also He went and preached to the spirits in prison, who formerly were disobedient, when once the Divine longsuffering waited in the days of Noah, while the ark was being prepared, in which a few, that is, eight souls, were saved through water" (1 Peter 3:18–20).

(1) "By whom also He went and preached" (v. 19) suggests Jesus, by the agency of the Holy Spirit ("by the spirit" [vs. 18]), communicated the message in Noah's day through Noah himself. While this interpretation fits the context and is legitimate by current standards, it does require some juggling of one's natural understanding of the text.

(2) The alternative interpretation is to understand that while Jesus was in the grave, He descended into hell and preached to the spirits in Hades. Jesus didn't preach to get them saved, but to announce His victory. This interpretation has problems too. For example, the content of the preaching is supposed to be an announcement of victory rather than the preaching of the gospel message, but the word used (Greek *kerysso*) definitely means "preach the gospel" or "evangelize" (Greek *euangelizomai*).

(3) It is thought by some that these spirits were the sons of God described in Genesis 6. The reason for their iniquity was a satanic attempt to corrupt human flesh and thus prevent the promised Incarnation (Gen. 3:15) from taking place. Here Peter describes Christ telling them their foul plan didn't work!

In conclusion it should be noted that a *fourth* view has been advocated in recent times that says the sons of God were indeed fallen angels who totally controlled and possessed all the evil men living before the Flood.

An exact identification of the "spirits in prison" is not possible. Because a reference is made to Noah, however, very likely they are either supernatural spirit creatures connected with the terrible conditions that led to the deluge Flood or the people to whom Noah preached while preparing the ark.

What does the Bible teach about the resurrection of Jesus?

The Resurrection involved much more than reviving the physical body of Jesus. The body and spirit that had separated at death once again were reunited. Jesus was now subjecting the powers of Satan, based upon the authority of the Cross. Before His death, He was subjected to the limitation of humanity, but in His resurrected body He once again enjoyed access to heaven. Jesus applied the spiritual authority and position of His new life to all believers. So the issues concerning the Resurrection of Christ are certainly much more than the mystery of a missing body.

What does the Bible teach about how Christians receive eternal life?

Every Christian has eternal life; this is what Jesus came to give (John 3:16). The basis for eternal life is the Resurrection. Jesus said, "I am the resurrection and the life. He who believes in Me, though he may die, he shall live" (John 11:25). He also said, "He who hears My word and believes in Him who sent Me has everlasting life, and shall not come into judgment, but has passed from death into life" (John 5:24). Paul stated, "The gift of God is eternal life in Christ Jesus our Lord" (Rom. 6:23).

What does the Bible teach about how Christians get power from the Resurrection?

Paul prayed that the Ephesian Christians would understand "what is the exceeding greatness of His power toward us who believe, according to the working of His mighty power which He worked in Christ when He raised Him from the dead" (Eph. 1:19–20). If Christians understood and applied the Resurrection and Ascension of Christ, it would radically change much of the work done for God by them. Christians need not be defeated. The same power that raised Jesus from the dead, works not only to save us but also to assist us in our Christian lives and service.

What does the Bible teach about the Ascension of Christ?

The disciples who witnessed the Ascension of Christ probably did not completely understand what they were seeing. It involved more than His physical return to heaven. The Ascension meant that Christ was returning to His former place of authority in heaven. He was reclaiming His former place of glory, and was beginning a new ministry for believers in heaven—He would be their (and our) Intercessor (Heb. 7:24–25).

What does Jesus do for us in heaven today?

The Bible teaches, "He is also able to save to the uttermost those who come to God through Him, since He always lives to make intercession for them" (Heb. 7:25). As our High Priest, Jesus is constantly interceding for us. He understands the problems we encounter in life, having experienced the same when He lived on earth. "For we do not have a High Priest who cannot sympathize with our weaknesses, but was in all points tempted as we are, yet without sin" (Heb. 4:15).

QUESTIONS
ABOUT
PRAYER

217

What should my attitude be in prayer?

Prayer is communication with God, requiring neither wisdom nor experience. The weakest believer, like a simple child, can talk to the heavenly Father. The poorest sinner, like an impoverished beggar, can reach out to God in prayer. The ability to call on God is one of the attributes that distinguishes men from animals. We are not merely biological beings. We are spiritual beings, created in the image of God.

As you commune with God in prayer, thank Him in advance for answering your prayers. Let Him know that you are confident that He will answer you according to His will. Praise Him for who He is, for what He has done for you, and for what He is going to do in the future.

How often should a person pray for a particular need?

In answer to this question, look to the teachings of Jesus Christ concerning continuous prayer: "So I say to you, ask, and it will be given to you; seek, and you will find; knock, and it will be opened to you. For everyone who asks receives, and he who seeks finds, and to him who knocks it will be opened" (Luke 11:9–10). The words *ask, seek, and knock* are in the continuous Greek tense, suggesting continuous asking, seeking, and knocking.

As Jesus taught His disciples how to pray (Luke 11:1–4), He gave an illustration of a man whose friend came to him at midnight and requested three loaves of bread (Luke 11:5–8). In this, Jesus was explaining the principle of importunity, or continuous asking. *Importunity* is a translation of the Greek *anaideian,* or "shamelessness." The idea is not badgering God into action, but rather that God responds to the open, confident praying of His children.

The Scriptures give us another illustration in which a woman of Canaan came to Christ stating, "Have mercy on me . . . my daughter is severely demon-possessed" (Matt. 15:22). Jesus did not respond to her request immediately, but after her persistence her request was granted. Our Lord's attitude was intended to test the woman's faith. She was rewarded by the miraculous healing of her daughter. Thus, we may conclude that often our prayers are not answered immediately simply because God may be testing our faith. God may desire that we repeat with persistence our requests for specific needs before He answers those needs.

What is meant by the "priesthood of the believer"?

In the Old Testament God called the nation of Israel to be His chosen people: "And you shall be to Me a kingdom of priests and a holy nation" (Ex. 19:6). In 1 Peter 2:5, Peter says, "You also, as living stones, are being built up a spiritual house, a holy priesthood, to offer up spiritual sacrifices acceptable to God through Jesus Christ." Peter is speaking of the born-again believer as part of a priesthood *to offer up sacrifices acceptable to God.*

In Revelation 1:6, the Word of God again describes the priesthood of the believer, that God has made us kings and priests unto God. In Revelation 20:6, He says that those priests (born-again believers) of God and of Christ shall reign with Him a thousand years.

As believers, in relationship to our priesthood, we need to realize that we have a responsibility to each other—to pray for one another, to assemble ourselves unto God, to worship together. God has set aside the church today, local assemblies of born-again believers, that we might in every aspect be priests through that church to reach out to a lost and dying world. We have a responsibility to the lost—to tell them about Christ. Of course, as believers in Christ, the ultimate responsibility should be our love for the Lord, and our worship of Him.

Should every prayer be ended "in Jesus' name"?

Most Christians use the phrase "In Jesus' Name" for prayer closure. Jesus said, "Whatever you ask the Father in My name He will give you. Until now you have asked nothing in My name. Ask, and you will receive, that your joy may be full" (John 16:23–24). Until Jesus instructed the disciples, prayer had been made directly to God. Now they were to pray in the merits of the finished work of Christ . . . prayer made in Jesus' name.

Also, the use of the phrase "for Christ's sake" as a prayer closure is not to take away from any work or quality of Christ but the phrase is simply recognizing that because of Jesus Christ we are privileged to come to God the Father with our prayers.

It should be noted that simply the utterance of a prayer formula ("in Jesus' name") does not guarantee that the person's prayer will be granted or even heard by God the Father. "Many will say to Me in that day, 'Lord, Lord, have we not prophesied in Your name, cast out demons in Your name, and done many wonders in Your name?' And then I will declare to them, 'I never knew you; depart from Me, you who practice lawlessness'" (Matt. 7:22–23).

Is there a technical "gift of healing" today?

No, I do not believe that anyone has the gift of healing. However, I do believe that God heals in answer to prayer, and I have seen great healings in answer to prayer. At Liberty University on April 25, 1985, over five thousand students fasted all day. All students committed themselves to pray one hour for the healing of cancer in the life of Vernon Brewer, the dean of students at the university. God healed Vernon Brewer, and each year on April 25, I phone Vernon to praise God with him because God still heals. Vernon needed both chemo and radiation for stomach cancer, plus an operation during which the doctors removed a five-pound cancerous growth. But everyone knows what happened, and agrees that it was not medical technology or anything that doctors did; it was a miracle of God!

But even in the healing of Vernon Brewer, there are several principles that you ought to recognize and follow in healing. (See the next question for further explanation.) However, even as I say, "There is no gift of healing today," I believe that there are certain people that God leads to pray for the healing of others, and for some reason God hears their prayers more than others. They have the spiritual gift of faith that leads to healing, and they have successfully exercised that faith over the years, so it appears that they have the "gift of healing."

Does God heal every person who prays?

No, it is not God's will to heal everyone who is sick. When Timothy had stomach problems, Paul did not heal him, nor offer to heal him (1 Tim. 5:23). Paul had a thorn in the flesh and prayed three times for it to be removed, but God did not remove it (2 Cor. 12:7–10). Paul had to learn to glorify God through his sufferings. Also, Paul didn't heal one of his friends, but said, "Trophimus I have left in Miletus sick" (2 Tim. 4:20).

Some people are confused about healing because the Bible says in James 5:14, "Is anyone among you sick?" People apply this to themselves. Also, they see that Jesus went about "healing all manner of sickness and all manner of disease among the people" (Matt. 4:23 KJV). In another place it says, "Great multitudes followed Him, and He healed them all" (Matt. 12:15). However, in some Scripture, the word *all* is not intended to mean everyone was healed. "At evening, when the sun had set, they brought to Him all who were sick . . . then He healed many who were sick . . ." (Mark 1:32, 34). Notice He healed *many*, but He did not necessarily heal *all*. Again in Mark 3:10 it says, "For He had healed many." Remember, there are some that God wants to be a testimony through their sufferings. The will of God is that they suffer, not that they are healed. What can we say about our sufferings? "Even we ourselves groan within ourselves, eagerly waiting for the adoption, the redemption of our body" (Rom. 8:23).

How can we know it is God's will to be healed?

This is a very difficult question to answer, especially since it is usually asked by someone very concerned about healing for himself or others. At that point, the questioner hangs on every word of your answer.

No one can know instinctively that it is God's will to be healed, nor can anyone know absolutely that it is God's will to heal. The first step to being victorious is to be yielded to God's will, and wait for Him simply to give you clear leading how to pray for healing, or whether to pray for "special grace" for others.

However, it is always right to pray for healing, because you don't always know the will of God. And when you can't pray in deep faith for healing, you should pray like the father in the Bible who said, "Lord, I believe; help my unbelief" (Mark 9:24).

However, when God encourages you to pray for healing, then your faith should be bold to pray for answers. However, if your heart has doubt, you could only pray, "Thy will be done." Sometimes when you are praying for healing, you may have doubt in your heart. Change your request to pray for yieldedness or for the grace to accept what He has given.

How much healing can we expect?

A person who has been healed by God does not receive a perfectly new body. We will not receive glorified, sinless, perfect bodies until after the Resurrection. All healing is temporary; people who have been healed will get sick again and eventually die. When a person is healed, it does not stop the aging process. It will not make young bones out of brittle ones, nor will it alleviate the infirmities of age. The Bible speaks about "the redemption of our body" (Rom. 8:23). In the future we will have sinless, painless bodies of perfect health.

Can sickness be caused by a demon or the devil?

There are some occasions in the Bible when a demon was cast out and the patient was restored to full health. There was the story of the boy who could not speak or hear, and when the demon was cast out, he was able to speak and hear. Apparently his physical problems were associated with the demon. However, that is no indication that all sickness is caused by a demon or devils.

There may be a few cases—very few—where sickness is caused by demons. Most sickness comes from disease, poisons, rotten food, germs, or other external causes.

God controls everything, and no disease can attack your body except by God's permission. Sometimes those who are outstanding Christians, living model lives, have been subjected to poor health or sickness simply because it is God's will. While we can't understand why that happens, God uses it to bring glory to Himself.

Is anointing oil essential for healing? (James 5:14–15)

It is not the oil that heals, but "the prayer of faith will save the sick" (James 5:15). The oil is intended to be an expression of our faith, and sometimes it motivates our faith.

Some in the Bible were healed when oil was used. And they "anointed with oil many who were sick, and healed them" (Mark 6:13). On the other hand, there were many occasions of healing in the Bible when they were not anointed with oil.

If you don't know whether to use oil or not, pray and ask God what you should do. Sometimes I have prayed for the sick and used oil; sometimes I have not.

What does "oil" mean when used while praying for the sick?

The Bible speaks about "anointing him with oil" (James 5:14). Some believe it is not literal oil, but oil as a symbol of the Holy Spirit who will heal. Other people think that oil was/is medicinal, as was the view of John Calvin. There were medical doctors in the early church who anointed with oil to cleanse a wound, or oil was taken internally to heal the sick person. A third view is that oil *is* literal oil. Obviously, the oil did not heal and the oil did not guarantee healing. The oil was an expression of the faith of the person who was praying, that the Holy Spirit, who is symbolized by oil, would come to heal the body.

Should you lay hands on people when you pray for them to be healed?

There are many occasions where Jesus touched those that He was going to heal, for example, Jairus's daughter, blind Bartimaeus, etc. However, there were others that Jesus healed whom He did not touch. He only spoke to Lazarus to come forth from the grave, and he did. Jesus spoke miracles on many occasions without touching.

I have laid hands on people as I have prayed for them, and they were healed. At the same time, I have laid hands on other people as I have prayed for them to be healed, but they were not healed. Laying on of hands, in my case, was not a deciding factor for the sick to be healed. I believe people are healed by prayer, faith, and the power of God. It is not the laying on of hands that heals people, but the power of God.

Should people today take up deadly snakes or drink poison to demonstrate the power of God?

There are very few churches where snakes are handled or where they drink poison to demonstrate faith. Those who do ("snake handlers") are trying to demonstrate that God can protect them. They quote the following Scripture as proof of their endeavors: "And these signs will follow those who believe: In My name they will cast out demons; they will speak with new tongues; they will take up serpents; and if they drink anything deadly, it will by no means hurt them; they will lay hands on the sick, and they will recover" (Mark 16:17–18).

Some claim that this verse is not in the two most ancient Greek manuscripts, the Sinaiticus and Vaticanus, and that other manuscripts have included it with partial omissions and variations. They claim this promise is not in the Bible; however, it was quoted by Irenaeus and Hippolytus in the second and third centuries, so it must be part of the authentic Word of God. We do not say it is not Scripture, and we do not use that basis to deny these activities.

Others say there was a transitional time between the death of Christ and the end of the book of Acts when these miracles (picking up snakes or drinking poison) happened; but these miracles do not happen today. We do not take that approach.

The entire Bible is for today, but every promise in the Bible must be interpreted within the parameters of what is promised. As an illustration, we do not circumcise to keep the Jewish Law, we do not offer animal sacrifices, and most Christians do eat pork and shellfish. Should someone pick up a poisonous snake accidentally or be forced to drink a poisonous liquid, it is within the power of God to keep that person alive. While not technically a healing, the same God who heals cancer can keep a person from dying from snake venom. And when Christians are fed poison in an attempt to assassinate them, God can protect their lives. The same God who heals them can keep them safe from poison.

However, to pick up a snake or take poison intentionally is contrary to the rest of Scripture. This seems to be tempting the Lord God to display His power, when it is not His will to show Himself powerful. We know that Paul was bitten by a deadly serpent and it did not hurt him (Acts 28:3–5), but we do not know that anyone drank poison and lived. We do know that if God promised it, and if God did it in the past, He can do it today. But that does not mean that people should foolishly swallow poison or pick up snakes just to prove that it would not hurt them.

Is the day of miracles passed?

There are some who would foolishly say that the day of miracles has passed. Every person who is born again experiences a miracle. Every answer to prayer is a miracle. Every time the Holy Spirit gives you supernatural insight to read and understand the Bible is a miracle. It is the ignorant or those with hearts of unbelief who say the day of miracles has passed.

God has promised, "Whatever you ask in My name" (John 14:13), and "Whatever things you ask when you pray, believe that you receive them, and you will have them" (Mark 11:24). These are promises that God has made, and He will not go back on His promises.

However, there are some things that God does not do today. God is not inspiring more of the Bible, because the Canon is closed. God is not creating new things or adding to creation because God is resting from all His Creation (Gen. 2:1–2). And Jesus is not revealing Himself in the flesh today, as He did when He was on earth. You should never say that God is not doing miracles today. However, there are some types of miracles that He is not doing.

What about faith healers today?

There are those who go from church to church or hold crusades in tents or civic centers and offer healing for the multitudes. However, the Bible teaches that the sick are to call for the elders to pray over them, not that the faith healers are to call for the sick (James 5:14).

Some are actually healed at meetings where faith healers have healing lines. I believe this happens because God honors the faith and prayers of those who come to the meetings. Sometimes God honors the faith and prayers of the faith healer. So it is not "the gift of healing" that brings about the healing of the sick person; it is faith.

Some who claim to be "faith healers" do so to make money, as a racket. Because of their sensationalism and sinful practices, they bring disgrace upon the cause of Christ. They have even caused physical and spiritual problems to the people who listen to them and believe in them. Some sick people have stopped taking treatments or medicine and have become permanently harmed.

The Bible claims that the sick should call for the elders of the church (James 5:14), and they shall pray over him. Why elders of the Church? Because the elders know the spiritual condition of the sick person. The elders may even know if sickness is a judgment of God for sin in one's life. If not, then the elders can pray together for healing. If there are any "faith healers," they should probably be the elders of the church.

What is Christian fasting?

Fasting is a nonrequired discipline that alters your diet or eliminates food and/or drink for a biblical purpose that is accomplished by prayer.

Should Christians fast today?

Jesus gave the challenge of fasting when He said, "When you fast do not be . . . with a sad countenance . . . that [you] may appear to men to be fasting . . . Anoint your head and wash your face, so that you do not appear to men to be fasting" (Matt. 6:16–18). While some think that fasting is only an Old Testament custom or discipline (that is, the Yom Kippur fast), the New Testament church also fasted. "As they ministered to the Lord and fasted, the Holy Spirit said, 'Now separate to Me Barnabas and Saul for the work to which I have called them'" (Acts 13:2).

What are the various types of fasts taught in the Bible?

First, there is the *normal fast*, which is going without food for a certain period of time, but drinking liquids (water and/or juice). Second, there is the *absolute fast*, in which no water or food is taken. The *partial fast* omits certain foods on a schedule of limited eating, for example, only one meal a day, only vegetables, and so forth. The *John Wesley* fast is eating only bread (whole grain) and drinking water. The *supernatural fast* is what Moses followed when he went to meet the Lord on Mt. Sinai, forty days without food or drink (Ex. 24:18). A person can only go approximately seven days without drinking water before he dies, therefore this is called a supernatural fast.

What is a private fast?

A private fast is when a person is burdened about a certain request and does not tell anyone else, but fasts as he or she continues normal life. This is usually a very personal request about which one fasts and prays, "that you do not appear to men to be fasting" (Matt. 6:18).

What is a joint fast?

There are times when people join together in a fast, an entire church, church staff, or any other group of people. In the Bible, Ezra challenged over four thousand people to join him in a fast for safety on a journey from the Euphrates River back to Jerusalem.

What is the Yom Kippur fast?

That is a one-day fast that extends from sundown the first day until sundown the second day. This fast follows the biblical designation of a day: "Evening and the morning were the first day" (Gen. 1:5). *Yom Kippur* stands for the Day of Atonement. On that day God commanded every Jew, "On the tenth day of the seventh month of each year, you must go without eating to show sorrow for your sins" (Lev. 16:29 CEV).

What fast is best when a Christian fasts for the first time?

A Christian should not begin with an extended fast. When fasting for the first time, a Christian should follow the Yom Kippur (one-day) fast. Also, rather than taking a seven-day fast, I suggest a Christian fast one day a week for seven weeks.

What day of the week is best to fast?

Monday is recommended because it is possible to start the fast on a Sunday, the Lord's Day. The Christian has been to church, has been challenged with the reading of God's Word and singing of hymns, and is prepared to trust God for bigger things in the fast on Monday.

How long can an absolute fast be planned?

A person cannot go more than three days without water before he begins to permanently harm his body. Since the body is made up of 80 percent water, among the first things to suffer are the membranes within the brain, and when they are permanently lost, they cannot be restored.

Are there some people who should not fast?

Yes, those who have certain medical problems should not fast. That is why fasting is called a "nonrequired discipline." Those with medical problems should (a) treat food as medicine, and not miss their medicine, (b) remember that God would not have you harm your body (the Christian life is not measured by aestheticism), (c) enter into the *spirit* of fasting and prayer, while not actually going through the physical withdrawal of food.

When is it proper to publicize a fast?

When one publicizes a fast, he has committed himself to a certain diet for a certain length of time. Technically a fast is a vow to God, but the public commitment motivates a person to carry the fast through to the end. It is also a statement of faith that he is trusting God to see him through to the end of the fast, and for God to grant the thing for which he is fasting.

What steps should I follow when leading a group in fasting?

First, gather your group together so they may feel your heart and passion for the project for which you are fasting. Second, challenge your group to the biblical purpose for which you are fasting. Third, start fasting together and end together. Many groups start their fasts at the Lord's Table, and if stretched over a long period of time (perhaps forty days), end their fasts at the Lord's Table.

What can a person drink during a normal fast?

I have interviewed many people who have fasted, and find that many drink juice, Slim-Fast, Ensure (nutritional supplements), and coffee. Others are opposed to drinking any type of liquid other than water during a fast. But remember that God does not measure the success of your fast by what you withhold, but rather what comes out of your heart in faith, prayer, and sacrifice.

When drinking liquids other than water, make sure the drink is not chosen for its enjoyment value. Some drink juice because it has a certain amount of nutrients to keep one's elimination system going. However, when thinking about what to drink during a fast, remember the law of silence: "When God hasn't spoken, don't make rules." There is not much said in the Bible about what people drink when fasting, so don't make rules about what a person can or cannot drink during a fast.

Is the forty-day fast possible today?

Yes, I have fasted for forty days.

Is fasting legalism?

To some people, fasting is legalism because they bargain with God, "If you answer my prayer, I will go without food." Also, tithing, baptism, or church attendance can be legalism. The purpose of any fast is not to bargain with God or manipulate God into answering a prayer because you have gone without food. A Christian should "hunger and thirst after righteousness" rather than hunger and thirst after food and drink.

Does God speak to us through dreams today?

On certain occasions God spoke to people through dreams. He spoke to both unbelievers, such as Pharaoh (Gen. 41:1–44) and Nebuchadnezzar (Dan. 2:11–49), and to His own children, such as Joseph, the husband of Mary (Matt. 1:20; 2:13), and the wise men (Matt. 2:12). He even gave men of God (Joseph and Daniel) the ability to interpret those dreams according to God's meaning. However, when Peter on the day of Pentecost said, "Your young men shall see visions, your old men shall dream dreams" (Acts 2:17), did he mean that dreams are an avenue of divine communication?

When there was the office of prophets, God spoke to them through dreams, visions, and many other symbolic actions. However, the day of prophets who received a message from God has passed. All that we need to know from God about salvation and Christian living is found in the Word of God. The Word of God is complete and is the final Word of revelation. God does not speak new messages to us today through dreams or visions.

We do have dreams, and they are usually the products of our *recessive memories*. Because of this, many people have religious dreams, because thoughts about God and the Bible are on their minds. Some people have nightmares because of fears, and other people have pleasant dreams about their desires in life.

While God does not communicate new revelation through a dream(s), God may use a dream, just as He uses our memories or our thought patterns to lead us to do His will or to remember certain things. The problem is, some people mistake the leadership of God through dreams with the communication of a new revelation by God. Sometimes people have quirks of theology that they get in dreams, and then try to make their theological quirks authoritative because their ideas came through a dream.

When Peter says, "Your young men shall see visions, and your old men dream dreams," this has a twofold meaning to us. Because a passage has only one interpretation, that passage applies to the future when Christ shall come back. When Jesus Christ returns, sign miracles shall be reintroduced and reactivated. God will speak through dreams in the future.

While a passage has one *interpretation*, it also has many *applications*. In applying *dreams* to the church today, a young man's vision may be what he wants to do with his life. Others apply this passage to mean the vision or dream that church leaders have for ministry. For more information, see *The Power of Vision* by George Barna (Ventura, CA: Regal Books, 1997).

Just as God may use a dream in the life of a Christian, Satan or demons can also use dreams to torment people—dreams about a death, an accident, or calamity to a loved one. Base your life and ministry on the Word of God, not on dreams.

Does anyone have the gift of interpreting dreams?

There are some con artists who claim they have the ability to interpret dreams. But these first want you to tell them the content of your dream before they will interpret it. Then they will ask more questions about your life, looking for "bridges" between your life and your "dream." Sometimes they sense what your fears or ambitions are, then relate your dream to that interpretation.

Notice the same thing happened when Nebuchadnezzar had a dream: The wise men wanted to know about the dream before they interpreted it. But Nebuchadnezzar would not tell them the content of this dream. Because Daniel had the ability to interpret dreams, he first told Nebuchadnezzar the content of the dream (demonstrating God had given him supernatural knowledge), and then Daniel interpreted the dream (with supernatural cred-ibility, predicting what was going to happen).

People who interpret dreams today (from Freudian psychologists to occult religious leaders) always point to symbols, explaining their meanings. They use symbols to lead people away from God. The Christian should always go to the Bible to lead people to Christ.

What should my response be when God doesn't answer the prayers that I pray?

There are many conditions to getting your prayers answered. One of them is asking according to the will of God. God will not answer a prayer that is against His will or His laws. You cannot ask God for the sun to turn cold, nor can you ask for something rolling off the table to float or fall upward. God will not go against the laws of gravity.

Even Jesus didn't get everything He wanted. On the night before He died He prayed, "O My Father, if it is possible, let this cup pass from Me" (Matt. 26:39). This prayer was not answered, because several hours later, Jesus was nailed to the cross.

The apostle Paul prayed, "Brethren, my heart's desire and prayer to God for Israel is that they may be saved" (Rom. 10:1). Despite his prayers, many Jewish people continued to reject Jesus Christ as their Messiah and/or Savior. God cannot save a person apart from his or her wanting to be saved. Paul prayed three times for God to remove his thorn in the flesh (2 Cor. 12:7–9), but God did not do it. God had other lessons to teach Paul.

Why does God not answer our prayers?

Sometimes it's because we are asking for things that God has not promised to give us. God has not promised long life to every person, though a few people may live long. So God may not answer your prayer for a long life. God may also not answer your prayer because you ask God to take away things that He doesn't want removed. As an illustration, God promises trouble to every person (Job 5:7), so we should pray for wisdom in the midst of our troubles for how to solve them or live with them (James 1:5). But God may not answer your prayer to *take away* your troubles.

God does not answer prayers when you ask Him to go against His nature. God cannot erase history or make a square circle. God will not make a stone too heavy for Him to lift. A student taking a test cannot pray for an answer if he has not studied and the answer is not in his mind. God doesn't communicate out of a vacuum.

Sometimes you don't get your prayers answered because you quit praying too soon. Perhaps God began answering your prayer, but you did not continue asking, so you didn't get an answer. At other times we don't get an answer to prayer because we don't have faith (Mark 11:24). Sometimes, we don't ask in Jesus' name (John 14:14), don't abide in the Word of God (John 15:7), or don't pray according to His will (1 John 5:14–15).

What should our response be when God is silent?

First, we should submit to His will and pray, "Nevertheless, not as I will, but as You will" (Matt. 26:39). Second, we should learn patience and that God is working His plan in the world. And third, we must live our life based on what we understand in the Bible. When God is silent, then live your life by what you already know from the Bible; don't seek what you don't know.

Since the Bible says, "Thou shalt be saved and thy house," why are members of my household not saved even though I pray for them?

First of all, the promise of "household salvation" might be taken out of context. They are not automatically saved because you believe in Christ. The command was, "Believe on the Lord Jesus Christ, and you will be saved, you and your household" (Acts 16:31). A careful study of the verse says that you must believe to be saved, and so every member of your house must believe to be saved. But when you are saved, they are much more likely to be saved because they hear the gospel from you, they see your changed life, and they see how the Bible is working in your daily life. So claim this promise for the salvation of all in your family.

QUESTIONS ABOUT PROPHECY

Why should I study prophecy?

Perhaps the most obvious reason is because there are prophecies in the Bible. As a matter of fact, much of the Bible was prophetic when it was originally written, and of course, some of it has been fulfilled (the coming of Jesus Christ, His life, and His death). Also, the Old Testament prophets predicted a coming judgment by Babylon against Israel—the nation's captivity. These prophecies have all been fulfilled, so you should study prophecy to see how God has fulfilled His past predictions. It will tell you how God will fulfill His future prophecies.

God has planned a future for this earth and all the people on it. Since you will be a part of that future plan, you ought to study prophecy to learn what will happen to you and to the earth. Some of the predictions are good, and you will want to be a part of them: "Where I am, there you may be also" (John 14:3). There are other predictions that He will judge the world with fire (2 Peter 3:10). When you study prophecy, you can properly prepare for the future. While much of prophecy describes the coming blessings of those in Christ, there are enough warnings in prophecy to tell those who are not saved to prepare for the coming judgment.

How has prophecy been abused?

Some people have fallen into the trap of always seeking new truth or trying to find something that is new in the Bible. Others have become proud of their knowledge of prophecy, or they've used prophecy as a tool to make money or promote their organizations. Some people have made the mistake of fixing dates or identifying personalities, such as the identity of the Antichrist. Still others have let their views of prophecy become major divisions of fellowship with other Christians. And then some have become so focused on prophecy that they have forgotten the central focus of Scripture, which is Jesus Christ. The first verse in the book of Revelation gives the focus of all prophecy, "The Revelation of Jesus Christ" (Rev. 1:1), which is a good guide to keeping prophecy properly focused.

Why have some Christian leaders taught there are no signs before the rapture?

They teach that Jesus is coming unexpectedly as a "thief in the night." They teach that if there were signs, they would take away from an "any moment" rapture.

What are some signs before the rapture?

There are no signs to tell us exactly when the rapture will come. "But of that day and hour no one knows, not even the angels of heaven, but My Father only" (Matt. 24:36). Travelers realize a town is near when they are crossing the countryside because they see an abundance of signs. Likewise, we should know that the Lord's coming is near (not the exact time) because there is an appearance of certain signs.

First, the seven church epistles (Rev. 2–3) seem to reflect seven periods of time between the Lord's first coming and His next coming. We seem to be living in the times described by the last of the seven churches, the church of Laodicea (Rev. 3:14–22). If this view is accurate, it tells us that we are in the last times.

Next, the Lord indicated that before the end, Israel would return to the land in unbelief and set up a nation. God told Ezekiel (Ezek. 37:11–14) that He would bring Israel back to the land in unbelief (the valley of dry bones). Then God would reestablish David upon the throne of Israel. The nation Israel was established in 1948, and during the Six-Day War in 1967, Jerusalem and other parts of the homeland were conquered and became part of the nation. But Israel does not believe in Jesus as their Messiah today; they live in Israel in unbelief. There is coming a time in the future when Israel will be regenerated; the Bible says, "All Israel will be saved" (Rom. 11:26).

During the end times, especially during the Tribulation, the world will have one leader, one government, and a short period of international unity. We should realize that the end is near as we see the growth of internationalism, a one-world monetary system, a global communication system (the Internet), a worldwide economic system, and potentially a one-world banking system.

Also, during the Tribulation period there will be a one-world religion headed by Antichrist. There is a strong ecumenical spirit in the world today that is dominated by tolerance and unity, even though there is a diversity of religions. This one-world concept of religious tolerance lays the groundwork for a "one-world church" at the return of Christ.

There seem to be other ecological, atmospheric, and societal signs that point to the soon coming of Jesus Christ. "For nation will rise against nation, and kingdom against kingdom. And there will be famines, pestilences, and earthquakes in various places" (Matt. 24:7); "many shall run to and fro" (Dan. 12:4); "knowledge shall increase" (Dan. 12:4); "you will hear of wars and rumors of wars" (Matt. 24:6); "evil men and impostors will grow worse and worse" (2 Tim. 3:13); "some will depart from the faith" (1 Tim. 4:1); "they will not endure sound doctrine" (2 Tim. 4:2–4); "there will be scoffers who doubt the second coming of Jesus Christ" (2 Peter 3:3–14); "mockers in the last time who would walk according to their own ungodly lusts" (Jude 16–18); "heaping treasures to themselves" (James 5:3–6); "false prophets" (Matt. 24:11); "perilous times" (2 Tim. 3:1); "disobedient to parents" (2 Tim. 3:2) "lovers of pleasure more than lovers of God" (2 Tim. 3:4 KJV); and "having a form of godliness but denying its power" (2 Tim. 3:5).

What will be the next event on God's prophetic calendar?

"For the Lord Himself will descend from heaven with a shout, with the voice of an archangel, and with the trumpet of God. And the dead in Christ will rise first" (1 Thess. 4:16). This is when the physical bodies of saved believers will be raised at the return of Christ. He will bring with Him their souls. "For if we believe that Jesus died and rose again, even so God will bring with Him those who sleep in Jesus" (1 Thess. 4:14). At the rapture their bodies and souls will be reunited.

"Then we who are alive and remain shall be caught up together with them in the clouds to meet the Lord in the air. And thus we shall always be with the Lord" (1 Thess. 4:17). Note what will happen. We will be "caught up." The Latin word for "caught up," *rapto,* is the source for the word rapture. We will meet Jesus in the air, and we will go live with Him forever.

At that time we will receive glorified bodies. "The dead will be raised incorruptible, and we shall be changed" (1 Cor. 15:52). How long will this take? "In a moment, in the twinkling of an eye" (1 Cor. 15:51–52).

Why is the restoration of Israel to the promised land a sign that Jesus is coming soon?

God told Ezekiel that He would bring His people back into the land (Ezek. 37:11–14). That promise included both the restoration of the Jews to the land that God gave Abraham, and the regeneration of that people in the land. During the past century, we have seen maps drawn outlining the boundaries of David's kingdom (following World War I) and that kingdom in part given to the Jews (1948). During the Six-Day War of 1967, Jerusalem and other parts of the Jewish homeland were conquered and became a part of the national geography of Israel. When Israel declared Jerusalem her capital during the summer of 1980, yet another step had been taken toward the ultimate fulfillment of those prophecies concerning the restoration of the Jews in Israel.

Why is our present growth toward internationalism a sign that Jesus is coming soon?

Daniel described the progress of world history in terms of four beasts representing kingdoms. "Thus he said: 'The fourth beast shall be a fourth kingdom on earth, which shall be different from all other kingdoms, and shall devour the whole earth, trample it and break it in pieces'" (Dan. 7:23). That beast was the Roman Empire, which will be revived before Christ returns. This revived empire appears to be a world government that will have international control and influence.

John also described the ruler of that kingdom, observing, "It was granted to him to make war with the saints and to overcome them. And authority was given him over every tribe, tongue, and nation" (Rev. 13:7).

These two writers expected a world leader who would establish a world government. Today, our society appears to be moving to that end. With many major and minor crises that have confronted world leaders in recent years, an internationalist view of world politics is becoming more popular. Some have cited organizations such as the United Nations and the European Common Market as possible patterns for an international government. It is generally agreed that such a government would demand a strong leader. As we move closer toward conditions that will exist when Jesus returns to earth, we consider these conditions as "signs" that His coming is near.

What are some general signs that suggest Jesus is coming soon?

There are some conditions in the Scripture that imply the return of the Lord. However, it is difficult to give an objective identification to them, so some are not sure they are "signs." Paul noted,

"In the last days perilous times will come: for men will be lovers of themselves, lovers of money, boasters, proud, blasphemers, disobedient to parents, unthankful, unholy, unloving, unforgiving, slanderers, without self-control, brutal, despisers of good, traitors, headstrong, haughty, lovers of pleasure rather than lovers of God, having a form of godliness but denying its power." (2 Tim. 3:1–5)

Some of these conditions have been true in every age, as they were in Timothy's day. But others seem more evident in these last times, such as the pleasure seekers, those with a form of godliness but no power, and those disobedient to parents. These supportive conditions are only mentioned by inference and should not be considered strong arguments for the signs of the times. But their appearance in Scripture meant they could not be left off the list.

How do we know the rapture could occur at any given time?

One cannot read the New Testament and conclude the writers believed in anything but an imminent return of Christ. Christ can return at any moment. Christians are exhorted to keep watching for His return (1 Thess. 5:1–8; 2 Pet. 3:8–10) and waiting for it (1 Cor. 1:7; 1 Thess. 1:9–10; Titus

2:13). These commands were as meaningful and applicable to the first century as they are today.

When will the physical bodies of New Testament believers be resurrected?

Paul told the Thessalonian Christians not to grieve for their dead relatives and friends. The Greek present tense makes possible the translation, "Lest you sorrow as others who have no hope" (1 Thess. 4:13). Christians should take hope in the fact that Paul said the saved dead would be raised. The Christian's hope has always been the Resurrection.

"But I do not want you to be ignorant, brethren, concerning those who have fallen asleep, lest you sorrow as others who have no hope. For if we believe that Jesus died and rose again, even so God will bring with Him those who sleep in Jesus. For this we say to you by the word of the Lord, that we who are alive and remain until the coming of the Lord will by no means precede those who are asleep. For the Lord Himself will descend from heaven with a shout, with the voice of an archangel, and with the trumpet of God. And the dead in Christ will rise first. Then we who are alive and remain shall be caught up together with them in the clouds to meet the Lord in the air. And thus we shall always be with the Lord." (1 Thess. 4:13–17)

The certainty of the resurrection for the Christian is based upon the Resurrection of Christ. That Christ arose according to the Scriptures is an indisputable truth. There is a relationship between the Resurrection of Christ and of Christians in 1 Corinthians 15:23: "Christ the firstfruits, afterward those who are Christ's at His coming." Therefore, since Christ arose from the dead, so we shall rise at His coming.

The words *caught up* (1 Thess. 4:17) denote the resurrection of the body of those believers who have died, whose spirits are already with the Lord. "Then we who are alive and remain shall be caught up together." It is from the word for "caught up" (Greek *harpazo*) in the Latin translation that we get our word *rapture*. The word in the original means "snatch," or "seize." The result of this snatching away, of course, is that we meet the Lord and He catches us away.

Does the soul "sleep" after death until the resurrection?

There are some Scriptures that seem to teach that the soul sleeps after death. After Jesus was told of Lazarus's death, He waited before going to visit Mary and Martha. Finally Jesus told His disciples, "Our friend Lazarus sleeps, but I go that I may wake him up" (John 11:11). Here is a straightforward statement by Jesus that Lazarus was "sleeping," and that Jesus would "resuscitate him" out of his sleep. Later when Jesus was invited to the home of Jairus to heal his daughter's sickness, He told them after her death, "The child is not dead, but sleeping" (Mark 5:39).

Finally, as Paul speaks of the coming rapture of those who are dead, he describes them as "those who have fallen asleep," (1 Thess. 4:13). Paul further said, "For if we believe that Jesus died and rose again, even so God will bring with Him those who sleep in Jesus" (1 Thess. 4:14). He describes those dead believers as "asleep," in contrast to those who are "alive and remain until the coming of the Lord" (1 Thess. 4:15). Paul's plain teaching is that "the Lord Himself will descend from heaven with a shout, with the voice of an archangel, and with the trumpet of God. And the dead in Christ will rise first. Then we who are alive and remain shall be caught up together with them in the clouds to meet the Lord in the air" (1 Thess. 4:16–17).

These Scriptures do not teach that the soul is asleep, but rather that the body is in the grave, and that death is a metaphor to describe asleep. Paul describes the moment of death: "To be absent from the body and to be present with the Lord" (2 Cor. 5:8). At death a Christian instantly enters the presence of the Lord. Jesus told the story of a beggar named Lazarus who died: "So it was that the beggar died, and was carried by the angels to Abraham's bosom. The rich man also died and was buried" (Luke 16:22). The unrighteous rich man did not go into "soul sleep," because the Bible says, "And being in torments in Hades, he lifted up his eyes" (Luke 16:23). The rich man had a conscious existence in hell. And what about Lazarus? "He saw Abraham afar off, and Lazarus in his bosom" (Luke 16:23). Lazarus was not in "soul sleep," but was enjoying fellowship with Abraham in heaven.

On another occasion Jesus said to the repentant thief on the cross, "Today you will be with Me in Paradise" (Luke 23:43). This does not sound like the soul went to sleep.

In the case of the Scriptures that some use in support of "soul sleep," when Jesus referred to Lazarus or the daughter of Jairus being asleep, He was not referring to their souls sleeping, but their bodies sleeping in the grave until the Resurrection. This is the teaching of 1 Thessalonians 4:13–18.

Will backslidden Christians be taken in the rapture?

Some teach a partial rapture theory, saying only Christians in fellowship with the Lord will be taken in the rapture. They teach that sinning or unbaptized Christians will be left behind. Those who hold this position teach that sin or disobedience will be punished in the Tribulation period. But this position is not correct. Jesus paid the price for sin. "The blood of Jesus Christ His Son cleanses us from all sin" (1 John 1:7). That means all Christians stand equal before God—forgiven. Those who think backsliders will not be taken in the rapture have confused rewards and forgiveness of sin.

What will happen to the children of Christians at the rapture?

Technically, children before the age of accountability are not "saved" in the sense of going through a regeneration experience. However, they are "safe" (2 Sam. 12:23; Matt. 18:3–6; 19:13–14). All children who die before the age of accountability go into the presence of God at death. Therefore, those children that belong to Christians would be taken with their parents into the presence of the Lord at the rapture. Why? Because a God of love would not leave their children to be reared by the ungodly and suffer the wrath of God in the Tribulation. Also, the rapture marks the end of the period of grace. As their parents were under grace, so their children would also be dealt with in grace.

What will be the response of the unsaved when Christians are missing because of the rapture?

The Antichrist will rise to a position of power at this time and will have an answer for the disappearance of Christians. "And for this reason God will send them strong delusion, that they should believe the lie" (2 Thess. 2:11). The Antichrist will have a *lie* to explain what happened to Christians, and the unsaved world will believe him. The Bible says, "For this reason God will send them strong delusion," which is the Antichrist's own "spiritual blind-ness" to keep people from believing the truth, just as "the god of this age has blinded the minds, who do not believe, lest the light of the gospel of the glory of Christ, who is the image of God, should shine on them" (2 Cor. 4:3–4).

What will the Antichrist do at or after the rapture?

1. The Antichrist will arrive on the scene and overcome a death wound. "And I saw one of his heads as if it had been mortally wounded" (Rev. 13:3),

and "whose deadly wound was healed" (Rev. 13:12). Some believe he will be killed, but arise from the dead. The word *Antichrist* means "substitute Christ," so he will do what Christ did—arise from the dead. Others believe only God can raise from the dead, so the Antichrist will not come back from the dead. They say this resurrection from a "death wound" is a picture of a nation coming back together and back into power, or "coming back from the dead."

2. The Antichrist will reveal himself as a world ruler: "The lawless one will be revealed" (2 Thess. 2:8).

3. He will gain worldwide leadership power as he brings the nations of Europe (the revived Roman Empire) into realignment, and with them there will be a confederation of the nations of the rest of the world (Rev. 13:1; 16:13–16).

4. The Antichrist will do great miracles in the power of the false prophet, including bringing "fire come down from heaven" (Rev. 13:13). Because the Antichrist is a substitute Christ, he will do what happened when the church began (fire fell on pentecost). The Antichrist will duplicate that type of miracle.

5. The Antichrist will have great powers of speech, persuasion, and conciliation: "And he was given a mouth speaking great things" (Rev. 13:5). The Antichrist will persuade people to accept his leadership and program. Everyone will believe in him and follow him.

6. The Antichrist will make a covenant (peace pact) with Israel that will ensure the Jews' safety (Dan. 9:27).

7. He will also solve the financial problems of the world and/or offer a solution to the financial problems of the world that all will accept (Rev. 13:15–18).

8. The Antichrist will register all people of the earth into a financial system and give them a number (666) (Rev. 13:16–17).

9. The Antichrist will set up a unified religion of the world with himself as its head to receive veneration and worship. The false prophet will then cause all "to worship the first beast" (Rev. 13:12).

10. The false prophet will cause people to make images and replicas of the Antichrist in loyalty and worship to him (Rev. 13:14).

Will the Antichrist be a Jew?

Many think that the Antichrist will be a Gentile, because in Revelation 13 he comes up out of the sea (the sea is a symbol of the nations of the world).

He is also believed to be a Gentile because he rules the Gentile nations of the world.

However, those who believe he is a Jew identify Antichrist with Jewish heritage based on Daniel 11:37: "He shall regard neither the God of his fathers." Second, the Antichrist will set up "a god of fortresses; and a god which his fathers did not know he shall honor with gold and silver, with precious stones and pleasant things" (Dan. 11:38). This verse suggests that the Antichrist is a Jew, because it again identifies him with his "fathers," that is, the Jewish heritage. Third, the Antichrist not only *opposes* Jesus Christ, but wants to be a *substitute* of Jesus Christ. To be a substitute Jesus, he would have to be a Jew, as was Jesus.

How does the Antichrist try to establish a false religion?

First, there is the Trinity of the Father, Son, and Holy Spirit (Matt. 28:19) that is reflected in the trinity of Satan, Antichrist, and the false prophet (Rev. 20:10). Just as Jesus is the second Person of the Godhead, Antichrist is the second person of the unholy trinity. And as Jesus came performing miracles, so Antichrist will come performing miracles (2 Thess. 2:9). Because Jesus appointed apostles (Matt. 10:1), Satan has false apostles (2 Cor. 11:13). Just as God wants to put a mark on His servants (Rev. 7:3), so will Antichrist put the mark of the beast on his followers (Rev. 13:16). Just as the followers of Jesus Christ study to understand the mystery of godliness (1 Tim. 3:16), so the Antichrist has his mystery of iniquity (2 Thess. 2:7 KJV).

Who will the Antichrist be?

Actually, no one knows who the Antichrist will be. Some believe the Antichrist will be a Gentile, since he comes from the sea (Rev. 13:1), which is often a symbol for Gentiles and heathen nations. Also, he rules over Gentile nations. Some believe the Antichrist will be a Jew (Dan. 11:37–38) because he is likened to the god of his "fathers," in other words, the Jews. This view also says he is a Jew because he tries to take the place of Jesus as a substitute Christ.

On the basis of Revelation 13:3 and 17:8, some believe the Antichrist will be a resurrected individual. As such, some think he will be Judas Iscariot (John 6:70–71; Luke 22:3; John 13:27; 17:12; 2 Thess. 2:3; Acts 1:25). Some also have thought he might be others who have hated God and fought against Christians or the Jews, perhaps Nero, Dioclatian, Hitler, Stalin, Saddam Hussein, or Osama Bin Laden.

What will characterize the Antichrist's rule?

The Antichrist will be an intellectual genius (Dan. 8:23), an oratorical genius (Dan. 11:36), a political genius (Rev. 17:11–12), a commercial genius (Rev. 13:16–17; Daniel 11:43), a military genius (Rev. 6:2; 13:4), and a religious genius (Rev. 13:8; 2 Thess. 2:4). He will have the qualities to become a world ruler.

What is the strategy of the Antichrist during the Tribulation?

The Antichrist will begin by controlling the Western power bloc (federation of nations, that is, Revised Roman Empire) (Rev. 17:12), then making a seven-year covenant with Israel, and breaking it after three and a half years (Dan. 9:27). He will then attempt to destroy all of Israel (Rev. 12). He will also set up a false religious system and use this system to give him authority to rule unhindered (Rev. 17:16–17). Ultimately the Antichrist will set himself up as God (Dan. 11:36–37; 2 Thess. 2:4, 11; Rev. 13:5). He will rule briefly over all nations (Ps. 2; Dan. 11:36; Rev. 13:16), but will be utterly crushed by the Lord Jesus Christ at the Battle of Armageddon (Rev. 19), and will be thrown into the lake of fire (Rev. 19:20).

The Antichrist will be identified with the number 666 (Rev. 13:16–17), which is the mark of the Beast. He will require people to have this number if they are to buy or sell. The mark reflects a deep commitment to him, and all who accept this number will go to hell (Rev. 14:9–11). No saved person will accept the mark of the Beast, even if it costs him his life to reject it.

What is the "Seventieth Week," and what is its relationship to Prophecy?

Daniel provided a key to understanding Bible prophecy in his vision of seventy weeks (Dan. 9:24). More accurately, a week was "sevens of years," therefore, the last week is seven years long. A gap of some unspecified duration exists between the sixty-ninth and seventieth week, but the final week (seven years) is described in terms of a single unit. Several other passages describe this week as a single unit, the entire week having the same characterization. It is a time of wrath (Rev. 14:19), judgment (Rev. 15:4), and punishment (Isa. 24:20–21). The week will be marked with darkness (Joel 2:2) and destruction (Joel 1:15). The week is identified as an "hour of trial" (Rev. 3:10).

What is the "seven-year Tribulation period"?

After saints have been raptured from the earth to be with the Lord, there begins a seven-year period called the "Tribulation." The Bible uses various names for this period, such as the day of the Lord (Isa. 2:12), the time of the end (Dan. 12:9), and the end of this world (Matt. 13:40, 49 KJV).

The Tribulation period is divided into three eras, the first era being approximately three and a half years; the brief middle period being perhaps only a few weeks; and the last era, called the Great Tribulation, being approximately three and a half years.

A powerful ruler will rise to power, led by Satan and referred to as the Antichrist. He will make a treaty with Israel that will allow them to build a temple in Jerusalem. He will lead the nations to form an alliance to help preserve the world system, primarily an economic alliance. After three and a half years, the Antichrist will break the treaty with Israel and be responsible for persecuting the nation of Israel.

During the Tribulation, God will pour out His wrath upon the earth and mankind unlike anything that has ever taken place before. It will be a terrible time of persecution and suffering. The Antichrist will perform miracles and set up an alternate church made up of a vast number of religions. He will require everyone to worship himself.

Those who become Christians during the Tribulation will be terribly persecuted. Judgments from God upon the natural elements of the earth and upon the inhabitants of the earth will be severe. Even in the midst of suffering, people will still be unwilling to turn to God and will blaspheme Him (Rev. 16:21). For further reference, see Matthew 24:11; 2 Thessalonians 2:3–11; and Revelation 13:16–18; 14:14–20.

The Tribulation ends when the Antichrist leads the world to attack Israel. Those in opposition to God and Israel will be destroyed in the battle of Armageddon. Then Jesus Christ will return to earth victoriously to set up His earthly kingdom that will last one thousand years.

Will the church go through the seven-year Tribulation period?

The answer to this question is, No! Although the word *rapture* is not found in the Bible, it is indeed an event in prophecy taught in the Scriptures. First Thessalonians 4:14–17 is actually the next prophecy to be fulfilled (see also 1 Corinthians 15:51–57, when all Christians, living and dead, will be caught up "to be with the Lord in the air"). First Thessalonians 5:9 says, "God hath not appointed us to wrath" (KJV). Revelation 3:10 is also an indication that the church will not suffer the terrible days of the Tribulation. From the first chapter through the third chapter of Revelation, there are several references to the church. However, from the fourth chapter until the nineteenth chapter, as the Tribulation is discussed, the church is not mentioned. From this argument of silence, it is assumed the church is not on earth.

There will be many people converted and saved during the Tribulation. These are Jewish believers in Jesus who will have to suffer during the days of the Tribulation and about whom the Bible speaks in Revelation 20:4. These Christians will suffer terrible persecution, primarily because they have refused the mark of the beast.

What is the "mark of the Beast"?

The Scripture teaches that there will be a "mark of the Beast": "He causes all, both small and great, rich and poor, free and slave, to receive a mark on their right hand or on their foreheads, and that no one may buy or sell except one who has the mark or the name of the beast, or the number of his name. Here is wisdom. Let him who has understanding calculate the number of the beast, for it is the number of a man: His number is 666" (Rev. 13:16–18). This passage informs us of the universal influence of the Antichrist and the false prophet. They will position their mark in the most conspicuous place on the bodies of their followers, the forehead or right hand. The "mark" (Greek word *charagma*) means an impression made by a stamp, like a brand used on slaves and animals, or a stamp placed on an official document. During those terrible days known as the Great Tribulation, people without the mark of the Beast will be unable to buy, sell, or trade. Life will come to a grinding halt without that mark. The False Prophet will ration commodities only to those who have the mark of the Beast.

Some think the mark of the Beast will be a triple six—"the number of a man," that is, 666, each digit falling short of the perfect number seven. Six, in the Scriptures, is man's number. The number 666 applies this title to the first beast, Antichrist.

Others don't think the mark of the Beast will be 666, but will be an identifying number assigned to each individual, like a social security number or a student ID number at a large university. This ID number will be invisible to the naked eye but discernable to an infrared reader. This number will be the means to buy in a "cashless" society.

What is the judgment (Bema) seat of Christ?

The Bema seat of Christ occurs at the time immediately following the translation, or "rapture" of the church (1 Thess. 4:14–17; 1 Cor. 15:51–52). The place of the Bema seat of Christ is in the sphere of the heavenlies.

From 2 Corinthians 5:10, John 5:22, and Romans 14:10, we are told that the judge at the Bema seat is Christ Himself. One day all the saved dead of the church will be raised to stand before Christ (those saved from the Cross to the rapture). The unsaved will stand before God at the Great White Throne Judgment (John 5:29; Rom. 14:10–12; Rev. 20:11–15).

Only those who are born-again believers will stand before the Bema seat of Christ (2 Cor. 5:1–19). The purpose of the Bema seat is to make a public manifestation of the essential character and motives of the individual Christian. The believer's works are brought into judgment, called "the things done in the body" (2 Cor. 5:10), that it may be determined whether they are good or bad. This judgment is not to determine what is ethically good or evil, but rather that which is acceptable and that which is worthless/unprofitable to the work of Christ.

"Each one's work will become clear" (1 Cor. 3:13–15). While it is possible to hide the true quality of one's service for Christ in this life, there will be a time of reckoning for the Christian. There is coming a time when all will be openly displayed for what one's true motives were.

The results of the judgment are twofold: (1) a reward received, or (2) a reward lost. If a man's work remains undamaged by the fire, then he receives rewards (Greek *misthos*). If a man's work does not endure and is consumed in the fire, then he shall "suffer loss."

What are the future events between the rapture and the Great White Throne judgment?

The next great event that we can expect on God's calendar of prophecy is the appearance of Christ in the air, when He comes to take all Christians up to heaven: "The dead in Christ will rise first. Then we who are alive and remain shall be caught up together with them in the clouds to meet the Lord in the air. And thus we shall always be with the Lord" (1 Thess. 4:16–17). This event is known as the *rapture*. Immediately following the rapture, the Bema Judgment (or the Awards Judgment) occurs.

The seven years following the rapture is known as the Great Tribulation. During this time, the terrible judgments and events described in the book of Revelation will transpire. Those who were left behind at the rapture because they were not saved will suffer terrible persecution. Judgments from God upon the natural elements of the earth and upon the inhabitants of the earth will be severe during this seven-year period.

At the end of this period, the Second Coming of Christ will occur. Jesus will touch down upon the Mount of Olives (Zech. 14:4–8). Accompanied by the holy angels and the church (including those who were raptured), Christ will march toward Armageddon (Isa. 34:6; 63:1).

Satan's forces (the Antichrist and the world's nations assembled at Armageddon) will be destroyed by Christ (Rev. 19:17–21). Satan will be bound for one thousand years (Rev. 20:1–3).

Then, all other believers not resurrected in the rapture (Old Testament and Tribulation saints) will be resurrected just prior to the Millennium (Rev. 20:4). These events will usher in the thousand-year reign of Jesus Christ known as the Millennium. Christ will personally rule the earth during this glorious period. The inhabitants will be saved: Israel, saved Old Testament and Tribulation Gentiles, the church, and the elect angels. The Lord Jesus Christ will, of course, be the King supreme, but the vice-regent will be David (Jer. 30:9; Hos. 3:5). David will once again sit upon the throne in Israel. He will be aided in his rulership by the church (1 Cor. 6:3); the apostles (Matt. 19:28); nobles (Jer. 30:21); princes (Isa. 32:1; Ezek. 45:8–9), and judges (Zech. 3:7; Isa. 1:26).

Concerning the geography of the Millennium, Palestine will be greatly enlarged and changed (Isa. 26:15; Obad. 1:17–21). For the first time Israel will possess all of the land promised to Abraham in Genesis 15:18–21. A great fertile plain will replace the mountainous terrain. A river will flow east to west from the Mount of Olives into both the Mediterranean and the Dead Seas (Zech. 14:4, 8, 10; Joel 3:18; Ezek. 47:8–9, 12). Jerusalem will become the worship center of the world (Mic. 4:1; Isa. 2:2–3). The city will occupy an elevated site (Zech. 14:10). It will be named *Jehovah-Shammah*, meaning "the Lord is there" (Ezek. 48:35) and *Jehovah-Tsidkenu*, meaning "the Lord our righteousness" (Jer. 23:6; 33:16). Although this city has been called by many titles in the Bible, these two will be the final names for God's beloved city.

There will be babies born to the mortal Israelite and Gentile parents who survived the Tribulation and entered the Millennium in that state of mortality. Many in the Millennium, although their outward acts will be subjected to the existing authority, will only give lip service to the Savior. Outwardly they will conform, but inwardly they will rebel against God.

Satan will be loosed for a season at the end of Christ's thousand-year reign. Those who are rebellious will make up Satan's army in his final revolt at the end of the thousand-year reign (Rev. 20:6–9). This army will be devoured by fire from heaven (v. 9).

Satan will then be "cast into the lake of fire and brimstone where the beast and the false prophet are. And they will be tormented day and night forever and ever" (Rev. 20:10). Following this event will be the "Great White Throne" judgment (described in Matt. 25:41–46 and Rev. 20:11–15. See also Dan. 7:9–10; John 5:22, 27; 12:48; Acts 10:40, 42; 2 Tim. 4:1; and Ps. 9:17). Only unsaved people will stand before this throne; after that, all believers will enter the new heaven and the new earth, as described in Revelation 21, to live forever with God.

When will the "Tribulation" begin?

The prophet Daniel prophesied concerning the seventy weeks in which God would deal with the nation Israel. As in the case of other Old Testament writers, the mystery of the church was kept hidden. Daniel did accurately predict the death of the Messiah and the destruction of the city of Jerusalem; he said that, after the sixty-ninth week, "Messiah shall be cut off, but not for Himself; and the people of the prince who is to come shall destroy the city and the sanctuary" (Dan. 9:26).

Most historians agree that Jesus was crucified about A.D. 30, and the Romans destroyed Jerusalem in A.D. 70. This ended the sixty-nine weeks that were predicted by Daniel. Then the prophet describes a gap between that time and the beginning of the Tribulation. The church age fits into that gap and has lasted almost two millennia. There is no indication of the length of the church age, also called the "age of grace." At the end of this age, "he shall confirm a covenant with many for one week; but in the middle of the week he shall bring an end to sacrifice and offering. And on the wing of abominations shall be one who makes desolate, even until the consummation, which is determined, is poured out on the desolate" (Dan. 9:27).

God still has a future for Israel. There is coming a period of about seven years when Israel will once again be the chief focus of God's activity. Unfortunately, much of that "week" will be devoted to judgment, and the world will be in a continual state of chaos. But the period is coming. It is as certain as the promises of God (Dan. 9:24–27). The Great Tribulation is as certain as the return of Christ Himself (2 Thess. 2:2–4).

Will the Jews accept Jesus as Messiah?

After the rapture, the judicial blindness of the Jews (Acts 28:25–28; 2 Cor. 3:13–15) will be removed from Israel. They will be able to perceive the true identity of Jesus as their Messiah. The gospel will be preached to the Jews and thousands will be saved.

Revelation 7:4 tells us that twelve thousand Jews from each of the twelve tribes of Israel—144,000 in all—will again preach the gospel of the kingdom to all the earth. We believe that God will manifest Himself to the Jewish nation at that time and that according to Romans 9–11, the book of Revelation, and the Old Testament books of Zechariah and Ezekiel, the Jewish nation will believe on the Messiah. Some have used the phrase to describe this was "a nation to be saved in a day." However, during the coming millennium, "all Israel will be saved" (Rom 11:26–27).

What is the identity of the 144,000 individuals of Revelation?

"And I heard the number of those who were sealed. One hundred and forty-four thousand of all the tribes of the children of Israel were sealed" (Rev. 7:4). Dr. John F. Walvoord, president of Dallas Theological Seminary, in his book entitled *True Revelation of Jesus Christ,* gives the following comments as to the identity of the 144,000 of Revelation 7:4:

There is a great deal of controversy surrounding the identity of the

144,000 individuals of Revelation 7. Many people are perplexed by the conflicting views and theories regarding the 144,000. It should be noted there are many unscriptural and often positively heretical sects and cults that identify themselves as the 144,000. The Seventh-Day Adventists apply it to the faithful of their communion, based on their faithful observing of the Jewish Sabbath at the Lord's return. The Jehovah Witnesses teach that the 144,000 include only their own "overcomers," a teaching of the system commonly called "Millennial Dawnism."

Besides these cults, there are many other groups who consider their peculiar followers to be the 144,000 sealed ones at the time of the end. All of these, however, overlook a very simple fact that, if observed, would save them from their folly. That is, the 144,000 are composed of 12,000 from each tribe of the children of Israel! There is not a Gentile among them, nor is there confusion as to the identification of their tribe. Therefore, a proper question to ask anyone identifying themselves as one of the 144,000 would be, "Which tribe do you belong to?"

First, that they are of Israel is manifest from their identity (vs. 4); they are from all the tribes of the children of Israel. Second, they cannot be reckoned as the church; for that body is never called Israel. Third, they cannot be Israel in general; for God would not place His seal upon unbelievers for service. Finally, these servants are from the twelve tribes of Israel, literally so, redeemed by God and sealed after the Church has been raptured to heaven (see Revelation 14:4).

The 144,000 Jews (12,000 from each tribe) will be wonderfully converted to Christ during the Tribulation after the exodus of the church (rapture).

Who are the two witnesses in Revelation 11, and what do they do?

During the first half of the Tribulation, two special witnesses begin to preach. Although they are not clearly identified, they do have the power of God to perform miracles similar to those of Moses and Elijah (Rev. 11:6). Some have speculated that these witnesses may be Enoch and Elijah, as they have not yet died, and every man has an appointment with death (Heb. 9:27). These men are killed by the beast, and their bodies are left lying in the streets of Jerusalem (Rev. 11:7). For three-and-a-half days their bodies will lie on the streets while the world celebrates their deaths. Then they are resurrected and raptured into heaven (Rev. 11:12–8). Despite the evangelistic efforts of these witnesses and the 144,000 Jews, the world will continue in its sin.

What is the battle of Gog and Magog?

During the latter half of the Tribulation, an alliance between Gog and his allies will invade Israel from the north. These nations will fail in great confusion in their attempt to destroy Israel. It will take seven months to bury the dead (Ezek. 38:1–19; 39:12). The geographic regions included in Ezekiel's vision of the allies are occupied by the Russian and the former Soviet-bloc countries in Eastern Europe today. This battle may be fought with allies attacking from the east (Rev. 16:12–16). Today, mainland China is the only nation in the world with an army or militia the size of that identified by John.

When will the battle of Gog and Magog take place?

There are several reasons to believe this battle will take place during the Tribulation: (1) The invasion takes place at a time when Israel is dwelling in their own land (Ezek. 38:8). (2) The invasion takes place when Israel is dwelling in peace in the land (Ezek. 38:11). (3) Ezekiel uses two expressions in chapter 38 that may give an indication as to the time of this invasion. In verse 8 the expression "latter years" and in verse 16 the expression "latter days" is related to the tie of Israel's glorification, salvation, and blessing in the kingdom age (Isa. 2:2–4; Mic. 4:1–7). The term "latter days" or "latter years" is related to the last days (the "Millennial Age"), which would be the Tribulation period.

The conclusion, then, since Ezekiel uses these expressions, is that events described by that prophet must take place within the Seventieth Week. Daniel 11:40 seems to have reference to the same period, for the prophet places these events "at the time of the end." This expression seems to separate this event from the end itself.

What is the battle of Armageddon?

The battle of Armageddon involves the nations of the world converging on the Middle East and surrounding the city of Jerusalem to destroy the Jews and the Jewish nation (Ezek. 12:2; 14:2–3, 12; Rev. 19:11–21). The nations will be led by the Antichrist and will be gathered together into a place called in the Hebrew tongue *Armageddon* (Rev. 16:16). This place is presently known as the valley or plain of Jezreel. In the middle of the battle, Christ will return and touch His feet on the Mount of Olives (Zech. 14:4; Acts 1:9–12). He then will destroy the Antichrist and the armies gathered at Armageddon (Rev. 19:11; Isa. 34:6; 63:1). The Beast and the false prophet will then be cast alive into the lake of fire forever (Rev. 19:20).

The armies of the East—that is, China, India, and other Asian powers— will march toward Jerusalem, and the Euphrates River will dry up (Rev. 16:12). The Euphrates River has been known as the boundary between the peoples east and west of it. History frequently refers to the great hindrance the Euphrates has been to military movements and to the differences between the peoples living to its east and those to its west.

What is the difference between the rapture at the beginning of the Tribulation and the return of Jesus Christ at the end of the Tribulation?

In the rapture Jesus meets people in the air (1 Thess. 4:17), while He returns to the earth and stands on the Mount of Olives at the end of the Tribulation (Zech. 14:4). The rapture can happen imminently at any moment (Phil. 4:5), while there are many signs that are necessary before Jesus comes the second time in His revelation. Following the rapture, the believers are judged (2 Cor. 5:10), while unbelievers are judged after the return of Jesus to the earth (1 Thess. 5:4). In the rapture, nothing happens to creation; it is not transformed by supernatural occurrences. But when Jesus returns to the earth, nature will be changed and the curse removed (Matt. 24:29–30). The rapture is called the "blessed hope" (Titus 2:13) and is a message of comfort to Christians (1 Thess. 4:18), while the return of Jesus Christ is called the "glorious appearing" (Titus 2:13), and is a message of judgment to the unsaved (1 Thess. 5:4–9).

What is the nature of the Millennium?

The word *millennium* does not appear in the Bible, but again the idea is taught. This word is derived from two Latin words meaning "thousand years." That expression is used six times in Revelation 20. When we talk about the millennial reign of Christ, we are talking about the thousand-year period when Christ personally sits on the throne of David and reigns over the earth from Jerusalem.

The Millennium is more than an era in history. It will be characterized by the restraining of Satan and the universal recognition of Christ as the

King. The land of Palestine will in that day be the focal point of attention, particularly Jerusalem as its political capital. Nature will be released from the bondage it has experienced since the fall of man. Righteousness will permeate all society. By anyone's definition, this kingdom will be desirable for its joys and comforts as well as the absence of sickness and death.

How will Christ rule in the Millennium?

The Millennium has been called the "theocratic kingdom" because it is a kingdom ruled directly by God in the person of Christ. Years before the first advent of Christ, Isaiah wrote, "For unto us a Child is born, unto us a Son is given; and the government will be upon His shoulder. And His name will be called Wonderful, Counselor, Mighty God, Everlasting Father, Prince of Peace" (Isa. 9:6). This Prince of Peace was prophesied to reign on the throne of David in an unending kingdom (Isa. 9:7). This will be accomplished in the Millennium. Christ will be the authoritative Leader and will rule in a way that all past rulers have failed to accomplish.

How does Palestine relate to the Millennium?

God chose the land of Palestine to be the focal point of His concern in the history of the world. The Jews are God's chosen people, and He gave that land to them. Throughout the years, the Jews have spent comparatively little time in the land, and much of the time they lived there was filled with uncertainty. Concerning the future, God has promised, "Then they shall dwell in the land that I have given to Jacob My servant, where your fathers dwelt; and they shall dwell there, they, their children, and their children's children, forever; and My servant David shall be their prince forever" (Ezek. 37:25). This land will be the Jewish homeland during the Millennium.

Where will the capital city of the world be during the thousand-year reign of Christ?

"And it shall come to pass that everyone who is left of all the nations which came against Jerusalem shall go up from year to year to worship the King, the LORD of hosts, and to keep the Feast of Tabernacles" (Zech. 14:16). Jerusalem will be a truly international city. The vast numbers of tourists to that city in the past is nothing in comparison with the crowds that will converge on the city during the reign of Christ. The city of Jerusalem will be the universal capital of the theocratic kingdom.

How will the world be changed during the Millennium?

An additional blessing of this golden era will be the liberty once again experienced in nature. The apostle Paul talked of a future day when "the creation itself also will be delivered from the bondage of corruption" (Rom. 8:21). At the Fall, even the creation that God had perfectly created was made subject to the bondage of sin. At the return of Christ, rescue from that bondage will be a part of the deliverance that Christ brings. Life in the Millennium is pictured thus: "The wolf also shall dwell with the lamb, the leopard shall lie down with the young goat, the calf and the young lion and the fatling together; and a little child shall lead them" (Isa. 11:6). There will be no destructive vengeance in nature. There will not be "survival of the fittest," but survival of all. And children will enjoy all of nature with no threat of danger to them.

What does the Bible teach about the rebuilding of the temple during the Millennium?

One of the things done in the Millennium will be the rebuilding of the temple. The Old Testament prophets wrote, "After this I will return and will rebuild the tabernacle of David, which has fallen down; I will rebuild its ruins, and I will set it up" (Acts 15:16). Several chapters in Ezekiel deal specifically with the rebuilding of the millennial temple and the conducting of memorial sacrifices (Ezek. 40–48).

When will Satan be judged?

When, in history, was Satan cast out of heaven? There are two important passages in the Word of God concerning the origin and fall of Satan. The first is found in Ezekiel 28:12–19 where Ezekiel describes the beautiful creation and severe judgment of an angel whose name we find out later to be Lucifer. The second passage relating to Satan's fall is found in Isaiah 14:12–14. Satan has already been judged in the past by God for his sins and will be further judged for his continued sins. There are at least six judgments associated with Satan:

1. He was barred from his original privileged position in heaven (Ezek. 28:16).

2. He was judged for his temptation of Adam and Eve (Gen. 3:14–15).

3. He was judged at the cross of Calvary (John 12:31).

4. Satan will be barred from heaven during the Tribulation period (Rev. 12:13).

5. He will be confined to the abyss during the Millennium (Rev. 20:2).

6. At the conclusion of the Millennium, Satan will be cast into the lake of fire for all eternity (Rev. 20:10).

What is the nature of the "Great White Throne" judgment?

At the end of the millennial reign of Christ, those who died unsaved will have to stand before the throne of God to be judged. "And I saw the dead, small and great, standing before God, and books were opened. And another book was opened, which is the Book of Life. And the dead were judged according to their works, by the things which were written in the books" (Rev. 20:12). This judgment does not suggest these people may enter into heaven or hell on the basis of their works. All those who are judged at the Great White Throne are already consigned to hell because they have rejected the gospel. The saved have already been resurrected and are enjoying fellowship with Christ. The Great White Throne judgment will determine the degree of punishment they will endure based upon the nature of their evil work. When the book of works is opened (Rev. 20:12), a sentence of the severity of their punishment will be determined. All those sentenced will be consigned "into the lake of fire" (Rev. 20:14), where they will suffer according to their personally assigned sentences.

QUESTIONS

ABOUT

SIN

If God is all-powerful so that He could prohibit sin, and all-loving so that he doesn't want to harm people, then why does He allow sin?

You have two alternatives. Either God is not all-powerful, or His motives are not all pure, yet the answer is that God is all-powerful *and* He is all-loving.

To be tempted is not the same as sinning. God created Adam and Eve to be free so that they could worship Him freely. God did not want coerced worship; He wanted authentic worship. So God gave Adam and Eve a free will to worship Him. If they were forced to worship God, it would not have been authentic worship; that is not true freedom.

For Adam and Eve to be free, they had to have the ability to both reject God and worship Him freely. Adam and Eve fully understood what God expected of them. And if they had never been tempted concerning their loyalty to God, they would have remained in immaturity. God did not give them an arbitrary insignificant demand. God said they could eat from all the trees in the garden *except* "the tree of the knowledge of good and evil." This tree was the *only* one that they could not eat from. If the fruit of this tree in the midst of the Garden were the only available thing to eat, then God would have been guilty of coercion to sin. But God created all of the trees and said that they could eat freely of all of them *except* the one in the middle of the Garden. Since sin is an *act*, *attitude*, or *response* toward God, Adam and Eve sinned by denying God's rulership over them and going contrary to the one and only thing that He requested.

The answer: God allowed Adam and Eve to sin because freedom was a requisite for authentic worship of God. God gave human beings the freedom to either worship Him or reject Him.

What is *sin*?

Sin is an act, attitude, or response against the Person or law of God.

What happens to our judicial standing before God when we sin?

God attaches *criminality* to our accounts, which is a moral worth attached to the acts of our rebellion.

What happens to us physically when we sin?

"For the wages of sin is death, but the gift of God is eternal life in Christ Jesus our Lord" (Rom. 6:23).

Does God tempt us to sin?

"Let no one say when he is tempted, 'I am tempted by God'; for God cannot be tempted by evil, nor does He Himself tempt anyone" (James 1:13).

What happens to us internally when we are tempted?

"But each one is tempted when he is drawn away by his own desires and enticed. Then, when desire has conceived, it gives birth to sin; and sin, when it is full-grown, brings forth death" (James 1:14–15).

Is "temptation" the same as "sin"?

No. Martin Luther said that temptation is the open door, and sin is walking through it. Temptation is not sin. Jesus was tempted in all parts of His being (Heb. 4:15), yet He did not sin.

What are the steps of temptation?

First, one *desires* something that God has prohibited. The person desires it because it is before him. Second, the person *intends* to have the sinful object or wants to do the wrong action. Third, the person develops a *plan* to get the object. When the person *willingly puts the plan into action*, (fourth step), sin happens. In the fifth step, physical movement is made to *get the object*. Finally, in the sixth step, the person *gratifies* himself or herself through the object.

What are the different kinds of sin?

A *presumptuous sin* is a willful, premeditated, rebellious act by a person to purposely deny or disobey God's clear command. A *sin of ignorance* is breaking God's law without being consciously aware that one is sinning against God.

A *sin of commission* is something done contrary to the law of God; it is *committing* the act of sin. The *sin of omission* is failing to do something that God has commanded we do.

Apart from what the Bible teaches about sin, what can we know practically about sin?

First, we realize that man dies physically, and when we look to the Scriptures, we see that the cause of death is sin. Second, we know that people get sick and suffer physically, and when we look to the Scriptures, again we see the cause is sin. Third, we see the inherent selfishness of babies, which is an unlearned response, and know that selfishness is inborn. Babies are born with their hands clenched and have strong unlearned desires that center around self. We know from the Bible that sin is attached to selfishness. Fourth, we know the propensity of men to lie. Satan is the father of lies, and the Bible teaches that all *men* are liars (Ps. 116:11). And finally, we can know that the tendency of one person to desire or actually harm another comes from a sin nature.

What is the "age of accountability"?

When a child is old enough to be aware of or responsible for his or her sin, that child is now responsible for his spiritual destiny. This age comes to some children much younger, perhaps at the age of three, and to other children much later, perhaps after they enter elementary school.

Do children who die before the age of accountability go to heaven?

Yes, God would not send a person to hell without that person having an opportunity to choose eternal life. When Jesus gathered the little children around Him, He said, "Let the little children come to Me, and do not forbid them; for of such is the kingdom of heaven" (Matt. 19:14). In this statement, Jesus was saying that little children are related to heaven, and He revealed His love to them. David prayed and fasted for seven days that his little baby boy might not die. However, the baby died. David said, "Now he is dead; why should I fast? Can I bring him back again? I shall go to him, but he shall not return to me" (2 Sam. 12:23). David was suggesting that his baby was in the presence of God and that upon his death, he would go to be with his son *in heaven.* Most conservatives do not consider a baby to be "saved" because it cannot pray the sinner's prayer; however, babies are considered *safe* and enter the presence of God upon death.

QUESTIONS
ABOUT
THE BOOK OF
GENESIS

What does the word *genesis* mean?

The word *genesis* means "beginning," and this book shows how everything began with God: "In the beginning God created the heaven and the earth" (Gen. 1:1 KJV).

Who wrote the book of Genesis?

The book of Genesis does not directly name Moses as the author, but the Jews of the Old Testament, as well as the early church and Jesus, all identify Moses as the author. If Moses did not write the book of Genesis, but Jesus said he did, then Jesus would either have been mistaken or misled the people. However, since Jesus is God, He cannot be mistaken, and since He is perfect, He knows all things; Moses wrote Genesis. Because of the credibility of Jesus Christ, most evangelicals believe Moses wrote the book of Genesis.

How was Moses prepared to write Genesis?

Some critics have said that there was no writing during the time of Moses, so he could not have written a book. However, scholars know better. The Bible says Moses was "learned in all the wisdom of the Egyptians" (Acts 7:22). When he was taken (adopted) by the daughter of Pharaoh and raised in the palace, he would have been taught how to read and write Egyptian, plus he would have been given the highest university training of his day. He would have been able to read and write other languages, including Hebrew, his mother's native tongue, and he would have been well able to write the book of Genesis.

What language was used to write Genesis?

Moses wrote the book of Genesis in the Hebrew language. Actually, Hebrew is one of the oldest and first phonetic languages used in civilization. Up until the time of Moses, most languages (Chaldean, cuneiform, Egyptian, and others) were pictorial based. The Phoenicians (modern-day Lebanon) were great tradesmen, and had influenced Egypt, where Moses was trained. Their language was based on an alphabet, as was the Hebrew language. The book of Genesis was one of the first books written using an alphabet.

What is the structure of Genesis?

Moses wrote the book around eleven different units, each one beginning with the word *generations,* using the phrase, "these are the generations," or "the book of the generations." These include the following sections:

(1) the introduction (1:1–2:3)

(2) the generation of heaven and earth (2:4–4:26)

(3) the generation of Adam (5:1–6:8)

(4) the generation of Noah (6:9–9:29)

(5) the generation of Noah's sons (10:1–11:9)

(6) the generation of Shem (11:10–26)

(7) the generation of Terah (11:27–25:2–11)

(8) the generation of Ishmael (25:12–18)

(9) the generation of Isaac (25:19–35:29)

(10) the generation of Esau (36:1–37:1)

(11) the generation of Jacob (37:2–50:26)

What is the key word in Genesis?

The key word in Genesis is *beginning.*

What is the key verse of Genesis?

"Now the LORD had said to Abram: 'Get out of your country, from your family and from your father's house, to a land that I will show you. I will make you a great nation; I will bless you and make your name great; and you shall be a blessing. I will bless those who bless you, and I will curse him who curses you; and in you all the families of the earth shall be blessed.'" (Gen. 12:1–2)

What does the name *Adam* mean?

Adam means "earth man" or "dust." The word comes from the root "red" suggesting Adam was formed out of red clay.

What does the name *Eve* mean?

Eve means "mother of all living."

Where is the Garden of Eden located?

Many believe the Garden of Eden is located in the Mesopotamian area (modern-day Iraq). This locality is east of Palestine, which may be the meaning of Genesis 2:8, "The LORD God planted a garden eastward in Eden." The Garden of Eden lies between the Tigris and the Euphrates Rivers. These rivers are actually united for a short distance as one stream before entering the Persian Gulf. Therefore, the Garden of Eden would have been located close to the Persian Gulf. The area watered by these two rivers would have been extremely fertile. This certainly fits the description of what we would think of today as an ideal agricultural location for the magnificent Garden of Eden.

Could Adam talk, read, and write?

Many secular historians explain that the first people were "cavemen" who communicated with grunts and sign language. However, Adam talked with God, probably using the language that God spoke. Adam probably wrote a family tree: "This is the book of the genealogy of Adam. In the day that God created man, He made him in the likeness of God" (Gen. 5:1). The word *generations* (*toledoth*) suggests something like a family tree or genealogy written on a tablet. This implies that Adam wrote down the names of his children that are recorded in Genesis 4. The Jewish rabbis of the Old Testament even suggested that Adam had written a book on carpentry.

Why are there two different accounts of the Creation story?

Many believe God wrote the first section, Genesis 1:1–2:4: "These are the generations of the heavens and of the earth when they were created, in the day that the LORD God made the earth and the heavens" (Gen. 2:4 KJV). Adam wrote the second account: "This is the book of the generations of Adam. In the day that God created man, in the likeness of God made he him" (Gen. 5:1 KJV). The first section explains *what was created* and the second section emphasizes *how God created:* "And the LORD God formed man of the dust of the ground, and breathed into his nostrils the breath of life; and man became a living being" (Gen. 2:7).

Is God presently adding to His creation (creating new things) today?

No, because "God ended His work which He had done" (Gen. 2:2). The word *ended* means "finished," so the creation of man was the final act of Creation.

Why did God rest on the seventh day? Was He tired?

After six days God had completed all He had intended to create, and He rested on the seventh day (the word *Sabbath* means "rest"). Notice the word is in the past tense: God rested in the past, but He is not resting now.

God rested on the seventh day as an example to us and for our benefit. It is a day of rest and rejuvenation, a day to get a new start in life. Then God blessed and sanctified the day; He made it "holy" or "hallowed." This means God set the Sabbath apart as our day to worship and have fellowship with Him. Some believe that God came to fellowship with Adam in the cool of the garden on the Sabbath day. Others believe God came every day.

We may not be sure today which is the exact seventh day, or Sabbath, because chronologists have lost track of the exact designation. But the Sabbath does not depend upon the movement of the sun, stars, or moon, but it is a memorial to the Creation week. When we rest on one day, the Sabbath (Saturday) in the Old Testament or Sunday in the New Testament, we are recognizing what God has done.

What was the Garden of Eden like?

The word *Eden* means "delight" or "fertile plain." But we would not find the area where many traditionally think the Garden of Eden is located to be fertile today. Technically, the Tigris River (Hiddekel) and the Euphrates River were located in the Garden. Therefore, the Garden of Eden was probably located in modern-day Iraq. (The biblical designation was Babylon or Mesopotamia.) Some think that the Garden might have been from fifty to two hundred miles wide, because that would encompass the modern-day Tigris and Euphrates Rivers. However, others think that the two rivers (the Pishan and Gihon) represent the Indus River of India and the Nile River of Egypt. If this is true, then the Garden of Eden stretched from Egypt to India—that is, the "Fertile Crescent."

What happened to the Garden?

First of all, God put cherubim at the gate of the garden to keep people out. Without human care it would naturally degenerate. During the Flood in Noah's time, the Garden would also have disappeared. Today, that part of the world is characterized by desert, rock, and sand, with very little vegetation.

Has the Garden of Eden ever been found?

Apparently the area between the Tigris and Euphrates was once very fertile and green, but today it is very dry and desertlike. Whereas people before the Flood knew where the Garden of Eden was and that they were not to go there because angels guarded its gates, its location since the Flood has remained unknown, so no one has *knowingly* found the Garden of Eden.

What were the "two trees" in the Garden?

The first was the Tree of Life, which would have given them eternal life, had Adam and Eve eaten of it. The second tree was the Tree of Knowledge of Good and Evil. Until the couple sinned, they did not understand experientially the concept of evil; they probably did not even know about sin in theory. But when they ate fruit from this tree, they understood sin in both theory and practice.

What was Adam's task in the Garden?

Adam was "to tend and keep it" (Gen. 2:15), which implies that he was to cultivate the garden and perhaps keep it tidy and clean. Some people think the word *keep* meant to protect it from Satan, who had sinned in heaven, so that he might not enter the Garden.

Why did God have Adam name the animals?

"Out of the ground the LORD God formed every beast of the field and every bird of the air, and brought them to Adam to see what he would call them" (Gen. 2:19). By giving them names, Adam exercised dominion over all the animals. Adam also learned that the animals were different from him, a human. This demonstrated to Adam that an animal was not a sufficient companion for him. After he named the animals, "there was not found a helper comparable to him" (Gen. 2:20).

What was the penalty for eating the trees that were prohibited?

God warned Adam, "Thou shalt surely die" (Gen. 2:17 KJV); the Hebrew language meant, "in dying thou shalt die." First death was to be gradual; through germs, bacteria, infection, and the process of decay, man would gradually get older until he died. The second death was spiritual. Individuals would be separated from their bodies, and in physical death they would meet God in judgment. If they believed in God, they would be ushered into heaven; if not, they would be judged in hell.

What does the word *helpmeet* mean?

Technically, a "helpmeet" is a helpmate, someone to help Adam. This would imply a physical, social, psychological, and spiritual helper. It also meant companionship because of loneliness (Gen. 2:18 KJV).

Why did God put Adam in a deep sleep to create Eve?

This was not an anesthetized sleep to prevent pain. God was choosing to withhold the mystery of divine creation of human beings, from Adam and from us. All we need to know is "we are wonderfully made."

What does the phrase "one flesh" mean?

Christians have differed on the interpretation of this phrase over the years. Some feel that "one flesh" meant sexual intimacy between Adam and Eve; that they acted, felt, thought, and responded as one. Others see this as a picture of the physical birth, when the semen of the man joins the eggs of the woman, forming the cell of the new baby. As the baby continues to grow by the dividing of cells, so each cell of the baby represents the original cell of the father and mother. The phrase "one flesh" also suggests that a couple should not corrupt their relationship by adultery, divorce, polygamy, or homosexuality.

What does the phrase "They were not ashamed" mean? (Gen. 2:25)

In some heathen tribes all members are naked, without apparent embarrassment. Likewise, some on the stage seem to undress in public without shame. As a result, some non-Christians think nudity among the sexes is normal. However, Christians have a different view toward modesty versus nudity. Those who have no embarrassment over nudity have hardened consciences. Adam and Eve had tender consciences toward God. They knew they were divinely created in accordance to God's purpose, and they knew that God had brought them together and told them to be fruitful and multiply; therefore, there was no embarrassment or shame of their nudity.

The nudity of man or woman had not been poisoned by their responses to sin, but immediately after their transgression, they realized they were naked before God. Why? Because of their moral guilt (Gen. 3:7).

What did the serpent look like?

"Now the serpent was more cunning than any beast of the field which the LORD God had made" (Gen. 3:1). The word *cunning*, Hebrew *machash,* possibly means a shiny, upright creature. The fact that the serpent was cursed to crawl on his belly on the dust of the ground implies that he previously traveled in a different manner.

"The serpent deceived Eve by his craftiness" (2 Cor. 11:3). Because Satan used the serpent, with time the devil has been given the name "that old serpent, called the Devil, and Satan" (Rev. 12:9 KJV).

Did the snake actually talk?

No, Satan used the snake's throat to talk to Eve. The conversation was between Satan, who was an angel, and Eve. She did not talk to a snake.

How did Satan get Eve to listen to him?

First, he cast doubt in Eve's mind by saying, "Has God indeed said . . . ?" (Gen. 3:1). Then he blatantly denied the word of God when he said, "You will not surely die" (Gen. 3:4).

How truthful was Eve's response to the serpent?

Eve said, "God hath said, Ye shall not eat of it, neither shall ye touch it, lest ye die" (Gen. 3:3 KJV).

First, Eve *omitted* part of God's commandment. God had said, "In the day that you eat of it . . ." (Gen. 2:17), but Eve didn't include the time factor. Second, Eve *added* to God's commandment when she said, " . . . nor shall you touch it" (Gen. 3:3). God had never said anything about touching the fruit. Third, Eve *altered* God's command by changing the word *surely* to *lest.* God promised Adam and Eve would surely die, but Eve added speculation to what God had said when she said "lest."

Where was Adam when Eve ate the fruit?

Some people believe that he was standing next to her, for Genesis 3:6 says, Eve "gave to her husband with her, and he ate." The phrase "with her" suggests he was there. He was responsible because he saw his wife disobeying God and apparently did nothing about it.

Why did Adam eat the fruit after Eve had disobeyed God?

Maybe Adam didn't want Eve to have knowledge superior to his. She knew something about "good and evil" that he didn't know. Or maybe he felt sorry for Eve and the consequences she would have. Because people do not like to sin alone, Adam joined with Eve in her transgression.

How long was it between the Creation week and man's fall into sin?

Since Adam and Eve were commanded to "be fruitful and multiply," and Eve had apparently not yet conceived, it was probably only a few days before Adam and Eve sinned. (Some have suggested the time was less than one menstrual cycle). Other people have said the time was long enough for Satan's rebellion in heaven and expulsion, so that he found his way to earth to tempt Eve.

What were the immediate consequences of Adam and Eve eating the forbidden fruit?

First, there was guilt; their eyes were opened. Second, they were shamed; they knew they were "naked." Next was fear; they "hid from God." (There was also the first finger-pointing: Adam blamed his wife, Eve.) Finally, there was spiritual death. Their relationship to God was broken, and they needed a Savior to forgive their sins (Rom. 5:12).

What were the ultimate results of eating the forbidden fruit?

First was spiritual death (Gen. 5:5), second, expulsion from the Garden (Gen. 3:23), and finally, physical death (Rom. 5:12).

What were the physical consequences of eating the forbidden fruit?

The woman was to have pain in childbirth (Gen. 3:16), and the man was to work in difficulty (Gen. 3:19).

When God promised "enmity" between the offspring of the woman and Satan, what did the word *enmity* mean?

Enmity means hatred, variance, or animosity. Satan would hate God's people from that moment on because their sin was responsible for his ultimate judgment by God.

What is meant by the phrase "her seed"? (Gen. 3:15)

A woman does not have a seed; she has an egg. A man has a seed. Birth comes when man's seed makes contact with a woman's egg, and the first cell is formed. But here the woman has the seed, contrary to human nature. This implies that the Child of the woman would be born without the aid of a man.

There are two implications to the phrase "her Seed." First, the Child of the woman would not inherit the sinful nature that other children inherit. Therefore, the promised Child (who is Jesus Christ) could redeem man from sin because He was sinless. Second, the phrase, "her Seed" is a predication of the virgin birth (compare Isaiah 7:14).

Who were the cherubim placed at the entrance to Eden? (Gen. 3:24)

Cherubim was one of the names for angels, and they were a specific class of angels. They kept man from returning to the Garden so he wouldn't have access to the Tree of Life (eternal life).

If the woman ate the fruit first, why was the man held responsible?

Adam should have told Eve about the tree, and we don't know that he didn't. The Bible teaches, "And Adam was not deceived, but the woman being deceived, fell into transgression" (1 Tim. 2:14). This means the woman sinned, but she didn't realize what she was doing. She was partially blinded to her acts. The Bible says, "Adam was not deceived," meaning he fully understood what he did. He sinned with his eyes wide open. Therefore, God came in the cool of the day, calling for Adam, not Eve. It has been God's plan that the man be the responsible head of the family, and Adam was the responsible head of the human race. Adam was condemned: "Because you have heeded the voice of your wife" (Gen. 3:17). The New Testament holds man responsible: "Just as through one man sin entered the world, and death through sin, and thus death spread to all men, because all sinned" (Rom. 5:12).

What does the name *Cain* mean?

Cain was the first child born. His name means "acquired" because Eve said, "I have gotten a man from the LORD" (Gen. 4:1 KJV). She probably thought this was the man who was to be their Redeemer.

What does the name *Abel* mean?

Abel was the second child born to Adam and Eve. His name means "keeper." He was a keeper of the sheep.

Why was Cain's offering rejected?

Cain brought vegetables, which were later a part of the peace offering to God in the tabernacle and temple, but he did not bring a *blood* sacrifice for the redemption of sin. His brother Abel brought a blood sacrifice and was accepted by God. Because he disobeyed God, Cain was rejected by God (Gen. 4:1–15). A few have suggested Cain was rejected because he worshiped pagan deities, but there is no proof for that.

What did God mean when He told Cain, "Sin lies at the door"? (Gen. 4:7)

The words *sin* and *sin offering* are the same. Some interpret this to mean God might have suggested that a sin offering (a lamb for sacrifice) was just outside the front door to Cain's house. Others interpret this to mean God was warning Cain that there was sin judgment against him on the other side of the door of opportunity. The door was Cain's opportunity.

Where did Cain get his wife?

There are three possible answers to this question: (1) Cain married a younger sister, a daughter of Adam and Eve. (2) Since God created a wife for Adam, He could also create a wife for Cain. (3) Cain married a woman from another unknown family.

We have to admit that there is no biblical answer to this question; however, it seems very unlikely that God would create a wife for Cain, as God rested from all of His creative activity (Gen. 2:3). Also, it's unlikely that there was another family besides Adam and Eve, because all of Scripture indicates Adam was the first created person. Cain probably married a daughter of Adam and Eve, although a few people think that he might have married a niece or a daughter of his murdered brother, Abel. However, there were no genetic problems with marrying within the family, as it might be today. The spread of pollution into the human bloodstream would not have been complete, and family intermarriage would not have produced physical maladies.

When the Bible says, "the sons of God saw the daughters of men," who were the sons of God? (Gen. 6:1–2)

Many contemporary evangelical scholars believe the sons of god were a godly line of Seth who compromised their faith by marrying women from the ungodly line of Cain. As a result of the corruption of the faith, God sent the Flood to destroy the world.

However, Jewish teachers in the Old Testament and most of the early church fathers believed the sons of God were angels who came down and cohabited with women on the earth. The results were, "There were giants on the earth" (Gen. 6:4). The giants were abnormal human beings, so God judged the unbelief of the world, saving only the people who were righteous, Noah and his family.

Why did people live longer before the Flood than today?

Originally people lived about a thousand years (Gen. 4–5), but with time the average life span dropped to 120 years during and after Noah's day: "Yet his days shall be an hundred and twenty years" (Gen. 6:3 KJV).

Today, the average length of life is seventy to eighty years. "The days of our lives are seventy years; and if by reason of strength they are eighty years . . ." (Ps. 90:10).

God originally warned Adam and Eve, "You shall surely die" (Gen. 2:17), if Adam and Eve sinned. The original Hebrew says, "In dying thou shalt die." The process of dying began with the gradual spreading of germs, bacteria, and disease into the human race, resulting in shorter lives, and eventually physical death. The more the germs spread, the shorter the average life became. By the time of the Flood, man's life was approximately 120 years long. Today, an average life is between seventy and eighty years long.

Since God never changes, how could He change His mind?

It is said of God, "I am sorry that I have made them [humans]" (Gen. 6:7). Obviously God doesn't change His mind: "And I relented not" (Zech. 8:14 KJV). The unchangeable nature of God teaches that He always loves without condition, and He will always judge sin without condition. When man sins, God cannot look on him with mercy, but with judgment. When man repents and changes his condition, it appears as though God is changing because He deals with man according to the "changed" condition of men. This is described as God "repenting." But God doesn't repent or change his mind. God deals with us one way when we sin, and He changes His relationship when we repent and believe.

What was Noah's ark like?

The word *ark* means "box." The boat that Noah built was a huge barge, 450 feet long, 75 feet wide, and 45 feet tall. This is about the size of a huge three-story dormitory on a college campus. And the ark was three stories tall: "You shall make it with lower, second, and third decks" (Gen. 6:16).

What is *gopher wood*?

Gopher wood is only mentioned in the Bible in connection with Noah's ark. It is a tight-grained type of hardwood that would resist rotting and have strength to hold the animals on the three stories of the ark. Gopher wood is similar to modern-day oak.

Was the Flood the result of a natural rainstorm?

No, the Flood was the result of the judgment of God. The Greek word *cataclysmas,* found in the Scriptures, is the word used in the Bible to describe the judgment of God. It had never rained before the Flood; there was only mist on the earth (Gen. 2:5–6). Yet it rained forty days and nights (forty is the number of judgment). Genesis 7:11 also says that the "fountains of the great deep were broken up." Apparently there were underground caverns of water that were released, as well as the tremendous rain when the mist or cloud of vapor that surrounded the earth all came down at one time.

Was it a local flood of the Tigris-Euphrates valley or a universal flood?

A few Bible scholars believe the Flood only covered the Tigris-Euphrates River valley. But universal terms are used to describe the Flood: "And *all* the high hills, that were under the *whole* heaven, were covered" (Gen. 7:19 KJV, emphasis mine). Genesis 6:17 says, "I . . . bring a flood . . . to destroy *all* flesh . . . from under heaven; and *every thing* that is in the earth shall die" (KJV, emphasis mine). Also, the size of the ark suggested it must have been a universal flood because it was large enough to save all the animals. And since the nature of the Flood was judgment, that is, *kataklumos,* from which we get our word *catastrophe,* then the Flood was a judgment on all the earth; it had to be a universal flood.

The fact that the Flood lasted one year also suggests it was more than a local flood. Had it been a local flood, waters would have receded within three or four weeks. But all the mountains were covered (*kosah*, meaning "overwhelmed"). The fact that all the animals and all peoples on the earth died also suggests it was a universal flood. Finally, the nature of the Noahic Covenant—that is, God promises to never repeat it again—suggests that it was a universal flood.

What happened to the atmosphere after the flood?

Many feel that God tilted the earth on its axis after the Flood, accounting for part of the earth being closer to the sun at certain seasons and farther away from the sun at others; hence, making the hot and cold seasons on earth. "While the earth remains, seedtime and harvest, cold and heat, winter and summer, and day and night shall not cease" (Gen. 8:22). Prior to this, the vapor cloud surrounded the earth and produced a mild climate year-round. The earth's perpendicular axis to the sun would have also produced an even, year-round climate. The change may account for why jungle vegetation has been found in solid ice in Siberia.

How many animals were brought aboard the ark?

Bible scholars suggest that there may have been approximately 35,000 individual animals in existence when the Flood came. However, probably far fewer than that were on the ark. Obviously, all the fish and aquatic creatures did not need a place aboard the ark. And while there may have been 35,000 animal species at that time, it was not necessary to bring every species onto the ark. As an illustration, not every type of dog was brought into the ark. In fact, perhaps as few as two thousand animals were on the ark. However, when you look at the size of the ark, it had a total volume of 1,518,000 cubic feet. This is roughly equivalent to 569 railroad boxcars. So the ark could have easily accommodated sixteen thousand animals. But those animals who were brought on the ark were probably not the largest in each specimen. Also, there are only a few very large animals such as dinosaurs, elephants, hippopotamus, etc. Even these could have been young ones. Probably the average size of the animals on the ark was about the size of a goat. Someone has estimated that three trains hauling approximately seventy cars each could have accommodated all the animals on the ark, but the ark was twice that size. That would have given ample space for Noah and his family, plus food and luggage.

Were dinosaurs real?

Yes, we have found many remains of dinosaurs—bones, teeth, claws, horns, and eggs (sometimes with unborn babies). Some remains are fully mineralized (petrified), but most are bones.

How did Noah breathe when the ark lifted above the mountaintops?

Today, when mountain climbers go to the top of Mt. Everest (the tallest mountain in the world), they need special training and/or oxygen tanks to make the trip because of the lack of oxygen at those high altitudes. However, as the rain gradually lifted the ark higher, Noah and his family would have been conditioned to live with less oxygen as certain mountain climbers learn to condition themselves. Second, the breakup of the subterranean oceans and the change in the topography of the earth during the Flood may have produced mountains that are higher now than were in existence when Noah lived. Third, the vapor canopy that surrounded the earth prior to the Flood would have been sustained by oxygen, so Noah and his family could have breathed.

What changed after the Flood?

First there was a drop in the lifespan of man. Mankind lived only 120 years. Second, there were seasonal changes (Gen. 8:22), which meant that tropical areas would be limited. Eventually the dinosaurs became extinct, and the polar caps began to emerge. Third, there probably was a geographical land restructuring, meaning landmass separated, mountains became higher, ocean canyons were created, and some of the continents began shrinking.

What was the result of the covenant that God made with Noah after the Flood?

God promised that there would not be another universal flood: "I will never again curse the ground for man's sake, although the imagination of man's heart is evil from his youth; nor will I again destroy every living thing as I have done" (Gen. 8:21). God also added meat to the diet of human beings; apparently before this time they were only vegetarians. "Every moving thing that lives shall be food for you. I have given you all things, even as the green herbs" (Gen. 9:3). Also as a result of this covenant, God instituted capital punishment for those who killed a human being: "Whoever sheds man's blood, by man his blood shall be shed; for in the image of God He made man" (Gen. 9:6). Finally, God put a rainbow in the sky to seal His covenant with Noah: "The rainbow shall be in the cloud, and I will look on it to remember the everlasting covenant between God and every living creature of all flesh that is on the earth" (Gen. 9:16).

Has anyone ever discovered Noah's ark?

In the past, many expeditions have traveled to the Ararat region of Eastern Turkey to explore the mountains where the ark landed after the Flood. There have been many who have claimed to see it from the land and the air, and some have even said, "I touched it." However, there is no solid evidence that anyone has found Noah's ark.

What was Noah's sin in his old age?

Some say that when Noah got drunk (Gen. 9:21) he didn't know the truth of fermentation, but only stumbled upon it. That's because before the Flood Noah was a carpenter, but after the Flood he became a farmer.

However, the reference by Jesus in Luke 17:27 suggested that Noah preached against drunkenness, so there would have been knowledge of fermentation before the Flood. As a result, when Noah became old, he gave up the standards he held as a young man and began to drink alcohol, ending up in drunkenness.

What was the sin of Canaan? (Gen. 9:25)

Some suggest it was some sexual or homosexual act. Whatever Canaan did, he did more than look upon the nakedness of his grandfather. One of the sons of Noah, "Ham, the father of Canaan, saw the nakedness of his father." Ham would have probably been blameless just for looking, but he "told his two brothers" (Gen. 9:22). Whatever Canaan did, we don't know, but it was serious enough to be cursed by his grandfather Noah, who said, "Cursed be Canaan" (Gen. 9:25).

What was the "curse on Canaan"?

Some have said the curse on Canaan was the servitude of black people to white people, since Scripture says, "A servant of servants he shall be to his brethren" (Gen. 9:25). However, history and geography do not reinforce this false theory. Ham went to Africa and was the fountainhead for the African nations. Canaan settled in what is known as the "promised land," or Palestine. When Joshua led the Israelites to conquer the nations living in Palestine (the Canaanites, who were the children of Canaan), he was in fact fulfilling the curse upon Canaan. The children of Canaan became servants to the children of Shem.

Is there any modern evidence of the Tower of Babel?

A few miles from the ancient town of Babylon and modern Baghdad, Iraq, is the ziggurat, where tradition to this day says that "people lost their speech." Oddly enough, it is a pyramid that was half completed and near the original site of Babylon, where tradition claims the Tower of Babel was located.

Was there only one language before the Tower of Babel? What was it?

When man was made in the image of God, he received God's personhood—intellect, emotion, and will. Part of that intellectual ability was the rational use of language (the ability to assign meaning to word symbols, call them to mind when necessary, and use them in communication with others). When Adam spoke with God, he used the language that God had been speaking throughout eternity, the same language the Trinity spoke among Themselves. So before the Tower of Babel, all people spoke the same language, the language of God. There were probably word derivations that different people created, though. For instance, cursing was invented by man to express his frustration or rebellion or sin.

When God changed men's languages at the Tower of Babel, it was more than changing their database of words. It probably included changing their ways of thinking, cultures, values, and the meanings they gave to words.

Does anyone speak God's language today?

The story in Genesis 11 suggests that the languages were confused, that is, they were changed from their original expressions. Therefore, no one speaks God's language today, though some who claim to have the gift of tongues, for example, charismatic-pentecostal Christians who "speak in tongues," believe that they have received the gift of God's language. They base this on 1 Corinthians 13:1, which says, "Though I speak with the tongues of men and of angels . . ." indicating that this is how God speaks to angels today.

What else was changed at the Tower of Babel?

Most biblical teachers feel that the various races or ethnic divisions of people happened at Babel. First, because language is more than word symbols, and conveys motives, objectives, and values that people give to words, as different groups of "language-speakers" began to develop, different cultures developed. Second, as groups of "language-speakers" migrated to various parts of the earth, they adapted to certain environmental traits, such as the darkening of the skin by long exposure to sun or the bleaching of the skin in far northern locations where there is less sun. Third, because we are products of the things we eat, and all food has its origin from the ground, the mineral differences in the geographical locations eventually produced differences in skin and hair texture, as well as in the various appearances of individuals. As an illustration, the lack of iodine in the soil in certain locations produces differences in size and skin pigmentation.

Some Bible teachers feel that the original differences in the races were embryonically in the genes of Adam when he was created, and were passed on to succeeding generations. The differences between the races were simply *enhanced* by environmental and mineral influences after people were scattered across the earth. God originally intended different races—therefore, we cannot attribute the differences solely to environment—because God had a divine purpose in making each different ethnic group. Each race of people manifested a certain strength from the personhood of God, and a total view of God's personhood is seen by looking at Him through all the different races.

What was the "Tower of Babel"?

Many children's Bible stories falsely portray the Tower of Babel as a round tower, like those on a medieval castle. People mistakenly think it could be climbed until one got to heaven. The Hebrew word for *tower* is a "stepped ziggurat," in other words, a pyramid. It was not a tower to use in climbing to heaven, but was a religious center dedicated to the worship of heaven.

There are many archaeological remains of ziggurats in the Tigris-Euphrates Valley. These pyramids were used for worship, as were the pyramids in Central and South America built by the Aztec and Inca Indians. However, the pyramids built in Egypt during this same period of history were burial vaults for Egyptian leaders.

How did worshipers use the Tower of Babel?

The Jewish rabbis claimed that there was a zodiac chart at the top of the Tower of Babel, whereby the people worshiped the sun and stars. Judging from the exact position of ziggurats in a north-south line, they must have been able to chart the stars. During this time we know that Abraham's father was a moon worshiper.

Who was Abraham?

Abraham was from the line of Shem, as are all Jewish people (Gen. 11:10–26). His father was Terah, also identified as an idol worshiper. From tradition it is said that as a young boy Abraham believed in the God who created heaven and earth, and because of that, God called him (Gen. 12:1–3). God promised to make Abraham a great name, and as a result he is one of the revered names in Christianity, Judaism, and Islam. God promised that the Messiah would come from his line (Genesis 12:1–3, Matthew 1:1–17).

Where was Abraham born?

He was born in Ur of the Chaldeans, in the land today called Iraq.

Who was Lot?

Lot was a nephew of Abraham who left with him from Ur of the Chaldeans. He journeyed with Abraham until he decided to settle in the prosperous Jordan River valley and Abraham settled in the hill country (Gen. 13). Lot compromised his faith in the city of Sodom, becoming an official of the city and finally refusing to take a strong stand for Jehovah.

Was Lot saved?

While Lot compromised his testimony and destroyed his family, the Bible says he was saved, and called him "righteous Lot, who was oppressed by the filthy conduct of the wicked (for that righteous man, dwelling among them, tormented his righteous soul from day to day by seeing and hearing their lawless deeds)" (2 Pet. 2:7–8).

What does the Bible teach about Melchizedec?

Melchizedec only appears in Scripture in three places: Genesis 14:18–20, Psalm 110:4, and Hebrew 6:20–7:21. Some Bible scholars point out that

Melchizedec is an Old Testament type of Christ. This means that Melchizedec as a human king was a divine picture of the coming Messiah, Jesus Christ. The author of Hebrews is attempting to prove the superiority of the priesthood of Melchizedec to the Levitical priesthood. He also shows that Christ, as a priest after the order of Melchizedec, is superior to the Levitical priesthood.

Melchizedec is said to be "without father, without mother, without descent, having neither beginning of days, nor end of life; but made like unto the Son of God" (Heb. 7:3 KJV). This means there is no record in Scripture of the genealogy of Melchizedec. This does not conclude that he was not fully human. It does, however, show that human Melchizedec is a type of Christ, the Son of God, because he also fits the above description.

The name Melchizedec literally means "King of Righteousness." He was the king of Salem, or Jerusalem. Salem simply means "peace." Therefore, by his name and location, he was the king of both righteousness and peace, two attributes that further link him in type to Christ.

A second view is that Melchizedec is a *christophany*, an Old Testament appearance of Jesus Christ (some call this a *theophany*), because Melchizedec (1) received tithes, as does God; (2) provided bread and wine, in other words, the Lord's Table; (3) has the titles of "peace" and "righteousness," as does Jesus Christ; and (4) has no genealogy, implying He was never born, but just appeared.

Who was Hagar?

Hagar was an Egyptian servant girl in Abraham's camp that he took as a "wife," thinking he was fulfilling God's promise of having a son by her (Gen. 16).

Who was Hagar's son?

Her son was Ishmael, the ancestor of the modern Arabs. Throughout the life of Ishmael (his name means "wild horse"), he did not follow the faith of his father, Abraham, but persecuted Isaac, and eventually was dispatched from the camp of Abraham (Gen. 16, 17, 21).

How old was Abraham when Isaac was born to him?

Isaac was conceived when Abraham was ninety-nine and Sarah was eighty-nine. The conception was miraculous because of their physical inability to bear children. The birth of Isaac was normal, and he fulfilled the promise that God made to Abraham that he would have a son.

Why did God require "circumcision" as the sign of the Abrahamic covenant?

There are several reasons why circumcision was used. First, by placing the sign of the covenant on the male sexual organ, God was reminding each Israelite that his body was devoted to the Lord, that he should not intermarry with heathen nations, and that sex was to be dedicated to the Lord ("You shall not commit adultery" [seventh commandment, Ex. 20:14]). Second, by circumcising the male, God was recognizing patriarchal leadership in the Old Testament and male leadership in the family. Third, circumcision required the shedding of blood, and all covenants were confirmed with blood, including the New Covenant, where Christ shed His blood for the sins of mankind.

Where were the cities of Sodom and Gomorrah located?

Sodom and Gomorrah were two separate cities that many think now lie beneath the Dead Sea in the southern Jordan valley. The Lord brought fire— apparently brimstone, or sulfur—out of heaven upon Sodom and Gomorrah. Many scientists think that the vast amounts of sulfur that exist today in the Dead Sea area resulted from God pouring sulfur from heaven. Other scientists believe that the fire from heaven mingled with the sulfur that was already there, causing huge chemical explosions so that flying sulfur destroyed much of the area around the cities. (See the following question about Lot's wife.)

How did Lot's wife turn to stone?

In her disobedience God turned her to stone: "But his wife looked back behind him, and she became a pillar of salt" (Gen. 19:26). Some biblical scientists believe that flying sulfur actually hit Lot's wife, killing her in the judgment of God. They look at the Hebrew language where "she became a pillar of salt" and see that the word *pillar* is "a pile," and that the word *salt* also means "sulfur." So Lot's wife was encrusted in a pile of molten sulfur and/or salt, and when she died, she became hardened, or oxidized. Those who hold this view say they are not taking away from the supernatural; God indeed poured fire out of heaven, and when Lot's wife looked back and desired the civilization of Sodom and Gomorrah, she put herself in "harm's way." God used flying sulfur to judge her.

What was the fire that fell from heaven to destroy Sodom and Gomorrah?
Some say this was an intense or enhanced lightning storm. Others say God created "liquid fire" in heaven and poured it out on the two cities.

What do some people believe is the greatest trial in Abraham's life?
God asked him to offer up Isaac as a burnt offering: "Now it came to pass after these things that God tested Abraham, and said to him, 'Abraham!' And he said, 'Here I am.' Then He said, 'Take now your son, your only son Isaac, whom you love, and go to the land of Moriah, and offer him there as a burnt offering on one of the mountains of which I shall tell you'" (Gen. 22:1–2).

Why did God ask Abraham to offer Isaac as a human sacrifice?
The Old Testament clearly prohibits human sacrifice (Lev. 18:21). Anyone who sacrificed a child was to be executed (Lev. 20:2–5). As Moses, the author, described the event, he clearly wanted readers to know that God did not intend to sacrifice Isaac. Rather, this was a "test" (Gen. 22:1) to determine Abraham's obedience to God. Abraham passed God's test by obedient faith when he intended to offer up Isaac (Heb. 11:17, 19). But God, who never intended for Abraham to sacrifice his son, providentially arranged for a ram to be caught by its horns nearby. The ram was sacrificed in the place of Isaac on the altar.

Did Abraham take the life of his son?
No, God stopped him when He saw the obedience of his heart.

How old was Isaac when his father intended to sacrifice him?
He must have been approximately twenty-five years old; he was old enough to resist his father should he have so chosen. His age indicates the faith of Isaac when he submitted to his father's intentions.

How did God stop Abraham from offering his son?
The angel of the Lord spoke from Heaven, saying, "Do not lay your hand on the lad, or do anything to him; for now I know that you fear God, since you have not withheld your son, your only son, from Me" (Gen. 22:12).

Since God prohibits child sacrifice in other places, then why did Abraham proceed with the "test" to kill his son?

Abraham knew that even if he killed his son, God would raise him from the dead. "By faith Abraham, when he was tested, offered up Isaac, and he who had received the promises offered up his only begotten son, of whom it was said, 'In Isaac your seed shall be called,' concluding that God was able to raise him up, even from the dead, from which he also received him in a figurative sense" (Heb. 11:17–19).

Whom did Abraham marry after the death of Sarah?

Abraham married Keturah, a woman we know little about (Gen. 25:1). Some say that Keturah was actually Hagar, who came to share the blessing and inheritance of Abraham. But no, Keturah is not Hagar; their names are completely different. Also, the sons of Keturah did not share in the inheritance of Abraham, just as the son of Hagar (Ishmael) did not share in Abraham's blessing: "And Abraham gave all that he had to Isaac. But Abraham gave gifts to the sons of the concubines which Abraham had; and while he was still living he sent them eastward, away from Isaac his son, to the country of the east" (Gen. 25:5–6).

Whom did Isaac marry?

Abraham sent his trusted servant to Mesopotamia (the land between the Tigris and Euphrates River), now modern-day Iraq, to get a wife for his son. Abraham wanted a woman from his tribe to marry his son Isaac. Her name was Rebekah, and she became the mother of Jacob and Esau.

What do we know about Isaac when he was married?

Isaac was forty years old (Gen. 25:20). He was a shepherd, his wealth consisted of sheep and cattle, and he was a nomad, living in tents.

What miracle surrounded the births of Jacob and Esau?

Rebekah was barren (Gen. 25:21), and Jacob prayed for her to conceive. God answered his prayer. After the twins were conceived, they apparently struggled in her womb. As Rebekah prayed to the Lord about her difficult pregnancy, the Lord said to her, "Two nations are in your womb, two peoples shall be separated from your body; one people shall be stronger than the other, and the older shall serve the younger" (Gen. 25:23).

What was the difference between Jacob and Esau?

Jacob was a quiet man, working around the house, shrewd in business, and yet one who was a "trickster." The Bible calls him the *supplanter* (Gen. 27:36). Jacob pleased his mother. Esau was an outdoorsman, a hunter; one who pleased his father.

How did Jacob get the birthright from Esau?

The birthright gave Jacob the spiritual leadership of the family and the task of praying for the family. Through the one who received the birthright would come the Messiah. When Esau came home from hunting, the shrewd Jacob talked him into giving up the birthright for a mess of pottage (stewed lentils).

What is the difference between the "birthright" and the "blessing"?

The birthright gave Jacob the spiritual leadership of the family, and the privilege of being the direct ancestor of the Messiah. The blessing involved the larger portion of the family property and goods (Gen 27:37).

How did Jacob steal the blessing?

Isaac apparently didn't know that Esau had given the birthright to his brother, Jacob. So Isaac planned a feast to give the blessing to Esau (Gen. 27:1–4). When Rebekah heard about the feast, she schemed a plan (Gen. 27) whereby young Jacob tricked his father into giving him the blessing too.

What was Esau's reaction when he found out his brother had stolen the blessing?

He planned to kill him: "So Esau hated Jacob because of the blessing with which his father blessed him, and Esau said in his heart, 'The days of mourning for my father are at hand; then I will kill my brother Jacob'" (Gen. 27:41).

How did Jacob escape from the threat of his brother, Esau?

He went to Mesopotamia, the land of his mother, and married there.

What was "Jacob's ladder"?

When Jacob was running away from his brother, God gave him a vision of a ladder that reached from earth to heaven. He saw angels ascending and descending upon the ladder. The ladder was a type of Jesus Christ Himself. Later Jesus referred to this event: "Hereafter you shall see heaven open, and the angels of God ascending and descending upon the Son of Man" (John 1:51).

What dowry did Jacob give to his Uncle Laban to marry Rachel?

Jacob worked for seven years tending the sheep of his uncle Laban, but on the marriage night, the uncle substituted Leah, the older daughter, for Rachel. The uncle said that he had to give the oldest before the younger because of tradition.

What was Jacob's response when he didn't get Rachel?

Apparently he took Leah on a one-week honeymoon (Gen. 29:27), and then was given Rachel in marriage. However, he had to work a second period of seven years as a dowry for Rachel.

How long was Jacob in Mesopotamia?

Jacob stayed there twenty years, serving fourteen years as dowry for the wives, and working six years for his own flocks (Gen. 31:41).

How did Jacob accumulate a large possession of flocks and herds?

It was the blessing of God. God blessed Jacob's flocks more than the flocks of Laban, which Jacob was also tending. But the sons of Laban were greedy and fearful of Jacob (Gen. 31:1). Jacob, feeling the pressure of the sons, went back to the promised land.

How many sons did Jacob have?

Jacob had twelve sons. These eventually became patriarchs and leaders in the nation.

Are the "twelve sons" the same as the "twelve tribes of Israel"?

No. Two of the sons are not among the twelve tribes. Joseph did not become one of the twelve tribes of Israel. Another son, Levi, did not become one of the tribes either because he became the priest who served the twelve tribes. The two tribes that replaced Joseph and Levi were the grandsons of Joseph, named Ephraim and Manasseh.

To which of Jacob's sons was he most partial?
Jacob was most partial to his son Joseph (Gen. 37:3).

Why did Joseph's brothers hate him?
Joseph had dreams given to him by God that showed the eleven other sons bowing down in reverence to him. Also, Jacob made a "coat of many colors," which was a robe of honor worn by the revered prince, the one who would assume authority when the father died. The ten brothers who were older than Joseph became jealous of him and plotted to kill him.

How did the ten older sons try to get rid of Joseph?
First they put him into a pit, a dry cistern that usually holds water during the rainy season. They intended to kill him, all but Reuben, who intended to restore him to his father. But when Reuben was gone, the brothers sold Joseph as a slave for twenty pieces of silver to a caravan of Midianite merchants.

How did the ten brothers explain the disappearance of Joseph to his father, Jacob?
They told the father that they found Joseph's coat bloody, and that he had probably been killed by a wild beast.

What happened to Joseph in Egypt?
Joseph was sold to Potiphar, the captain of Pharaoh's guards (Gen. 39:1).

What happened to Joseph in Potiphar's house?
The Lord blessed Joseph (Gen. 39:2, 21) so that he became the ruler or "trustee" over all of the other slaves.

How did Joseph manifest his integrity and faith in Potiphar's house?
When Potiphar's wife tried to get him to lie with her, Joseph refused, saying, "How then can I do this great wickedness, and sin against God?" (Gen. 39:9 KJV). As a result, the wife lied about Joseph, and he was cast into prison.

How did God deliver Joseph from prison?
Again Joseph had favor with God, and rose to leadership over all of the prisoners. While in prison, Joseph was able to interpret the dreams of Pharaoh's chief

butler and chief baker and predict each of their outcomes. Joseph's predictions came true. Later, when the chief butler heard Pharaoh talk about a dream that bothered him, he told Pharaoh about Joseph's ability to interpret dreams.

What was the dream that Pharaoh had?

Pharaoh saw seven fat cows and seven lean cows come up out of the river; then he saw seven full ears of corn on a stalk and seven lean ears on a stalk. The thin cows swallowed the fat cows, and the poor ears of corn swallowed up the full ears.

How did Joseph interpret the dream?

Joseph said to Pharaoh, "It is not in me; God will give Pharaoh an answer of peace" (Gen. 41:16). Pharoah described his dream to Joseph and asked for his interpretation.

Then Joseph said to Pharaoh, "The dreams of Pharaoh are one; God has shown Pharaoh what He is about to do: The seven good cows are seven years, and the seven good heads are seven years; the dreams are one. And the seven thin and ugly cows which came up after them are seven years, and the seven empty heads blighted by the east wind are seven years of famine. This is the thing which I have spoken to Pharaoh. God has shown Pharaoh what He is about to do." (Gen. 41:25–28)

What did Pharaoh do for Joseph as a result of the interpretation of the dream?

Joseph was given authority over all of the land of Egypt (he was probably made minister of agriculture). Joseph was second only to Pharaoh and carried out plans to provide food for the Egyptians when the famine came (Gen. 41:38–57).

What happened during the famine?

The people came to Joseph, trading money, their cattle, and their land for food. Many who study the history of Egypt know that at this time there was a transfer of power in Egypt from the rich landlords to Pharaoh. Pharaoh centralized the government and increased his power, becoming the most powerful nation in the known world. After the famine was over, the people had to give 20 percent of their income to Pharaoh in return for using the land that they had sold to him (Gen. 47:14–26).

How did Joseph meet his ten brothers?

The famine extended into their land, and Jacob sent the ten brothers to Egypt to buy grain.

How did Joseph receive his brothers?

He spoke to them roughly (Gen. 42:6–28), wanting them to come to a realization of what God was doing. He accused them of being spies but eventually did give them food and also returned their money. Joseph told them that they could not return for more food unless they brought their youngest brother, Benjamin, with them.

Why did Joseph ask for Benjamin?

Both Joseph and Benjamin had the same mother, Rachel.

Did they bring Benjamin the second time they came for food?

Yes, but Jacob didn't want to let Benjamin go because he was the youngest of the sons, and Jacob was fearful of losing him. However, Judah vouched for Benjamin's safety.

What was Joseph's response when he saw Benjamin and his brothers?

When Joseph saw them, he realized his love for Benjamin, and he had to go in private to weep (Gen. 43:30–31).

How did Joseph reveal himself to his brothers?

At first he made a feast for them, and gave a bigger serving of food to Benjamin than to the other brothers. As the brothers planned to leave, Joseph had his cup put in Benjamin's sack of grain. Joseph then sent to have Benjamin arrested as a thief. He threatened to make Benjamin his slave for his crime. It was then that Judah volunteered to become a slave in place of Benjamin. He told Joseph that losing Benjamin would kill his father, Jacob (Gen. 43:16–44:34). When Joseph heard this, he was overcome with emotion. He then dismissed his servants and revealed himself to his brothers. It was then that they were united. Joseph sent his brothers back home to get Jacob and to bring all of the family and their possessions into Egypt (Gen. 45:1–15).

QUESTIONS ABOUT THE BOOK OF EXODUS

Who wrote the book of Exodus?

The majority of evangelicals believe that Moses wrote the book of Exodus
for many reasons. Biblical writers, such as Joshua, Malachi, Paul, John, and
finally Jesus, all said that Moses wrote this book. Since Jesus said that Moses
wrote Exodus (Mark 7:10, 12:26, Luke 20:37, John 5:46–47, 7:19, 22, 23),
then to say He was wrong would mean that Jesus as God made a mistake,
and could not die for the sins of the world. Therefore to deny that Moses
wrote the book of Exodus is to deny the deity of Christ and His sacrificial
death.

When was Exodus written?

Most evangelicals believe that the Jews left Egypt in 1445 B.C., and that
Moses wrote this book while leading the children of Israel in the wilderness.

Moses probably kept an account, or a diary, of what God was doing. This book was probably composed on the desert plains in front of Horeb, beginning around 1445 B.C.

What is the time of the book of Exodus?

The book begins when Jacob arrived in Egypt around 1875 B.C. and ends with the erection of the tabernacle 431 years later, near 1445 B.C.

What is the key word in Exodus?

Exodus is the book of *redemption*, which is the central concept of Exodus—that God was redeeming the nation from Egypt. Then God gave Israel the plans for the tabernacle where each individual was redeemed.

What is the key verse in Exodus?

"I am the LORD, I will bring you out from under the burdens of the Egyptians, I will rescue you from their bondage, and I will redeem you with an outstretched arm, and with great judgments" (Ex. 6:6).

Why is the book called "Exodus"?

The word *Exodus* means "exit," "departure," or "going out" (see Ex. 19:1). It tells of Israel going out of Egypt.

Why were the Israelites in Egypt?

When a worldwide famine threatened the world, God used a young Israelite slave—Joseph—to reveal to Pharaoh the imminent disaster. Pharaoh appointed Joseph as minister of agriculture, and gave him power to store food for the coming famine. Different ethnic groups came to Egypt for food, including a delegation of Jacob's sons who came seeking food from Egypt. Through a series of events, they discovered that Joseph was their brother, resulting in the entire family of Jacob (Israelites) moving to Egypt for safety during the famine.

What happened to the Israelites after Joseph died?

Because the Egyptians were afraid that the rapid growth of the Israelites would overwhelm them—or at least that the Israelites might side with an attacking enemy—the Egyptians put Israel in slavery and oppressed them (Ex. 1:6–14).

How did the Egyptians oppress the Israelites?
They forced them to make bricks and other building supplies for the cities of Raamses and Pithon (Ex. 1:11).

How did Egypt plan to get rid of the Israelites?
Through a process of child holocaust, the Egyptians killed all of the male Israelite babies that were born (Ex. 1:22).

How did God provide a deliverer for the Israelites from Egypt?
An Israelite mother hid her baby (Ex. 2:2). The baby was placed in a small basket in the Nile River where the daughter of Pharaoh found him. The princess—many people think she was Hetshepsut (1504–1450 B.C.)—retrieved baby Moses and raised him in the palace; thus he received the education of a king, while he still had the blood of an Israelite and a heart for God's people (Acts 7:20–23).

What caused Moses to leave Egypt?
When Moses saw an Israelite taskmaster beating an Israelite, he killed the Egyptian in anger. Later, when the murder was known, Moses fled to the Sinai Peninsula where he lived for forty years (Acts 7:29–30).

How did God call Moses?
While keeping sheep, Moses saw a bush burning with fire yet not consumed. Then God spoke to him from the bush and commissioned him to go bring the Israelites out of Egypt (Ex. 3:1–7).

Why did God send plagues on Egypt?
Moses and his brother, Aaron, went to Pharaoh asking for Egypt to release the Israelites. Instead, the Egyptians increased the workload of the Israelites. As a result, God sent ten plagues on the land as a warning and/or punishment.

What were the first nine plagues?
The plagues were (1) the water of the Nile River turning to blood, (2) frogs coming into the houses, (3) swarms of lice, (4) swarms of flies, (5) the cattle becoming sick, (6) boils and sores, (7) hail and lightning that destroyed the vegetation and cattle, (8) swarms of locusts, and (9) thick darkness for three days.

What was the response of Pharaoh to these plagues?
Rather than heeding the warnings, Pharaoh hardened his heart and refused to release God's people.

What was the tenth plague?
A death angel passed through the land, and the firstborn of all the Egyptians and their cattle died.

How were the Israelites delivered from the death angel?
God commanded each family of the Israelites to sacrifice a lamb and smear its blood on the doorposts and lintil. He promised that when the death angel saw the blood, he would "pass over" that house and not visit it with judgment.

What did the Israelites eat in the Passover feast?
They were to eat a roasted lamb and bitter herbs. They were also to eat unleavened (flat, yeastless) bread. Later, as they continued celebrating the Passover, other religious exercises were attached to the meal.

Why was the lamb important for the Passover?
The lamb was a symbol of Christ, the Lamb of God, who was slain from the foundations of the earth (John 1:29, 1 Peter 1:18–21). The lamb died so the family wouldn't have to die, and the blood was the symbol of the sacrificial death.

How did Israel leave Egypt?
When Pharaoh and the others found their firstborn children had died, they ordered the Israelites to leave quickly (Ex. 12:31–32).

Was it honest for the Israelites to borrow money and possessions from the Egyptians before they left? (Ex. 12:35–36)
The word translated "borrow" could also be translated "ask." These were not loans, but were "unpaid wages" that Israel deserved for the years of slavery and abuse. Israel left all of their property for the Egyptians, and in return they asked for and took away gold and silver from their neighbors.

How did God protect Israel after the nation left Egypt?

Pharaoh had a change of mind and sent an army with chariots to attack Israel. God had given a Shekinah-glory cloud (a pillar of cloud and fire) to guide Israel. This "cloud" went behind Israel and kept the Egyptians in darkness, preventing them from attacking Israel.

How did the Israelites cross the Red Sea?

There are many ways that God performs miracles, but here He used a storm to push the waters apart: "The LORD caused the sea to go back by a strong east wind all that night, and made the sea dry land, and the waters were divided" (Ex. 14:21 KJV).

If God used a storm, how do we know it was a miracle?

"So the children of Israel went into the midst of the sea on the dry ground, and the waters were a wall to them on their right hand and on their left" (Ex. 14:22). God providentially kept the waters back while Israel passed through, but when Pharaoh tried to follow their example, the wall of water collapsed on the Egyptian army, killing all of them.

How did God give Israel water to drink in the desert?

When the spring of water at Horeb failed, Moses struck the rock and water flowed from the rock (Ex. 17:1–7).

How was a rock a type of Christ?

Paul said, "That rock was Christ" (1 Cor. 10:4), meaning that when Christ was crucified on Calvary, He was a picture of the rock that was smitten and gave water. From Christ, too, has come water (eternal life) to quench and satisfy sin-sick souls.

What was God preparing Israel to be or do?

"And you shall be to Me a kingdom of priests and a holy nation" (Ex. 19:6).

Where did God give the Ten Commandments?

God invited Moses to come to the top of Mt. Sinai, and it was there that God gave him the Ten Commandments. The nation was to stay away from the mountain while the presence of God was upon the mountain. The people saw thunder, lightning, clouds, and darkness, and they heard a trumpet blast and an earthquake on the top of the mountain when God appeared.

How were the Ten Commandments divided?

They are divided into two sections. The first section lists the duties that man owes to God (the first through the fourth commandments), and the second group gives the duties that mankind owes to each other (the fifth through the tenth commandments).

What was the nation's response to the Ten Commandments?

Because Moses stayed such a long time on the mountain (forty days and forty nights), the people forgot about God and began to worship a golden calf, probably sculpted from some of the gold they got from the Egyptians. While they intended it to be an image to Jehovah, it was an idol, and prohibited in the first and second commandments.

What was the response of Moses?

When Moses saw the golden calf and the people dancing nude, he broke the stone tablets bearing the Ten Commandments, symbolically showing that the people had broken God's law.

Who interceded for God not to destroy the Israelites?

Moses was not only a lawgiver, but because he was a Levite from the priestly tribe, he was qualified to intercede for God to not destroy Israel.

What proof do we have that Moses' intercession was accepted?

Moses took two fresh tablets to the top of Sinai, where he received the Ten Commandments a second time.

How long was Moses on the mountain the second time?

He was again on the mountain for forty days and forty nights (Deut. 10:10).

How do we know that God forgave Israel?

Moses spoke with God face-to-face, and God showed Moses His glory. "But since then there has not arisen in Israel a prophet like Moses, whom the LORD knew face to face" (Deut. 34:10).

Did Moses actually see the face of God?
The Bible says, "No one has seen God at any time" (John 1:18), so Moses didn't actually see the face of God, but He saw the glory of God, and as a result his face shone for forty days.

What does it mean, "Moses' face shone"?
Because Moses had seen the glory of God, apparently his face was transformed so that it glistened or shone (Ex. 33:35), much as Jesus' face shone on the Mount of Transfiguration. Matthew 17:2 says, "His face shone like the sun, and His clothes became as white as the light."

What is a *tabernacle*?
The *tabernacle* (literally, "tent") was the tent where the presence of the Lord dwelt among Israel. As a result, the Israelites came to worship God in the tabernacle.

What plans did the Israelites use to construct the tabernacle?
God Himself showed them a blueprint or pattern of the tabernacle (Ex. 25:9, 40).

Where did the material come from to construct the tabernacle?
The people gave freewill offerings for the materials necessary to build the tabernacle. The gold and silver came from what the Israelites borrowed from the Egyptians as they left Egypt (Ex. 35:21–29; 36:3–7).

What was significant about the tabernacle?
It was not a place where people went inside to hear a sermon or to worship the Lord, such as a "tent meeting" of today. Rather, the tabernacle was a "sanctuary." The word *sanctuary* means "the place where God dwells." The Shekinah-glory cloud rested on and over the Holy of Holies, a room in the tabernacle. The tabernacle was a home for God among His people on earth.

What furniture was in the tabernacle?
As the Israelites entered the Tabernacle yard, they saw a brass altar for burning sacrifices to God. Second, they saw a large golden laver for washings and purification. Inside the Holy Place, they saw a table of shewbread, a symbol

of Jesus—the Bread of Life. Next they saw a golden candelabrum, approximately five feet tall, showing Jesus is the Light of the World. Between the Holy Place and the Holy of Holies was a golden altar of incense, standing for the eternal prayers to God. Finally, in the Holy of Holies was the ark of the covenant.

How do we know God accepted the tabernacle?
The first fire on the brass altar was kindled by God Himself (Lev. 9:24), suggesting that God, who is a purifying fire, came to dwell among His people and accept their blood sacrifices.

What was the *shewbread?*
This was bread that was offered to the Lord, twelve loaves symbolizing one offering from each tribe. It was eaten by the priest, symbolizing strength that comes from Jehovah.

Could the average Israelite go inside the tabernacle?
No, only the priests—from the tribe of Levi—could minister to God. Priests ministered for the people.

Who went into the Holy of Holies?
Only the high priest went into the Holy of Holies, and only once a year: "But into the second part the high priest went alone once a year, not without blood, which he offered for himself and for the people's sins committed in ignorance" (Heb. 9:7).

What was the meaning of the "Holy of Holies"?
It was the room where the actual presence of God sat on the "mercy seat," that is, the lid on the ark of the covenant.

What kept the people out of the Holy of Holies?
There was a beautiful heavy veil, finely embroidered of rich material. The veil was so thick that no one could see through it.

What meaning does the veil have in our lives?
When Jesus died on the cross, the veil in the temple (transferred from the

tabernacle) was ripped from top to bottom, symbolizing that every person now had immediate access to God (Heb. 10:19–22).

What was the "ark of the covenant"?

The word *ark* means "box," and it was a small box made of tightly grained shittim (oak) wood overlaid with gold (Ex. 25:10–11).

What was in the ark of the covenant?

Three things were in the ark: the two tablets of the Ten Commandments, a golden pot filled with manna, and Aaron's rod that budded (Heb. 9:4).

QUESTIONS
ABOUT
THE BOOK OF
LEVITICUS

Why is this book called "Leviticus"?

The title comes from an early Greek title in the Septuagint, "That which pertains to the Levites." The priest came from the tribe of Levi, and this book is primarily about God's plan for the Levites who led worship services in the tabernacle. It is also about the godly life of His people.

Who wrote the book of Leviticus?

Evangelical Christians say that Moses wrote the first five books of the Bible, which includes Leviticus. Fifty-six times in this book it is stated that God imparted these laws to Moses (Lev. 1:1; 4:1; 6:1; 8:1; et al.).

When did Moses write Leviticus?

Israel was not wandering in the wilderness when Moses wrote this book. Rather, they were camped at the foot of Mt. Sinai (25:1; 26:46). During this time Israel constructed the tabernacle, which took exactly one year (Ex. 40:17). Leviticus begins the first month of that second year (Num. 1:1), and Moses probably wrote much of Leviticus during that first month.

What is the key word in Leviticus?

The key word is *holiness*. This book centers on the holiness of God and how His people can approach God and walk in fellowship with Him. Through a blood sacrifice, they could attain true holiness.

What is the key verse in Leviticus?

"For the life of the flesh is in the blood, and I have given it to you upon the altar to make an atonement for your souls; for it is the blood that makes atonement for the soul" (Lev. 17:11).

What were the offerings or sacrifices that people gave to God? (Lev. 1–6)

They were the burnt offerings (Lev. 1), the sin offering (Lev. 4), the trespass offering (Lev. 5), the peace offering (Lev. 3), and the meat (meal or grain) offering (Lev. 2).

What was foreshadowed in all of these offerings?

These offerings were a prefigure of Jesus Christ, who would come and be offered for the sins of His people (Heb. 10:1–18).

QUESTIONS ABOUT THE BOOK OF NUMBERS

Why is the book called "Numbers"?

This book is called "Numbers" because twice in the book a census or "counting" of the number of Israelites took place. At the beginning of the book, the people who came out of Egypt were numbered (Num. 1). At the end of the book, they were again numbered as they got ready to enter the promised land (Num. 26).

Who wrote the book of Numbers?

Evangelicals believe that Moses wrote the book because more than eighty times in the book we find the statement "The LORD spoke to Moses" (Num. 1:1, and so forth). Also it is stated, "Now Moses wrote down the starting points of their journeys at the command of the LORD" (Num. 33:2). Moses was the central character in Exodus through Deuteronomy, and was more qualified than any other to write Numbers and the Pentateuch.

When was the book of Numbers written?

While the book of Leviticus covers only one month, the book of Numbers stretches almost thirty-nine years (1444–1405 B.C.). The book of Numbers begins with the last twenty days at Mt. Sinai (1:1; 10:11), and traces the Israelites' wanderings in the wilderness through the fortieth year (22:1; 26:3; 33:50; Deut. 1:3).

What is the key word in Numbers?

The key word is *wandering*. God's people wandered aimlessly until all of the generation that disobeyed God passed away in the wilderness.

What are the key verses in Numbers?
"Because all these men who have seen My glory and the signs which I did in Egypt and in the wilderness, and have put Me to the test now these ten times, and have not heeded My voice, they certainly shall not see the land of which I swore to their fathers, nor shall any of those who rejected Me see it" (Num. 14:22–23).

What would Israel look like when they camped for the night?
When Israel stopped for the night, their tents would have occupied several square miles because there were over two and a half million people, based on the census of Numbers 1:26. The tabernacle would have been at the center of the camp, and the twelve tribes would have surrounded the tabernacle, three tribes on each of the four sides.

The Jewish people didn't surround the tabernacle to protect God from the enemy. Rather, the Jewish people surrounded the tabernacle to be close to God. When an attack came from an enemy, God could take care of Himself, and did on many occasions.

How did Israel know when to march and where to stop?
The Shekinah-glory cloud moved before the people, and they followed it. When the cloud stopped, the people stopped. Whenever it lifted up, they prepared to follow the Lord (Num. 9:17–23).

What was Moses' prayer for protection of Israel as they traveled?
"Rise up, O LORD! Let Your enemies be scattered, and let those who hate You flee before You" (Num. 10:35).

What happened when Israel got close to the promised land?
They sent out twelve spies, one from each tribe, to bring back a report of what the promised land was like (Num. 13:3–16).

How long did they search out the land?
They searched out the promised land for forty days (Num. 13:25).

What report did the spies bring back?

All twelve of the spies said that the land was fertile, and flowed with "milk and honey" (Num. 13:26–33). However, ten of the spies felt that the inhabitants were giants and that the cities were fortifications that could not be breached. They said, "We be not able to go up against the people; for they are stronger than we" (Num. 13:31 KJV). But the remaining two spies, Joshua and Caleb, believed God. They said, "We are well able to overcome it" (Num. 13:30), and, "He [the Lord] will bring us into this land and give it to us" (Num. 14:6–9). These two spies eventually went into the promised land.

What was the effect of the report on the Israelites?

The multitude was fearful and wanted to go back to Egypt (Num. 14:1–4), choosing to embrace the report of the ten frightened spies rather than Joshua and Caleb.

How did God punish the people for refusing to go into the promised land?

They had to wander forty years in the wilderness and die there instead of entering the promised land (Num. 14:33).

What did Moses do that kept him from entering the promised land?

As Israel was wandering in the wilderness, they ran out of water in the desert of Zin. God commanded Moses to speak to the rock so water would come out. However in rebellion and out of frustration, Moses implied that he and Aaron would bring water out of the rock by their authority. So rather than obeying God and speaking to the rock, Moses struck the rock (Num. 20).

What was Moses' punishment?

He was not allowed to enter the promised land, though God did let him see it (Deut. 34).

What was the meaning of the brazen serpent?

The people rebelled and murmured against God, so God sent fiery serpents—they were fire colored or produced a burning inflammation after they bit—to judge the people. Moses made a serpent of brass and lifted it on a pole. When people looked in faith at the serpent, they were healed.

What is the type of the brazen serpent?

The brazen serpent is a type of Jesus Christ who took the sin of the world upon Himself. Those who look on Him will live. "And as Moses lifted up the serpent in the wilderness, even so must the Son of Man be lifted up, that whoever believes in Him should not perish but have eternal life" (John 3:14–15).

QUESTIONS
ABOUT
THE BOOK OF
DEUTERONOMY

What does the name "Deuteronomy" mean?

The Jewish people call this book *Mishneh Hattorah*, meaning "repetition of the law," which is translated in the Septuagint "second law." The word *deutero* means "two"—not a second law, but a repetition of the original law given on Mt. Sinai.

What is in the book of Deuteronomy?

It consists of a series of farewell sermons by Moses to a new generation who would possess the promised land. Because they did not hear the original law, or may not have learned it, Moses gave it in words and writing so the new generation would have the direction of God as they entered the promised land.

Who wrote the book of Deuteronomy?

Many critics have vigorously attacked the Mosaic authorship of Deuteronomy, but the majority of evangelical Christians believe that he wrote it because other writers of Scripture attest to his authorship. Deuteronomy is quoted more than eighty times in the New Testament; these citations say that Moses was the author. The book of Deuteronomy itself includes over forty claims that Moses wrote it (1:1–5; 4:44–46; 29:1, etc.).

When was the book of Deuteronomy written?

The action in this book takes place on the plains of Moab, east of the Jericho River, as Israel is preparing to enter the promised land (1405 B.C.). Deuteronomy was written at the end of the forty years after Israel wandered in the wilderness. It is written for a new generation that was on the verge of entering the promised land.

What is the key word in Deuteronomy?

The key word in Deuteronomy is *remember*. The Israelites were reminded of what God had said in the past.

What are the key verses in Deuteronomy?

"And now, Israel, what does the LORD your God require of you, but to fear the LORD your God, to walk in all His ways and to love Him, to serve the LORD your God with all your heart and with all your soul, and to keep the commandments of the LORD and His statutes which I command you today for your good?" (Deut. 10:12–13).

How does Moses predict the coming of Christ in the book of Deuteronomy?

Moses describes "the prophet" in Deuteronomy 18:15–19, which refers to Jesus Christ (see Acts 3:20–22).

Where did Moses die?

Immediately after Moses finished his work, he went to the top of Mt. Nebo (east of the Dead Sea) where he was to die (Deut. 32:48–52).

What did Moses see before he died?

God gave him a panoramic view of the promised land (Deut. 34:1–4). He was not allowed to go into the land, but God showed him the land from the deserts (Negev) of the south to Mt. Hebron in the north. He saw from the Jordan River to the Mediterranean Sea. That view is still available today from the top of Mt. Nebo.

What was the condition of Moses' health when he died?

"Moses was one hundred and twenty years old when he died. His eyes were not dim nor his natural vigor diminished" (Deut. 34:7).

What happened to the body of Moses?

"So Moses the servant of the LORD died there in the land of Moab, according to the word of the LORD. And He buried him in a valley in the land of Moab, opposite Beth Peor; but no one knows his grave to this day" (Deut. 34:5–6).

If Moses died on top of the mountain, who wrote the last few verses of Deuteronomy?

Obviously, a dead man cannot write about his death or the inability of people to find his body, so some believe that Moses actually wrote by prophecy of his death and the subsequent actions. God wanted him to write the entire book of Deuteronomy. Others believe that Joshua wrote the conclusion to the book of Deuteronomy at about the same time that he wrote the book of Joshua.

QUESTIONS ABOUT THE HISTORICAL BOOKS

JOSHUA, JUDGES, RUTH, 1 AND 2 SAMUEL,

1 AND 2 KINGS, 1 AND 2 CHRONICLES,

EZRA, NEHEMIAH, ESTHER

RUTH

2 SAMUEL

1 KINGS

QUESTIONS ABOUT
THE BOOK OF JOSHUA

Who was Joshua?

Joshua was born a slave in Egypt. His father was Nun, a worshiper of the gods of Egypt. Joshua's original name was *Hoshea*, meaning "salvation" (Num. 13:8), but apparently Moses changed his name to *Yehoshua* (Num. 13:16), which means "Jehovah is salvation." He is called *Yeshua,* which is Joshua in our English. The Hebrew equivalent of his name is *Iesous,* that is, Jesus. As an attendant to Moses, Joshua learned courage, faith, obedience, and dedication to God. He was one of the twelve spies sent to search out the promised land, and only he and Caleb brought back a good report. Joshua became the leader and general who conquered the promised land after Moses' death. He then provided leadership for the division of the land for the twelve tribes to inhabit.

Who wrote the book of Joshua?

Strong Jewish tradition, as well as the majority of conservative Christians, tells us that Joshua was the author. The book also makes it clear that Joshua wrote it: "Then Joshua wrote these words in the Book of the Law of God" (Josh. 24:26). Joshua even used the first person in one place (5:6), and the word *we* appeared in some manuscripts (Josh. 5:1).

What is the key word in Joshua?

The key word is the word *victory* or *conquest*. As Joshua obeyed the Lord, God helped him conquer the land, becoming victorious over his enemies. Joshua is a book that many people use to focus on the victorious Christian life.

What is the key verse in Joshua?

"This Book of the Law shall not depart from your mouth, but you shall meditate in it day and night, that you may observe to do according to all that is written in it. For then you will make your way prosperous, and then you will have good success" (Josh. 1:8).

How is the book of Joshua divided?

The book is divided into three sections, mostly geographical divisions. In chapters 1–5, Israel is at the Jordan River. In chapters 6–13:7, Israel is conquering the heathen nations in the promised land. The third division focuses on the twelve tribes settling into the promised land (13:8–24:33).

What is significant about the book of Joshua?

Joshua led his people through three major military campaigns: (1) conquering Jericho and the cities about the Jordan, (2) conquering the kings of the south, and (3) conquering the kings of the north. Joshua defeated more than thirty enemy armies, and he demonstrated that victory comes through faith and obedience to the Lord rather than just through military might and superiority.

Who made Joshua the leader of Israel?

The Lord commissioned Joshua when he said, "Now therefore, arise, go over this Jordan, you and all this people, to the land which I am giving to them" (Josh. 1:2).

What was the river Jordan like when Israel crossed it?

The Jordan River is a small river by the world's standards, but it was overflowing at the time of floods (Josh. 3:15). God challenged His people to cross Jordan with this added obstacle to demonstrate His power to them and prepare them to face and defeat their enemy.

Why was a miracle necessary to cross the Jordan River?

The enemies on the other side could have easily defeated Israel as they crossed in small bands or tried to swim the river, especially women and children.

Who was Rahab?

Joshua sent out two spies to survey the land. When they came to Jericho, Rahab protected them because she believed in the monotheistic God of Israel. Because of that, the Bible says, "By faith the harlot Rahab did not perish with those who did not believe, when she had received the spies with peace" (Heb. 11:31).

How did God stop the waters of the Jordan River?

The priests carrying the ark of the covenant walked into the water, and when their feet touched the water, the waters began to dry up. Upstream, the Lord caused the river to pile up, and all the waters in the river in front of Israel drained out of the riverbed so the people could cross on dry land (Josh. 3:15–16).

What directions did God give to Joshua to defeat Jericho?

God told them to march around the city each day for six days; the priests marched around the city with the ark of the covenant (Josh. 6:2–10). On the seventh day, they were to march around seven times (Josh. 6:3–4). On the seventh day, when they had finished circling the city seven times, all the people were to shout, and the walls fell down.

How did the walls of the city of Jericho fall down?

They fell when all the people shouted, as God had instructed them.

What caused the walls of Jericho to fall down?

God did a great miracle here, and conservatives have speculated about how it happened. Some think it was the sonic boom of the great shouts of the crowd mixed with the din of the ram's horn that brought down the walls. Others feel that God sent an earthquake to collapse the walls. Another group believes that "sappers" had dug underneath the walls to remove the foundation so that when the people shouted, the walls fell outward. Finally, other people, myself included, believe it was simply the power of God that drove the walls down.

What was special about the city of Jericho?

The people were commanded to treat the city and its possessions as a burnt sacrifice to God. They were to take all of the gold and silver and give it to God and then burn the rest of the spoils. In later battles, the warriors could keep spoils for themselves, but they were to give all of Jericho to God (Josh. 6:18–19).

Who disobeyed and sinned during the battle of Jericho?

Achan, of the tribe of Judah, kept some bars of silver and Babylonian garments. God punished the nation by a defeat at the next battle at Ai (the name Ai means "little one"). When they prayed before God, it was revealed that Achan had disobeyed God.

How was Achan punished?

All Israel stoned Achan, and he, his loot, and his family were buried underneath the pile of stones.

How do we know that God recognized the repentance of Israel after Achan's sin?

The city of Ai was taken and destroyed (Josh. 8).

What happened when Israel defeated the Amorites and the "sun stood still"?

First of all, Joshua and his men did an all-night "force march" to attack the Amorites the following morning in a surprise attack. Second, "The Lord cast down great stones from heaven upon them" (Josh 10:11 KJV)—hailstones large enough to kill many Amorites, giving Israel the victory.

Then Joshua commanded, "Sun, stand still over Gibeon; and Moon, in the valley of Aijalon" (Josh. 10:12). This is called "the long day." Apparently the sun "stopped" in the midst of heaven, presumably midday.

How did God cause this miracle to take place?

Since the earth rotates on its axis, the sun could only be made to "stand still" by stopping the earth's rotation. Actually, the sun didn't stop, but the earth stopped its rotation. Some believe that the earth continued to rotate, but that God bent the rays by the act of refraction, so that it continued to be noonday. Others think that God created light in the valley where the battle was going on so that the sun "appeared" to give light for Israel to defeat the enemy, but the earth did not stop upon its axis. This miracle of light was similar to the miracle when God created "cosmic" light on the first day of Creation.

What was the last public act of Joshua?

Joshua called Israel to Shechem where he delivered a sermon that reviewed the great victories that God had won for them. Joshua wanted Israel to renew their covenant with God (Josh. 24:23), because apparently they were settling in the land and turning from their devotion to God.

What was Joshua's challenge to the children of Israel?

"[C]hoose for yourselves this day whom you will serve . . . but as for me and my house, we will serve the LORD" (Josh. 24:15).

What are the details of Joshua's death?

He was 110 years old and buried on Mt. Ephraim with honor and dignity (Josh. 24:29–31).

Who wrote the last five verses of Joshua 24?

Obviously this passage was written after the death of Joshua. Only a few people believe that he wrote it prophetically, because it included many other details of Israel not necessary for prophetic prediction. Most people believe that Eleazer the high priest, son of Phinehas, wrote this section (24:33).

QUESTIONS ABOUT THE BOOK OF JUDGES

What is the book of Judges about?

Joshua, the previous book in the Bible, shows the victory of Israel over the heathen nations in the promised land. The book of Judges shows how God's people were disobedient and worshiped idols; hence, they were defeated by surrounding heathen nations and put in servitude to them.

The book of Judges has seven distinct cycles of how God's people sinned, were put into servitude, cried out in repentance, and were delivered by a deliverer raised up by God (a judge) to defeat the enemy.

What does the name "Judges" mean?

The Hebrew title for the book was *Shophetiam*, which mean "ruler," "deliverer," "savior," or "judge." A judge was more than one who decided legal cases; a judge was also a soldier, king (or queen), prophet, and an administrator of justice.

Who wrote the book of Judges?

The book of Judges does not tell us who is the author, but most conservatives believe it was Samuel. It is clear from Judges 18:31 and 20:27 that the book was written after the ark was removed from Shiloh (1 Sam. 4:3–11). Also, the repeated phrase "In those days there was no king of Israel" (17:6; 18:1; 19:1; 21:25) suggests that the book of Judges was written after Saul began his rule. Again, the book of Judges says, "But the children of Benjamin did not drive out the Jebusites who inhabited Jerusalem; so the Jebusites dwell with the children of Benjamin in Jerusalem to this day" (1:21), which means it was written before 1004 B.C., when David captured Jerusalem (2 Sam. 5:5–9). Therefore, most feel that Samuel compiled the book from oral and written materials, God putting His seal upon the work of Samuel because he wrote under the influence of inspiration.

What is the key word in Judges?

The key word is *cycles*. The word itself does not occur in Judges; however, the *cycle* of sin, judgment, and repentance is seen repeatedly throughout.

What is the key passage of Judges?

"Now Joshua the son of Nun, the servant of the LORD, died when he was one hundred and ten years old. And they buried him within the border of his inheritance at Timnath Heres, in the mountains of Ephraim, on the north side of Mount Gaash. When all that generation had been gathered to their fathers, another generation arose after them who did not know the LORD nor the work which He had done for Israel." (Judg. 2:8–10)

Did Israel completely conquer the Canaanites?

No, many of the cities of the promised land were not captured and inhabited, and parts of the country were also not captured (Judg. 3:1–3).

What was the result of Israel's incomplete obedience?

Israel was led astray by the heathen living among them. Israel followed their gods and intermarried with them, adapting to their heathen practices (Judg. 2:12–16).

When the heathen put Israel into servitude, what did God's people do?

They repented of their sins and called upon God to deliver them (Judg. 2:16).

How many complete cycles of deliverance are described in the book of Judges?

There are seven cycles; hence there are seven judges (Judges of the cycle) who were raised up by God to deliver Israel: Othniel, Ehud, Deborah, Gideon, Abimelech, Jephthah, and Samson.

How many total judges were there?

There may have been others, but at least fourteen are named in the book of Judges, in addition to Eli and Samuel mentioned in 1 Samuel. Many of these judges fought against Israel's enemies, but they did not deliver Israel.

Who was the first judge/deliverer?

Othniel was the first judge. He was the younger brother of Caleb, the other loyal spy with Joshua (Judg. 3:8–11).

Who was Deborah the Judge?

Deborah was a prophetess, and people came to her to know the will of God (Judg. 4:1–9). She predicted that Israel would escape the servitude of the Canaanites through the influence of a woman. She was responsible for rallying Israel to battle.

Who was Barak?

He was a leader of the tribes of Zebulun and Naphtali (Judg. 4:6–10). Barak was afraid to lead his army into battle because of the overwhelming odds of the Canaanites, so he asked Deborah to go to battle with him. Barak was then told that the enemy's general would be given into the hands of a woman, not him, when Israel won the battle.

How did Israel overcome such a formidable army?

The Canaanites had six hundred chariots, but as the battle began, a tremendous rainstorm was sent by God so that the chariots bogged down in the mud and were useless. Israel was rallied to battle and defeated the Canaanites, who were apparently confused without their battle strategies that included using the chariots.

Who killed General Sisera, the Canaanite?

When the Canaanites were defeated, Sisera fled on foot and sought refuge in the tent of Jael, the wife of Heber, a Kenite. While he was sleeping, Jael took a tent peg and drove it through his head, killing him.

Who was Gideon? (Judg. 6–9)

Gideon was from a poor family in Manasseh and was the youngest in his father's house. Yet God wanted to demonstrate His power through Gideon.

What was Gideon's first act when told he would deliver Israel?

At night he threw down his father's idol and sacrificed a bull to Jehovah (Judg. 6:25–32).

What nickname was Gideon given?

Because of his act of throwing down the idol of Baal, he was called Jerubbaal, or "Baal fighter."

How large was the army that gathered against Gideon?

The Bible says, "Now the Midianites and Amalekites, all the people of the East, were lying in the valley as numerous as locusts; and their camels were without number, as the sand by the seashore in multitude" (Judg. 7:12).

When faced with this great number, what was Gideon's response?

Gideon was fearful, so he asked God to give him private assurance that he could deliver Israel from the Midianites. He constantly asked for signs, and eventually asked for a "fleece" (Judg. 6:37). He first asked God to cause a *fleece* (the wool of a lamb) to become wet on dry ground. When God answered that night, Gideon was still not sure. The following night God gave him a dry fleece on wet ground.

Should a Christian put out a "fleece" today to determine the will of God?

Christians often raise the question today whether it is valid to use "fleeces," or signs, in determining God's will for their lives. The context of the entire story of Gideon, from which this idea comes, indicates that the fleece incident would have been unnecessary if Gideon had fully trusted the Lord. Using a fleece is depending on signs and circumstances to discern the will of God ("If it rains today, I will know that God doesn't want me to go to church"). Such a dependence on signs is the exact opposite of a clear exercise of faith. God wants us to obey His Word and act thereupon. A "fleece" is when we ask God to fulfill conditions to demonstrate His will. Some may ask "if" God is going to answer, then ask Him to demonstrate it by working out circumstances. While God gave Gideon the sign of a fleece to confirm victory in this unusual manner, God does not speak through "fleeces" today.

When Gideon gathered his army, how did God test him?

First, Gideon told all that were cowards or frightened to go home (Judg. 7:2–3). Then God told Gideon to have all of his army go to the stream and drink. Some of the men lay down and put their faces in the water; others scooped water with their hands to drink. These were the ones God chose, because they remained on guard for an ambush, and proved ready and quicker to serve God.

How many men did Gideon take into battle?

Gideon took three hundred men into battle.

How did Gideon win a battle with only three hundred men against a superior force?

Each of the three hundred warriors took a trumpet, a lighted torch hidden in a pitcher, and a sword strapped to his side. At a given signal, they all broke their pitchers and blew their trumpets, scaring the enemy and throwing them into confusion. The enemy ended up slaughtering themselves (Judg. 7:16–20).

Who was Jephthah?

He was a great warrior with Gilead in Gad (Judg. 11:1), who had been born when his father had sex outside of marriage (he was born of a harlot). The fact that God used Jephthah demonstrates the grace of God to use people where He finds them and to use those who are yielded to Him.

What was the vow that Jephthah made before he went to the battle?

Jephthah said that if God would give him the victory, then the first thing that came out of his house when he returned home would be offered up to the Lord (Judg. 11:30–40). But the first to come out to meet him upon his return was his only daughter. He did not, however, sacrifice her as a burnt offering to the Lord. Instead, he dedicated her to ministry in the temple, much as Samuel would later be dedicated for ministry in the temple. In other words, the family gave up their child for the use of the Lord. Jephthah's daughter and her friends "wept," not because she was going to be sacrificed, but because she would never marry, and the line of Jephthah would come to an end.

Who was Samson?

He was a judge born into the tribe of Dan. Apparently his mother was barren and could not have a son. After an angel appeared to her, she conceived and bore Samson. He was a Nazarite separated unto God.

What is a *Nazarite*?

The word *Nazarite* comes from the Hebrew word *nazar*, which means "devout" or "to vow." A Nazarite makes a vow (1) to not consume grapes or the fruit of the vine (grape juice), (2) to not cut his hair, and (3) to not go near a dead body, which includes not eating an animal that was killed. Some had a temporary Nazarite vow to show their dedication to God, as Paul apparently did in Acts 18. Others had a lifelong Nazarite vow, as did Samson and John the Baptist.

What was the source of Samson's strength?

Some people feel Samson was a man of great muscular strength, able to defeat many warriors in battle. Others think he had a natural physical build, and got his strength from the Spirit of God (Judg. 16:20).

How did Samson lose his strength?

A woman named Delilah—a member of the Philistines, who were the enemies of Samson—seduced him to reveal his strength. She then had his hair cut—the sign of his Nazarite vow—rendering him powerless (Judg. 16:17–21).

Was Samson ever restored after his sin?

Yes, after the Philistines captured him and put him in servitude, his hair began to grow again. But it was not the hair that gave him strength. Samson repented and asked God to use him (Judg. 16:28). He destroyed the temple of Dagon, and the Bible says, "So the dead that he killed at his death were more than he had killed in his life" (Judg. 16:30).

QUESTIONS ABOUT
THE BOOK OF RUTH

Who was Ruth?

Ruth was a Moabitess woman (outside the covenant of Israel) who married an Israelite man who moved to her country. Ruth forsook her pagan heritage and chose to go with her mother-in-law, Naomi, to live in Bethlehem after the death of her husband. But more importantly, Ruth chose to put her faith in the God of Israel. God rewarded her by giving her another husband, Boaz, a rich landowner, and a son named Obed, who was in the line of Messiah. Ruth became the great-grandmother of David.

Why was the book of Ruth written?

This is a cameo love story that shows the faithfulness of Ruth during the time of Judges (Ruth 1:1), when the nation was faithless.

What is the key word in Ruth?

The key word is *kinsman*, the Hebrew word *goel*, which occurs thirteen times in the book. The word means "one who redeems."

What is the key verse in Ruth?

"Entreat me not to leave you,
Or to turn back from following after you;

For wherever you go, I will go;
And wherever you lodge, I will lodge;
Your people shall be my people,
And your God, my God." (Ruth 1:16)

What is the kinsman redeemer?

This is a picture of Jesus Christ, who came to identify with us and died to redeem us. In Israel, whenever a close relative became a kinsman redeemer (*goel,* Ruth 3:9), he had to (1) be related by blood to those he redeemed, (2) be able to pay the price of redemption, (3) be willing to redeem, and (4) free himself so he could deliver his relatives.

Who was Elimelech?

He was a landowner living in Bethlehem of Judea, apparently a long-time occupant of Bethlehem living in the days of Judges (1:1–2).

Why did Elimelech go to Moab?

There was a famine in Bethlehem, and because it is possible to physically see Moab from Bethlehem, Elimelech migrated to that country because of its better economic position. He died in Moab.

How did Ruth become a part of Elimelech's family?

Elimelech had two sons, Mahlon and Chilion, who both married Moabitess wives, Ruth and Orpah (Ruth 1:5). Both men died, leaving their wives widows.

How did Ruth demonstrate her faith in the God of Israel?

When Naomi decided to return home after the deaths of her husband and her sons, she advised her two daughters-in-law to go back to their people and their god. However, Ruth chose to follow Naomi and the God of Israel. Ruth said, "Your people shall be my people, and your God, my God" (Ruth 1:16).

How did Naomi and Ruth provide for their needs when they returned to Bethlehem?

Ruth went into the fields to glean behind the reapers, a tradition that allowed the poor and widows to pick up grain that was fallen during harvest and keep it for their own use (Ruth 2:2–3).

Who was Boaz?

Ruth happened to glean in Boaz's field. He not only was a rich landowner, but was also kindhearted and had deep faith in God.

What did Boaz do for Ruth?

He not only allowed her to eat and drink with his reapers during the lunch breaks, but he also told his harvesters to leave extra grain for her (Ruth 2:14–20; 3:1–4).

Did Ruth commit an immoral act by going to Boaz at night when he had harvested his grain?

No, it was the tradition for the workmen and owners to sleep with their grain to protect it from thieves. During the night Ruth became Boaz's servant. She slept at his feet (servants allowed the master to put cold feet on them to keep warm in the night). When Boaz awakened, he realized it was a woman and asked who she was. Ruth answered, "Your maidservant. Take your maidservant under your wing, for you are a close relative" (Ruth 3:9). Ruth was asking for Boaz to exercise the kinsman redeemer prerogative, to buy the land of Elimelech out of debt, and to redeem her.

What was the result?

Ruth eventually married Boaz, had a child named Obed, and became the great-grandmother of King David. She is also in the line of Jesus Christ the Messiah (Ruth 4:17–22).

QUESTIONS ABOUT
THE FIRST BOOK OF SAMUEL

Who was Samuel?

Samuel was born to Hannah in answer to prayer. Hannah had been unable to bear a child, but asked God for a son (1 Sam. 1:11), and God heard her request. The name Samuel means "to ask" or "heard of God." As a priest from the tribe of Levi, Samuel assumed the position of head priest, although he is not called by the title "high priest." But he did sacrifice for all of Israel. Samuel was also called a judge and led the nation from a theocracy (rule by God) to a kingdom (ruled by a king). He was born about 1105 B.C.

Who wrote the book of 1 Samuel?

Most conservatives believe that Samuel wrote this book by his name, or at least the first portion of the book, before the record of his death in 1 Samuel 25:1. He obviously did not write the next few chapters and 2 Samuel. But Samuel did write a book (1 Sam. 10:25), and he led a company of prophets (1 Sam. 10:5; 19:20), which would have involved writing an account of their accomplishments. First Chronicles 29:29 refers to "the book of Samuel the seer" which suggests he wrote this book. Also, the unity of purpose and natural development of the theme suggest that one man, Samuel, wrote it.

When was 1 Samuel written?

The book of 1 Samuel covers about ninety-four years (1067 to about 1015 B.C.), from the birth of Samuel to the death of Saul. He probably finished his writing soon before his death, around 1015 B.C.

What is the key word in 1 Samuel?

The key word is *transition*. The word is not found in the text, but reflects its message. Israel was going through a transition from judges to kings. Notice the three stages in the book of 1 Samuel: from Eli to Samuel, from Samuel to Saul, and from Saul to David.

Who was Eli?

Eli was the high priest who also served as a judge (1 Sam. 1:9; 4:18). Eli refused to reprove his wicked sons and restrain them as a father and high priest should (1 Sam. 2:23–25; 3:13–14). As a result, God judged him and he died in an accident.

Was Eli entirely ineffective?

No, Eli tried to serve God faithfully, but apparently had a weak will. When he saw Hannah praying intently in the tabernacle, he thought she was drunk (1 Sam. 1:13–18). When he found she was not drunk, he had spiritual discernment enough to tell her to pray and trust God (1 Sam. 1:17–28).

How old was Samuel when his mother dedicated him to tabernacle service?

He was "very young," perhaps as young as five or six years old (1 Sam. 1:24). Each year Hannah took a new set of clothes to her son at the tabernacle. While this may seem unusual, it is no different than people today who send their children away to boarding school, except that Hannah did it as an act of service to God.

How old was Samuel when the Lord called him?

He was probably about twelve years of age.

How did God call Samuel into service?

As Samuel was sleeping in the Tabernacle keeping watch over the fire by night, the Lord called his name. When Samuel asked Eli, the old priest didn't recognize it was the call of God. Finally, when awakened three times, the old priest told Samuel to answer, "Speak, LORD, for Your servant hears" (1 Sam. 3:9).

What should a Christian's response be if he (or she) feels God is calling him into special service?

A Christian should answer just as Samuel: "Speak, LORD, for Your servant hears."

Why would God allow the Philistines to capture the ark of the covenant?

Some people question why God has allowed His work to be destroyed by evil men. One answer to that question is the same reason why God allowed the ark to be taken. The leadership of Israel was using the ark as a "lucky charm," because they said, "Let us bring the ark of the covenant of the LORD . . . to us, that when it comes among us it may save us from the hand of our enemies" (1 Sam. 4:3).

Notice what is missing: They did not repent of their sins. They did not cry out for God's deliverance, nor did they ask for God's presence in the battle or for Him to give victory over their enemies. Today people use the "things of God" in the same way without meeting God's spiritual requirements.

What happened when the ark of the covenant was put in the temple of Dagon?

God judged the Philistines with painful diseases and a plague of mice (perhaps bubonic plague) that brought destruction among the people. When they placed the ark of the covenant next to Dagon, the next morning they found their idol/statue on its face before the Lord God who dwelled in the ark of the covenant.

How was the ark returned to Israel?

The Philistines yoked two cows to a cart to see if it would carry the ark of the covenant back to the land of Israel. To make sure the cows were not following natural inclination, they separated them from their calves (1 Sam. 6:7–12).

Where was the tabernacle located after the Philistines captured the ark of the covenant, defeated Israel, and overwhelmed the promised land?

The Bible is silent as to where the tabernacle was located. Some believe the tabernacle was quickly dismantled and hidden until the time of David. Some feel it may have been hidden in one of the large caves that are found in southern Israel. Still others feel the Philistines completely overran the camp and destroyed the tabernacle. But when David became king, the tabernacle reappeared.

Why did Israel want a king?

The people of Israel rejected God's rulership over them. They demanded a king. The people said to Samuel, "Look, you are old, and your sons do not walk in your ways. Now make us a king to judge us like all the nations" (1 Sam. 8:5).

What was God's reaction to Israel's request for a king?

The Lord told Samuel to, "Heed the voice of the people in all that they say to you; for they have not rejected you, but they have rejected Me, that I should not reign over them" (1 Sam. 8:7).

Who was Saul?

Saul was the son of Kish, from the tribe of Benjamin (1 Sam. 9:1). He was tall, handsome (1 Sam. 9:2), and he was chosen by God and anointed by Samuel to be the first king of Israel (1 Sam. 9:15–17; 10:1–27).

What does the Bible say about Saul's character?

In a few ways Saul worshiped and honored God, but in other ways he was proud, disobedient, self-willed, and superstitious.

How was Saul's rebellion manifested?

When Israel and the Philistines gathered for a great struggle (1 Sam. 13:4–23), Samuel didn't show up when Saul needed him. Because Samuel didn't come for seven days, Saul entered into the priestly office and offered the sacrifices for Israel. Finally, Samuel showed up to rebuke Saul. Immediately King Saul regretted what he did, but it was a revelation of his disobedience and lack of trust in God.

In what other ways was Saul's character revealed?

When Saul defeated the Amalekites, he did not do what God commanded. God had told him to completely destroy all of the Amalekites (1 Sam. 15:3). But Saul disobeyed God, keeping the best of the spoils (v. 15:9). Because of this disobedience, God turned His back on Saul.

Whom did God choose to be king instead of Saul?

God chose David, a young boy from the tribe of Judah, living in Bethlehem (1 Sam. 16:1–13).

What does the Bible say about David's character?

David was zealous in his love for God and was respected by all of the people who followed him. He was a great warrior and a poet, but most of all, "a man after God's own heart" (Acts 13:22).

How could Saul have an "evil spirit from God"? (1 Sam. 16:23 KJV)

Obviously, God cannot create evil, nor can He allow evil in His presence. However, an evil spirit was described as being "from God." God will allow Satan to do a work that ultimately brings glory to Himself. In this case, God allowed an "evil spirit" or a "demon" to trouble Saul.

This was not demon possession; actually there is no word in the original language for demon possession. Rather, the original language describes *demonizing*, or the word *demonized*. This means the demon would influence, irritate, control, or work through a person.

Can a Christian be demonized?

That is not an easy question to answer. Many believe that Saul was not saved, so he could have been demonized. Those who think that Saul was saved think that he could have been demonized (tormented by a demon).

How did the evil spirit depart from Saul?

David was chosen to come and play his harp in the presence of Saul. Notice what probably happened: The presence of a spirit-filled man (David) caused the demon to leave. Also, the singing of Scripture from the poems that David wrote drove the demon away. David also probably used a positive message from God, and the demon could not stay in the presence of God's influence (1 Sam. 16:23).

What was Goliath's "challenge"?

Goliath was a Philistine warrior who was well over nine feet tall. The Philistines engaged in what is called "battle by championship." Rather than the entire army facing each other, each side would choose one representative to fight for their army. The issue was not one army completely destroying and killing the other army, but rather, the winning side gaining the right to inhabit the other side, collecting spoils and taxes from them, and ruling over them. If Goliath won the battle, the Philistines would continue to dominate Israel.

Did David kill Goliath with a stone from his slingshot?

No, David chose five smooth stones and hurled one of them at the giant, hitting him in the forehead. This stunned Goliath; then David ran, took Goliath's sword, and cut off his head.

What did David do with Goliath's head and sword?

David was a young sixteen-year-old boy, and as many young boys, he kept his trophy. Later that day, David appeared in the tent of Saul, "with the head of the Philistine in his hand" (1 Sam. 17:57). David did not immediately dispose of the head, but "took the head of the Philistine and brought it to Jerusalem" (1 Sam. 17:54). At that time Jerusalem was still a heathen city. But David knew that he was going to capture Jerusalem and make it his capital city. So he probably went to the wall of Jerusalem and held up the head of Goliath to warn the inhabitants of Jerusalem that one day he would do to them what he did to Goliath. David also took the sword of Goliath and put it in his tent. Later he used it in battle (1 Sam. 17:54).

Which of Saul's sons became a friend to David?

Jonathan, the oldest son of King Saul, became "knit with the soul of David" (1 Sam. 18:1 KJV, 20:17).

How did Jonathan demonstrate his friendship to David?

Jonathan gave David his robe and some of his armaments (1 Sam. 18:4, 13:22). This demonstrates that Jonathan recognized David would be king. The heir to the throne of Saul was recognizing that David was the heir to the kingdom.

Why did Saul hate David?

Even though David won a great battle for Saul, Saul became angry when the women began to chant in the villages, "Saul has slain his thousands, and David his ten thousands" (1 Sam. 18:6–16). Saul was jealous, and for the next thirteen years he tried to kill David.

What was David's attitude while Saul remained king?

David knew that he was going to be king, because Samuel had anointed him with oil. However, though he had several opportunities, he would not kill Saul, stating, "Touch not God's anointed" (1 Sam. 24:10).

What was Saul's final act of rebellion?

Saul visited the witch of Endor and asked to speak to Samuel, or the spirit of Samuel. God had strictly forbidden communication with spirits (Deut. 18:9–14). This process is called "channeling" by spirit mediums, and is a part of the New Age movement, not a Christian activity. When a spirit controls the body of a medium or a witch, essentially that person is demonized. Any "guidance" of a medium or psychic will inevitably be deceptive and dangerous for the Christian. The one who is deceived by a medium or psychic with a message from someone who is dead will probably be deceived even further in other areas.

Did Samuel actually come back from the dead?

The Bible says, "When the woman saw Samuel, she cried out with a loud voice. And the woman spoke to Saul, saying, 'Why have you deceived me? For you are Saul!'" (1 Sam. 28:12). Most Christians believe that the witch knew she couldn't bring someone back from the dead. However, this witch "cried out" because she saw something she didn't expect: Samuel actually came back from the dead. Many times a witch will deceive a customer by claiming the dead are saying things, which in fact the witch makes up. At other times the witch will actually hear a message from the "spirit" but it will not be a message from the deceased, but from a demon that was in that person or had special knowledge about that person.

Would God allow a person to come back from the dead?

This is highly unusual, and many Christians believe that Samuel didn't come back from the dead. The witch and Saul only saw a "spirit" of Samuel. However, other Christians believe that in this unusual circumstance, God allowed Samuel to return to life so he could predict the death of Saul. If this was really Samuel' speaking to Saul, it was probably God's last warning to Saul, and his last opportunity to repent and turn back to God.

How did Saul kill himself?

The account in 1 Samuel says, "Saul took a sword and fell upon it" (1 Sam. 31:4).

Did Saul go to heaven?

Apparently his death was a suicide. Many believe that a Christian who is honestly born-again cannot commit suicide. However, this raises the question, Was Saul saved? No matter his spiritual condition, it is possible for a born-again Christian to commit suicide. A Christian can become so depressed, feeling he has nothing to live for, that he (or she) takes his own life. Other Christians under physical distress or heavy sedation can also take their lives. The loved ones of a Christian who has committed suicide should not be discouraged, thinking that their loved one did not go into the presence of God. Nothing a Christian can do in this life will take away his or her relationship with the Lord Jesus Christ. Remember, the Bible says, "The blood of Jesus Christ His Son cleanses us from all sin" (1 John 1:7). That means the blood of Jesus Christ cleanses from the sin of suicide.

QUESTIONS ABOUT
THE SECOND BOOK OF SAMUEL

Why is the book called "2 Samuel"?

The Hebrew titles for both books were originally called Samuel, and the Greek title for 2 Samuel was *Basileion Beta,* which means "second kingdom." The book of Samuel was originally divided because it took more Greek letters than Hebrew letters, and the content couldn't fit on one scroll. The second book continues to carry Samuel's name.

Who wrote 2 Samuel?

Obviously Samuel didn't write this book that's named for him, because he was dead during the events that are recorded here. Many feel that the two prophets who served under David, Nathan and Gad, referred to in 1 Chronicles 29:29, were the authors of this book because 2 Samuel is referred to in this reference.

What is the key word in 2 Samuel?

The key word is *David,* because he is the central person around whom the entire book is written.

What are the key verses in 2 Samuel?

"David was thirty years old when he began to reign, and he reigned forty years. In Hebron he reigned over Judah seven years and six months, and in Jerusalem he reigned thirty-three years over all Israel and Judah" (2 Sam. 5:4–5).

How did David become a king?

After Saul was killed in battle, David sought the direction of God, then went up to Hebron, where he was anointed king over Judah. He remained king of Judah for seven years. Then David became king over both Judah and Israel for thirty-three years. He was king for a total of forty years.

When did the other tribes recognize David as king?

After seven years the other tribes recognized David, and he became king over all twelve tribes (2 Sam. 2:5–10).

What was David's first battle and conquest?
He went and attacked the Jebusites and captured the city of Jerusalem (2 Sam. 5:6–9).

How did David, as king, fulfill his passion for God?
He brought the ark of the covenant to Jerusalem.

What happened as David tried to bring the ark to Jerusalem?
Instead of having the Levites carry it on their shoulders, as was commanded in Scripture, David attempted to bring it on a new cart. When the cart pitched, Uzzah tried to steady the cart, and God judged him for disobeying the command to not touch the ark. David was afraid to take the ark any further and left it in the house of Obed-Edom, the Gittite (2 Sam. 6).

What motivated David to get the ark a second time?
The blessing of God rested upon the house of Obed-Edom (2 Sam. 6:12).

What did David do differently the second time he brought the ark to Jerusalem?
The Levites brought the ark on their shoulders, and made blood sacrifices along the way to seek the forgiveness and blessing of God upon their endeavor. They brought the ark to Jerusalem with joy, but humble thanksgiving (2 Sam. 6:12–20).

Why didn't God let David build a house for the ark of the covenant?
Because David had been a man of war and shed much blood, God told him that his son Solomon would build the temple (Solomon's temple). The prophet Nathan brought this message to David (2 Sam. 7:3–15).

What was David's great sin?
When David sent his army out to besiege Rabbah, the capital city of modern-day Jordan, David stayed home at Jerusalem. There he saw Bathsheba taking a bath, sent for her, and had sex with her.

What happened after David sinned?

Bathsheba became pregnant, and when she told David her condition, David tried to use human "negotiations" to hide his sin. He brought Uriah, Bathsheba's husband, back to Jerusalem. He tried to arrange circumstances so that Uriah would sleep with his wife, so the baby would be thought to be his, but it didn't happen. So he sent Uriah back to battle, telling general Joab to put him at the front of the battle, and to withdraw when the battle raged (2 Sam. 11:15).

Did David commit murder?

Yes. Even though David didn't do the actual task, he negotiated the circumstances that led to Uriah's death. David had "murdered" Uriah in his heart long before it happened by an enemy soldier.

Did the Lord pardon David?

Yes. Nathan the prophet confronted David with his sin (2 Sam. 12:1–12), and David repented deeply (read Psalm 51). The Lord pardoned David, but still punished him by the death of the child (2 Sam. 12:13–23).

What was the proof that the Lord completely forgave David and Bathsheba?

Their next son was Solomon, meaning "peaceful," and Solomon had a peaceful kingdom. It was through Solomon that the Messiah was to come.

What preparation did David make for Solomon's temple?

David had stone, silver, gold, iron, brass (bronze), and cedar prepared for the building of the temple (1 Chron. 22:2–5).

QUESTIONS ABOUT THE FIRST BOOK OF KINGS

What is included in 1 Kings?

The first part of 1 Kings is a history of the life and reign of Solomon. As king, Solomon brought the nation to its zenith in size and glory, accomplishing peace in his time. He signed treaties with Israel's enemy, built Solomon's temple, and brought worldwide fame and respect to Jerusalem. However, in Solomon's later life, his pagan wives turned his heart away from the Lord and the temple worship. The *king with a divided heart* ended up with a *divided kingdom.*

Why is the book called "1 Kings"?

The Hebrew title for this book was *Melechim,* "kings," which is taken from the very first word in the Hebrew Bible (1:1). Since the book of Kings was divided into two books, obviously the first book was called 1 Kings.

Why are there two books of Kings?

Originally in the Hebrew Bible, there was one book called "Kings." However, when the Old Testament was translated into Greek, these two books were artificially divided because the Greek language required a greater amount of scroll space than did the Hebrew language.

Who wrote the book of 1 Kings?

Technically we do not know who wrote the book of 1 Kings. Many conservatives believe that Jeremiah wrote the book, because he was a prophet-historian. As a prophet, Jeremiah exposed apostasy, which is the message of 1 Kings. As a historian, Jeremiah wrote of judgment on idolatry and immorality in the nation. Hebrew scholars see a similar style in 1 Kings and Jeremiah. Also, as you read 1 Kings, you find "the book of the acts of Solomon" (11:41), "the book of the chronicles of the kings of Israel" (14:19), and "the book of the chronicles of the kings of Judah" (14:29; 15:7). These were probably official court records from which Jeremiah gleaned in writing the book (2 Kings 18:18).

What is the key word in 1 Kings?

The key word is *division* because the kingdom that was united under Saul, David, and Solomon, is irrevocably divided in this book.

What are the key verses in 1 Kings?

"Now if you walk before Me as your father David walked, in integrity of heart and in uprightness, to do according to all that I have commanded you, and if you keep My statutes and My judgments, then I will establish the throne of your kingdom over Israel forever, as I promised David your father, saying, 'You shall not fail to have a man on the throne of Israel.'" (1 Kings 9:4–5)

"Therefore the LORD said to Solomon, 'Because you have done this, and have not kept My covenant and My statutes, which I have commanded you, I will surely tear the kingdom away from you and give it to your servant.'" (1 Kings 11:11)

Why did Solomon make alliances with his enemies?

Whereas David was a man of war and conquered his enemies, Solomon was a man of peace and made alliances with his enemies by taking a wife from the daughters of heathen monarchies. He married the daughter of Pharaoh as a political measure to guarantee peace, because Egypt was probably the most powerful nation in the world (1 Kings 3:1).

How is Solomon's wisdom demonstrated?

God appeared to Solomon in a dream soon after his father's death to ask what he would like. Solomon didn't choose wealth or power but chose wisdom (1 Kings 3:2–15). God answered his prayer and made him one of the wisest men in the world.

What was the architectural plan for the building of the temple?

The plan was originally given to David by "the Spirit" of God (1 Chron. 28:11–12). Solomon followed this plan when he built the temple.

Where was the temple originally built?

It was built on Mt. Moriah in Jerusalem (2 Chron. 3:1).

Is it true that Solomon's temple was built quietly?

The stone was prepared entirely before it was brought to Jerusalem. "The temple . . . was built with stone finished at the quarry, so that no hammer or chisel or any iron tool was heard in the temple while it was being built" (1 Kings. 6:7).

How did God respond to the temple?

Solomon celebrated a solemn feast and brought the ark of the covenant into the temple. Solomon made an eloquent plea for the presence of God to come dwell in the temple. When the Shekinah-glory cloud entered the temple and the house was filled with smoke, God proved that He had accepted the temple and would dwell there (1 Kings 8).

How else was Solomon's wisdom manifested?

He had great wisdom in deciding difficult questions. For example, two prostitutes argued over one baby, each saying it was hers. When Solomon said to cut the baby in half, the real mother objected (1 Kings 4:29–31; 3:12, 16–28).

What was Solomon's reputation among heathen monarchs?

When the Queen of Sheba (Ethiopia or southern Egypt) came to see Solomon's kingdom, she said, "The half was not told me" (1 Kings 10:7).

What was the besetting sin of Solomon?

It was the taking of heathen wives. He ended up following their idolatry, and they turned his heart from the Lord (1 Kings 11:1–10).

How long did Solomon reign?

Solomon reigned for forty years.

What does the Bible say about Solomon's son, who reigned in his stead?

Rehoboam was a foolish son (1 Kings 11:43), who followed the advice of his young court advisers instead of the advice of the older men. Rehoboam raised taxes and increased the burden on the people, and the people rebelled against his leadership.

What was the result?

The ten tribes who had voluntarily followed David now revolted against Rehoboam and established a separate kingdom under Jeroboam.

Who was Jeroboam?

He was not of royal blood from Solomon, but was the Nebat who had been a manager in Solomon's kingdom. Because he spoke against Solomon or "lifted up his hand against the king," he had been forced into exile in Egypt (1 Kings 11:26–40 KJV). The ten tribes brought Jeroboam back to be their king.

What happened to the worship of God in the ten tribes?

They did not have priests from the tribe of Levi to lead them, so they chose priests from the lowest of people, and their worship degenerated into idolatry, immorality, and eventually worship of evil spirits (1 Kings 13:1–16).

Who was Elijah?

He was a prophet from Gilead, considered one of the greatest prophets in the Old Testament. He was rugged, abrupt, and dressed in skins with a leather girdle and a long "mantle." The mantle was the symbol of his office. Elijah was a preaching prophet, not a writing prophet, and his message was primarily to the ten tribes of Israel. He ministered primarily during the time of King Ahab (1 Kings 16:29–22:40).

QUESTIONS ABOUT
THE SECOND BOOK OF KINGS

What is included in the book of 2 Kings?

This book traces two nations—the northern ten tribes of Israel and the two southern tribes of Judah. The author looks at the different kings in both nations, first looking at one nation, then retracing the same period for the other nation.

All kings in the northern ten tribes were evil, and they did not depart from the idolatrous calf-worship of Jeroboam, the first king of the north. However, there were some godly kings in the south who brought both reforms and revivals, so that the evil of the people of some previous kings and the evil of the people in general were dealt with. However, sin seems always greater than righteousness, and both the Northern and the Southern kingdoms were carried away into captivity.

Who wrote 2 Kings?

The writer of 2 Kings is probably the same author as that of 1 Kings, that is, Jeremiah. This book was written before the Babylonian captivity, "to this day" (17:34, 41). The book follows the literary style of 1 Kings and Jeremiah, and it is interesting that 2 Kings 24:18–25:30 is almost the same as Jeremiah 52. However, the last two chapters were evidently added by another author after the Babylonian captivity, because Jeremiah was forced into Egypt (Jer. 43:1–8), not to Babylon, which is the focus of the last two chapters.

When was 2 Kings written?
Second Kings was written prior to 586 B.C., the beginning of the Babylonian captivity.

What is the key word in 2 Kings?
The key word is *captivity*. There are two great captivities spoken of in 2 Kings: The ten northern tribes of Israel were carried away by the Assyrians (2 Kings 17), and Jerusalem and Judah were destroyed and carried into captivity by the Babylonians (2 Kings 25).

What are the key verses in 2 Kings?
"For the children of Israel walked in all the sins of Jeroboam which he did; they did not depart from them, until the LORD removed Israel out of His sight, as He had said by all His servants the prophets. So Israel was carried away from their own land to Assyria, as it is to this day." (2 Kings 17:22–23)

"And the LORD said, 'I will also remove Judah from My sight, as I have removed Israel, and will cast off this city Jerusalem which I have chosen, and the house of which I said, 'My name shall be there.'" (2 Kings 23:27)

How did Elijah end his ministry?
Second Kings tells the story of Elijah going up to heaven in a whirlwind. Apparently he did not die, but was translated into the presence of God. His prophetic mantle—symbol of office—was dropped as Elijah was carried into heaven. Young Elisha took the mantle and carried on his work.

What is the difference between the ministries of Elisha and Elijah?
Whereas Elijah was rough and ministered in the wilderness apart from society, Elisha went into the cities, spoke to the kings in their courts, and lived with a school of prophets. Whereas Elijah did seven miracles in his lifetime, young Elisha, his student, did fourteen miracles, probably because he asked for a "double portion of [Elijah's] spirit" (2 Kings 2:9).

What kind of "fire from heaven" did Elisha bring?

An army captain came to arrest Elisha, but the prophet called fire down from heaven that destroyed his arrestors (1:14). Elisha demonstrated the same thing that his mentor, Elijah, had done ten years earlier on Mount Carmel when he, too, brought fire from heaven. This "fire" was apparently more than lightning directed against Baal worshippers; it was specially created fire that had the same deadly effect as lightning.

Who are the sons of the prophets?

These were part of a school apparently established earlier by Samuel (1 Sam. 10:5–13, 19, 24), and were in the line of the prophets. They did the work of God, some copying Scripture, some teaching, and some preaching for God. Just because a person was a prophet did not mean he predicted the future. Rather, many delivered the Word of God to the people. Jezebel killed many of those in the school of the prophets, but some were hidden and preserved beyond the reach of Jezebel (1 Kings 18:4).

How did Elijah go up into heaven?

Just as Enoch walked with God during a time of deep apostasy "and was not," so Elijah, during a time of apostasy, was taken to heaven without dying. There was a fiery tornado that seemed to be accompanied by a flaming horse-drawn chariot as he went up into heaven and out of Elisha's sight.

Was it right for Elisha to curse young children?

Some people have said that Elisha did an unethical thing: "Then he went up from there to Bethel; and as he was going up the road, some youths came from the city and mocked him, and said to him, 'Go up, you baldhead! Go up, you baldhead!' So he turned around and looked at them, and pronounced a curse on them in the name of the LORD. And two female bears came out of the woods and mauled forty-two of the youths" (2 Kings 2:23–24).

The King James translates this as "little children" but the Hebrew word is young unmarried men, up to the age of thirty. This was a rebellious gang of young men who rejected Jehovah, probably because they worshiped Baal. They were not only ridiculing Elisha, but also his predecessor, Elijah. The phrase "go up" was used to ridicule Elijah's translation to heaven, indicating that they did not believe Elijah was taken to heaven. Apparently, they were insulting God Himself. God had promised that if His people turned against Him, He would "also send wild beasts" among them, which would "rob [them] of [their] children" (Lev. 26:22). Apparently the judgment of God was on these young rebels.

How did Elisha make the iron head "swim"?

This is not a miracle of creation, but rather, God redirected the energy in the laws of nature, similar to what He did when Christ walked on the water. According to the faith of Elisha, God redirected an antigravitational force (the law of gravity being superseded) so that an iron ax head rose to the surface of the water and floated (2 Kings 6:6).

What did Elisha's servants see when he saw the mountains full of horses and chariots? (2 Kings 6:17)

Elisha had said, "Do not fear, for those who are with us are more than those who are with them" (2 Kings 6:16). God has promised that there would be "an innumerable company of angels" (Heb. 12:22) that will serve God's people, "ministering spirits sent forth to minister for those who will inherit salvation" (Heb. 1:14). Apparently the servant had his spiritual eyes opened and saw angels surrounding them to protect them. So when you are in difficulty, think of what God did for Elisha's servant and remember, "He who is in you is greater than he who is in the world" (1 John 4:4).

Who was Jehu?

Jehu was the king of Israel who was commanded to destroy the entire house of Ahab (2 Kings 9:7–9). He did so by killing all of the children of Ahab. Unfortunately, Jehu's zeal to carry out God's command was more a "grab for power" than a love for God. He was not interested in just destroying Baal worship in Israel, but was also interested in power and might (2 Kings 10:20–28). Jehu could be described as one who wanted to build a good strong nation, but not necessarily a godly nation.

What does it mean when Ahaz made his son "pass through the fire"?

Perhaps the worse thing that any heathen can do is sacrifice his or her children to a false god. Even though Ahaz was an Israelite—a presumed child of

God—he followed "the abomination of the heathen." Evidences of his child sacrifices have been found in archaeology.

QUESTIONS ABOUT THE FIRST BOOK OF CHRONICLES

Why do 1 and 2 Chronicles repeat the material found in the books of Samuel and Kings?

Even though these two sets of books (Kings and Chronicles) cover the same events and periods of time, they are different in perspective. They are not a perfect repetition of the same material; rather, the books of Samuel and Kings give a political history of the ten northern tribes of Israel, with emphasis on rebellion, disobedience, and idolatry. The Chronicles describes Israel and the Davidic dynasty from a priestly and spiritual perspective. The Kings emphasize the ten northern tribes, while the Chronicles emphasize the southern tribes of Judah and Jerusalem. As a result of the different perspective, the books of Chronicles contain certain new records that describe the spiritual works of God, and omit many of the sins that were included in the books of Samuel and Kings. The books of Chronicles do not describe the rebellion by Absalom, Solomon's moral decline in his later years, and certain other sins.

Why do the first nine chapters of 1 Chronicles cover past genealogies?

To answer that question, look at the genealogies from the perspective of the exiles returning from Babylon. They needed to know that they had family ties with the work of God before the Babylonian captivity. They needed to tie their heritage to David and the plan of God all the way back to Abraham. Because Messiah had not yet come, they needed to know their family background so they could trace the lineage of Messiah when He finally came.

Why is the book called "1 Chronicles"?

Originally 1 and 2 Chronicles were one continuous book in the Hebrew scroll. The title meant "the words of the days," which became its title. Eventually, because of the extra space required for the Greek text, the books were separated when translated into Greek.

Who wrote 1 Chronicles?

Most conservatives believe that Ezra the priest was the author of the book. Ezra would have emphasized the temple, the priesthood, and the theocratic line of Messiah.

Who was Ezra?

He was an educated priest (Ezra 7:6) who led a group of priests back from the Babylonian captivity to reestablish the kingdom. The rabbis teach that Nehemiah brought back an extensive library that was available to Ezra for his use in writing the Chronicles.

Ezra refers to the writings of the prophets "Nathan and Gad" (1 Chron. 29:29), and in 2 Chronicles he mentions "the book of the kings of Judah" (2 Chron. 16:11), "the book of the kings of Israel" (2 Chron. 20:34), and "the book of the kings of Judah and Israel" (2 Chron. 25:26). He would have used these sources to write Chronicles. He also wrote the book of Ezra.

What are the key words in 1 Chronicles?

The key words are found in 1 Chronicles 17:14: "His [Messiah's] throne shall be established for evermore" (KJV).

What are the key verses in 1 Chronicles?

"And it shall be, when your days are fulfilled, when you must go to be with your fathers, that I will set up your seed after you, who will be of your sons; and I will establish his kingdom. He shall build Me a house, and I will establish his throne forever. I will be his Father, and he shall be My son; and I will not take My mercy away from him, as I took it from him who was before you. And I will establish him in My house and in My kingdom forever; and his throne shall be established forever" (1 Chron. 17:11–14).

QUESTIONS ABOUT
THE SECOND BOOK OF CHRONICLES

What is included in 2 Chronicles?

Second Chronicles parallels the material found in 1 and 2 Kings, but for the most part does not touch on the ten tribes of the Northern Kingdom because of its false Baal worship, its disobedience, and its ungodly ways. Perhaps the ten tribes are deemphasized because the northern tribes refused to acknowledge the temple in Jerusalem. Second Chronicles focuses on the temple and on the lives and reign of godly kings, such as David, Asa, Jehoshaphat, Joash, Hezekiah, and Josiah.

Who wrote 2 Chronicles?

Ezra is the author of 2 Chronicles. The closing verses of 2 Chronicles (36:22–23) are almost the same as the opening verses of Ezra (1:1–3). Ezra also wrote 1 Chronicles.

What is the key word in 2 Chronicles?

The key word is *Judah*. This book describes what God was doing through the Southern Kingdom of Judah, more than the Northern Kingdom. This is because Judah had the temple, the priestly line, and the line of Messiah through David.

What is the key verse in 2 Chronicles?

"If My people who are called by My name will humble themselves, and pray and seek My face, and turn from their wicked ways, then I will hear from heaven, and will forgive their sin and heal their land" (2 Chron. 7:14).

What was the amazing prophecy about the length of time God's people would be in the Babylonian captivity (seventy years)?

God had said that He would allow the land to rest for the time that Israel had not observed the Sabbath. Since Israel was in the land for 490 years, they had not observed the Sabbath for an accumulation of seventy years. "And those who escaped from the sword he carried away to Babylon, where they became servants to him and his sons until the rule of the kingdom of Persia, to fulfill the word of the LORD by the mouth of Jeremiah, until the land had enjoyed her Sabbaths. As long as she lay desolate she kept Sabbath, to fulfill seventy years" (2 Chron. 36:20–21).

QUESTIONS ABOUT
THE BOOK OF EZRA

What is the key word in Ezra?
The key word is *temple*, or the house of the Lord.

What is the key verse in Ezra?
"Who is among you of all His people? May his God be with him, and let him go up to Jerusalem which is in Judah, and build the house of the LORD God of Israel (He is God), which is in Jerusalem" (Ezra 1:3).

Who wrote the book of Ezra?
Ezra, the priest who came out of the Babylonian exile, wrote the book of Ezra around 438–433 B.C.

What is the book of Ezra about?
It describes the people who came from Babylon out of exile, about fifty thousand people with Zerubbabel, and about two thousand with Ezra. The book encouraged those who returned to the promised land to be faithful to the Lord, to restore temple worship, and to record the genealogical line that would lead to Messiah.

What motivated the decision to allow Israel to return from the Babylonian captivity?
After Cyrus of Medo-Persia captured the city of Babylon in 539 B.C., he signed a decree to send God's people back to the promised land. While God's people were in Babylon, they were a slave nation who needed food, housing, and clothing. But by returning to the land, they could work or pay taxes to Medo-Persia. Cyrus wanted Israel to resettle the promised land and become prosperous so he could tax them and make money off of them. So he sent Israel back to their land (Isa. 45:1).

What did the Jews do when they returned to the promised land?
First, an altar was built and the sacrificial system was reestablished (Ezra 3:1–3). Next, they observed the Feast of Tabernacles (Ezra 3:4). They then began work on the temple (Ezra 3:10), with a special ceremony when the foundation was laid (Ezra 3:10–13).

Why was the temple not built immediately?

Those who opposed Israel told lies to the king of Medo-Persia about the intentions of Israel. Immediately the work stopped on the temple (Ezra 4:18–24).

What happened to get the temple rebuilt?

The prophets Haggai and Zechariah began their preaching ministry sixteen years later, challenging the people to rebuild the temple. The new Persian king, Darius the Great, took interest in the work and ordered the temple to be completed. Darius even paid for the supplies to rebuild the temple (Ezra 6:1–12).

Did all Israel return to the land?

All Jews were encouraged to leave captivity, but many did not come back to the land because they had jobs, businesses, and children in Babylon. Instead they gave offerings to help support those who were returning to rebuild the temple (Ezra 7:11ff).

QUESTIONS ABOUT
THE BOOK OF NEHEMIAH

Who was Nehemiah?

He was the cupbearer to Artaxerxes, the king of Persia (Neh. 1:11).

Who wrote the book of Nehemiah?

Originally, the books of Ezra and Nehemiah were considered one book, and since Ezra was a contemporary of Nehemiah in postexilic Jerusalem, and there was much common ministry between the two, most think Ezra the scribe actually wrote Nehemiah. Others think Ezra wrote the first chapters and see strong internal evidence that Nehemiah wrote the rest of the book.

What is the key word in Nehemiah?

Walls. The key to this book was rebuilding the walls. The enemies who opposed the rebuilding of the walls knew the walls stood for national identity and purpose. The temple had been rebuilt, but the Jews did not consider their nation reestablished until the walls of their capital city of Jerusalem were rebuilt.

What are the key verses in Nehemiah?
"So the wall was finished on the twenty-fifth day of Elul, in fifty-two days. And it happened, when all our enemies heard of it, and all the nations around us saw these things, that they were very disheartened in their own eyes; for they perceived that this work was done by our God" (Neh. 6:15–16).

What was a "cupbearer"?
This was a high office that meant Nehemiah was favored by the king. The cupbearer was a protector of the king (to make sure he wasn't poisoned), as well as a confidant and adviser to the king.

What was Nehemiah's great burden?
As a Jew, Nehemiah was greatly concerned about the reestablishment of Jerusalem and the temple, specifically, rebuilding the walls that had been torn down.

Who was the Persian king?
Most Bible scholars believe he was Artaxerxes (the preface *arta* means he was the son of the great King Xerxes known for invading Greece).

What was Nehemiah's request of the king?
Nehemiah wanted the king to send him to rebuild the walls of Jerusalem.

How did the king answer Nehemiah's request?
Nehemiah was sent to lead the effort to rebuild the walls. Nehemiah had a royal decree that allowed him access to resources, supplies, and protection from the Persian Empire. Implied in the decree, Nehemiah was to be the royal governor of Jerusalem.

What was the reaction to Nehemiah's efforts by the nations surrounding Jerusalem?
They were angry because they distrusted the Jews, and felt that if Jerusalem were rebuilt, then the Jews would strengthen themselves to attack them.

Therefore, they undermined Nehemiah's leadership and sent conflicting reports to the king regarding Nehemiah's intentions.

What was the response of the Jews in Jerusalem?

Nehemiah was able to rally the Jerusalem residents to work on the walls. They said, "Let us rise up and build" (Neh. 2:18).

What was Nehemiah's tactic in rallying the people to rebuild the walls?

Each person was to rebuild the part of the walls in front of his own home, thus guaranteeing that the wall would be built strong and beautiful. By delegating the work to many people and involving many people the walls were rebuilt in fifty-two days.

What other problems did Nehemiah face in Jerusalem?

The rich Jews in Jerusalem were charging excessive interest for loans given to the poor (this is called *usury*). When Nehemiah confronted the leaders concerning their greed, they responded immediately to Nehemiah's request. Nehemiah demonstrated his support by not receiving his own allowance (salary) as royal governor. This was his way of relieving the poor of an additional tax burden.

Why is the genealogy of Israel in the book of Nehemiah so important?

The genealogy ties the line of Messiah from Abraham through the kings of Judah to the line of Jews who returned from the Babylonian captivity. This guarantees that the promise made to Abraham (Gen. 12:1–3) would be fulfilled in the Messiah, who was Jesus Christ (Luke 1:30–33).

QUESTIONS ABOUT
THE BOOK OF ESTHER

Who was Esther?

Esther was a young Jewish lady living in Persia. She was the cousin of Mordecai. Apparently Mordecai adopted Esther at the death of her parents (Est. 2:5–7). This may be why he is called "uncle" at times.

Esther entered a contest to determine who would be the next queen of Persia. She won and was crowned queen. In this position, Esther was able to deliver the Jews from a potential holocaust.

What is the key word in Esther?

Hidden. The name Esther means *star* or *myrtle*, both are hidden at times. A star can't be seen in daylight, and the myrtle flower hides under its leaves. In this book the providence of God is seen, but the name "God" is not mentioned, suggesting God is hidden. God's hand is seen by His people, but hidden from their enemies.

What is the key verse in Esther?

"For if you remain completely silent at this time, relief and deliverance will arise for the Jews from another place, but you and your father's house will perish. Yet who knows whether you have come to the kingdom for such a time as this?" (Est. 4:14).

Who was Ahasuerus?

Most Bible scholars believe he was Xerxes the Great, the king of Persia, known in secular history for his attempted invasion of Greece.

How did Esther become queen?

Xerxes' former wife had embarrassed him publicly, and after his failed invasion of Greece, he divorced her. Then in a national contest, Esther was chosen as queen and was taken into the palace (Est. 1:9–2:17).

Who was Mordecai?

Mordecai was a Jew who had an office in the king's palace, usually considered a lesser office. As the cousin of Esther, he was vitally interested in her becoming the next queen. When she assumed the position, he became her adviser and counselor.

Who was Haman?

Haman was the prime minister who directed the affairs of the kingdom for Xerxes. He was a descendent of Agag, King of Amalek. This is the nation that Saul was told to destroy but in disobedience did not obey the Lord.

Historically, the Amalekites were hated opponents of Israel since Genesis 21. Haman attempted to exterminate the Jews.

What fueled Haman's hatred of the Jews?
Mordecai was the only man who would not reverence and bow down to him (Est. 3:2–6).

How did Haman attempt to retaliate against the Jews?
He negotiated for the king to sign an edict declaring that anyone who destroyed or killed a Jew could keep his property and/or wealth.

How did Esther save the Jewish nation?
When Mordecai heard about the plot, he convinced Esther that she had to go to the king to solve the problem. Esther asked the Jews to fast and pray for three days. She then approached the king. This was especially dangerous because anyone approaching the king unsummoned could be put to death unless the king overruled the punishment. The king welcomed Esther. Esther invited King Xerxes and Haman to a meal at her house. It was there that the problem was eventually solved.

How did the sovereignty of God intervene by saving the Jews from a holocaust?
After the meal in Esther's home, King Xerxes could not sleep that night, and had a history of his reign read to him. There he found out that Mordecai had saved his life from an assassination attempt. The following day King Xerxes told Haman to honor Mordecai in front of all of the people in the capital city. This was especially degrading because Haman was planning to execute Mordecai. Esther held a second feast for King Xerxes and Haman. It was there that she petitioned the king to be delivered from the intended holocaust against the Jews.

How did Esther actually deliver the Jews?
When King Xerxes heard that Haman had conceived the plot against the Jews, he left the room in a rage. Haman fell at Esther's feet, begging for mercy. When the king returned, he thought Haman was making sexual advances on the queen and had Haman executed.

According to the law of the Medes and Persians, the king's edict for a Jewish holocaust could not be overturned. So Esther suggested a second edict that each Jew could defend himself and in so doing, take the property of those who attacked the Jews (Est. 8:9–11).

What great feast grew out of the book of Esther?
The feast of Purim (Est. 9:26) became a permanent celebration day for Israel. The name *Purim* came from *Pur*, or "the lot," referring to the time of destroying Jews. In gratitude, the Jewish nation still celebrates this feast.

QUESTIONS ABOUT THE POETIC BOOKS

JOB, PSALMS, PROVERBS,

ECCLESIASTES, SONG OF SOLOMON

QUESTIONS ABOUT THE BOOK OF JOB

Who was Job?

Job was an early patriarch who probably lived during the times of Abraham. He lived in the land of Uz (Job 1:1), which was either in Saudi Arabia or the Sinai Peninsula, south of the promised land.

Who wrote the book of Job?

Most people think that Job wrote it; however, a few people think that it was Elihu, one of Job's comforters. Some also think Moses talked to Job when he was exiled on the Sinai Peninsula, and that afterward Moses wrote the book.

When was Job written?

It was probably written before 1400 B.C. because there was no reference to Moses, the Law, or the sacrificial system. Also, the earlier title for God, "the Almighty," was the primary title used to describe God in the book of Job. There is very little emphasis on the other personal names of Jehovah in Job. Further, life spans mentioned in Job were long, which put Job closer to the Flood than to a later period. Finally, families were still governed by clan leadership, that is, patriarchal leadership, as Job demonstrated over his family.

What is the key word in Job?

The key word is the *Almighty*, the main name for God in the book of Job.

What are the key verses in Job?

"Behold, happy is the man whom God corrects; therefore do not despise the chastening of the Almighty" (Job 5:17). "Man who is born of woman is of few days and full of trouble" (Job 14:1).

What lessons can we learn from Job?

First, Satan can only touch a believer by the permission of God. Second, God is greater than our problems, even our physical problems. Third, our problems are not eternal but are limited by time and space. And finally, all of our problems are small in relationship to the loss of family and health.

How was Job restored after his trials?

First, the Lord accepted Job (42:9); then he was told to pray for his friends (Job 42:10). God gave him twice as much as he had before (Job 42:10, 12). He was seventy years old when the trial began, and he lived another 140 years. He was 210 years old when he died.

QUESTIONS ABOUT
THE BOOK OF PSALMS

What does the name *Psalms* mean?

It comes from the Hebrew word *tehillim*, which means "praise." The Greeks called the book of Psalms "the Psalter," which was also a musical instrument.

Who wrote the psalms?

There were several authors: David, Moses, Solomon, Asap, Hemon, Ethan, and the sons of Korah.

What is the key word in Psalms?

The key word in Psalms is *Praise*.

What are the key verses in Psalms?

Praise the LORD!

Praise God in His sanctuary;
Praise Him in His mighty firmament!
Praise Him for His mighty acts;
Praise Him according to His excellent greatness!
Praise Him with the sound of the trumpet;
Praise Him with the lute and harp!
Praise Him with the timbrel and dance;
Praise Him with stringed instruments and flutes!
Praise Him with loud cymbals;
Praise Him with clashing cymbals!
Let everything that has breath praise the LORD.
Praise the LORD! (Ps. 150:1–6)

What type of poetry is in the book of Psalms?

Some psalms are written in *synonymous parallels*, which means there are rhyming thoughts or dual ideas: "But his delight is in the law of the LORD, and in His law he meditates day and night" (Ps. 1:2). Other psalms are written in *antithetic parallels*, which put forth contrasting ideas such as, "The LORD knows the way of the righteous, but the way of the ungodly shall perish" (Ps. 1:6). Some psalms are *synthetic parallels*, which means a thought is progressively developed: "Blessed is the man who walks not in the counsel of the ungodly, nor stands in the path of sinners, nor sits in the seat of the scornful" (Ps. 1:1). Finally, there is *exemplar poetry*, poetry written as an exhortation: "Let the redeemed of the LORD say so, whom He has redeemed from the hand of the enemy" (Ps. 107:2).

What was the Megilloth?

These were five scrolls of Scripture that were read at certain feasts in the year. Song of Solomon was read at Passover; Ruth was read at Pentecost; Lamentations was read at the Feast of Ab; Ecclesiastes was read at the Feast of Tabernacles; and Esther was read at the feast of Purim.

How is the book of Psalms organized?

The ancient Jewish rabbis saw an outline in Psalms that parallels the message of the first five books of the Bible. Psalms 1–41 parallel Genesis; Psalms 42–72 parallel Exodus; Psalms 73–89 parallel Leviticus; Psalms 90–106 parallel Numbers; and Psalms 107–150 parallel Deuteronomy.

Why are the last five psalms called the "Hallelujah Psalms"?
(Psalms 146–150)
These are refered to as the "Hallelujah Psalms" because each Psalm both begins and ends with the word *Hallelujah*.

What do the various musical terms mean that are in the Psalms?
The term *chief musician,* which means "choir leader," occurs fifty times. The term *sons of Korah* occurs ten times. These sons of Korah were authors. The word *jedutham* occurs three times and meant a "guild of musicians." The word *neginot* occurs seven times and was a stringed instrument. Finally, the word *selah* occurs seventy-one times and means "lift up" or "be silent." In modern-day terminology it meant to stop singing and think about the message of the psalm.

QUESTIONS ABOUT
THE BOOK OF PROVERBS

Who wrote the book of Proverbs?
King Solomon is the author of the book of Proverbs: "The Proverbs of Solomon the son of David, king of Israel" (Prov. 1:1). This is supported by 1 Kings 4:32, which suggests that Solomon wrote three thousand proverbs. Agur wrote Proverb 30 and King Lemuel wrote Proverb 31 (though King Lemuel could be Solomon).

When did Solomon write Proverbs?
He was probably in his thirties. By this time he had demonstrated his wisdom, and his kingdom was one of the most powerful nations in the Near East. Therefore, his rule gave credibility to the wisdom that he wrote in Proverbs.

What is the key word in Proverbs?
The key word is *wisdom.* The word *wisdom* means more than being smart. Biblical wisdom is moral discernment, mental clarity, perception, and the discipline to do what you know to do.

What are the key verses in Proverbs?
"A wise man will hear and increase learning, and a man of understanding will attain wise counsel, to understand a proverb and an enigma, the words of the

wise and their riddles. The fear of the LORD is the beginning of knowledge, but fools despise wisdom and instruction" (Prov. 1:5–7).

What is a *proverb*?

A *proverb* is a summary statement of great universal truth expressed in simple thought. In American terms a proverb is like, "An apple a day keeps the doctor away." In Near East thought, "As cold water to a weary soul, so is good news from a far country" (Prov. 25:25).

What is the theme of Proverbs?

The book of Proverbs has no history, no emphasis of the law, no theory, and no explanation or presentation of theology (no systematic presentation of doctrine). It is a book that emphasizes practical application of the law; lessons learned from life; principles to guide everyday life; and reverence for God, respect for parents, and regard for the law.

QUESTIONS ABOUT THE BOOK OF ECCLESIASTES

What does *Ecclesiastes* mean?

Ecclesiastes is from the Greek word that means "convener" of an assembly. The book is often referred to by its Hebrew name, *qoheleth*, which means "preacher." The book of Ecclesiastes is an address or sermon by a speaker or preacher, that is, Solomon.

Who wrote Ecclesiastes?

Solomon wrote Ecclesiastes as an elderly man, past age forty, after he had accumulated wives and drifted away from God. The book reflects his frustration, sin, and emptiness. It is even a pessimistic book: "'Vanity of vanities,' says the Preacher; 'Vanity of vanities, all is vanity'" (Eccl. 1:2).

What is the key word in Ecclesiastes?

The key word is *vanity*, reflecting how empty Solomon's life had become because he didn't make God his first priority. The word *vanity* appears thirty-seven times.

What is the key phrase in Ecclesiastes?
The key phrase is "life under the sun" which occurs twenty-nine times. It means life is filled with injustice, dangers, uncertainties, and "chance."

What are the key verses in Ecclesiastes?
"And I set my heart to seek and search out by wisdom concerning all that is done under heaven; this burdensome task God has given to the sons of man, by which they may be exercised. I have seen all the works that are done under the sun; and indeed, all is vanity and grasping for the wind" (Eccl. 1:13–14).

What is the theme of Ecclesiastes?
The theme is "All is vanity." *Vanity* does not just mean selfish pride, as Americans use the word, but the emptiness of life apart from God.

What is the final admonition in Ecclesiastes?
"Fear God and keep His commandments" (Eccl. 12:13).

QUESTIONS ABOUT
THE SONG OF SOLOMON

What is the meaning of the "Song of Solomon"?
The title "Song of Solomon" identifies the book was written by Solomon. However, the Hebrew title is *shir hash-shiam*, which means "Song of songs" or "the best song of all."

Who wrote the Song of Solomon?
Solomon wrote it, *circa* 791 B.C. in his youth, before he fell into sin with his countless wives. Solomon wrote about the pure love he experienced as a young shepherd, perhaps before he was anointed king of Israel.

What is the key word in the Song of Solomon?
The key word is *love*.

What is the key verse in the Song of Solomon?
"I charge you, O daughters of Jerusalem, by the gazelles or by the does of the

field, do not stir up nor awaken love until it pleases" (Song 2:7). This verse could be interpreted by an expanded translation: "Stir not, nor awaken your passion for love, until you are the proper age or at the proper time."

What is the development of the story in the Song of Solomon?

The book begins as Solomon, one of the many sons of David, keeps sheep out in the pastures. He meets a young girl who is forced by her family to work in the vineyard. She falls in love with young Solomon, who promises to return for her and marry her. Solomon is taken from her (to become king), and she dreams about him in his absence. While Solomon is gone, the family criticizes her, saying she will never marry Solomon. Solomon returns as king to take her as his bride-queen. After he returns, the girl's family praises her for her beauty and virtue.

Is there a progression to love in the Song of Solomon?

First, the girl has the boy: "My beloved is mine, and I am his. He feeds his flock among the lilies" (Song 2:16). Second, the boy has the girl: "I am my beloved's, and my beloved is mine. He feeds his flock among the lilies" (Song 6:3). Third, they belong to each other: "I am my beloved's, and his desire is toward me" (Song 7:10).

What are the internal problems with the Song of Solomon?

First, there is sexually explicit language that creates mental pictures about sexual activities so that it cannot be used in mixed-age church settings. Second, Jesus never quoted from this book, and early-church fathers rarely quoted from it.

Who are the characters of the book?

First, there is the groom, who is Solomon. Second, there is the bride, who is a young Shulamite, a Gentile (a picture of the type of Christ). Third, there are the "daughters" of the bride, who are her friends and observers. There are also watchmen who keep the city, who are the men she sees in her dream. Finally, there is the mother of the groom, Bathsheba.

QUESTIONS
ABOUT
THE MAJOR PROPHETS

ISAIAH, JEREMIAH,
LAMENTATIONS, EZEKIEL, DANIEL

DANIEL

QUESTIONS ABOUT
THE BOOK OF ISAIAH

Who wrote the book of Isaiah?

Isaiah, a member of the king's court, was called by God to be a prophet and to deliver a message to the nation of Israel (chapter 6). Isaiah's name means *yeshuyahu*, "The Lord is Salvation." His ministry covered the reigns of Uzziah, Jotham, Ahaz, and Hezekiah.

What is the key word in Isaiah?

The key word is *salvation*, which occurs twenty-six times in the book, but only six times in all the other prophets. Even Isaiah's name means "Salvation is of the Lord," reflecting the key word.

What are the key verses in Isaiah?

For unto us a Child is born,
Unto us a Son is given;
And the government will be upon His shoulder.
And His name will be called
Wonderful, Counselor, Mighty God,
Everlasting Father, Prince of Peace.
Of the increase of His government and peace
There will be no end,
Upon the throne of David and over His kingdom,
To order it and establish it with judgment and justice
From that time forward, even forever.
The zeal of the LORD of hosts will perform this." (Isa. 9:6–7)

What are the major characteristics of Isaiah?

Isaiah is called the "prince of prophets," and demonstrates that the spiritual can influence the political. He emphasized personal redemption of individuals, while most of the other prophets emphasized national repentance and judgment.

Why do certain liberal scholars say that there are two Isaiahs?

The book of Isaiah is divided into two sections: Chapters 1–39 emphasize the enemy Assyria, and chapters 40–66 warn about the coming Babylonian captivity. Those who deny the authorship of Isaiah say the first Isaiah wrote the first thirty-nine chapters, and a second Isaiah wrote chapters 46–66. They say the predictions of chapters 40–66 couldn't be known by the first human writer, so the liberals say the second Isaiah wrote after the Babylonian captivity occurred. Because liberals deny the supernatural, they have to explain away the predictions of the future.

What proof is there that there was only one Isaiah?

Throughout the book there is one primary title given to God: "the Holy One of Israel." It occurs in both the first and second sections and reflects the unity of the book. The New Testament writers quoted both sections and credited both to Isaiah. Jesus Himself quoted both sections of the book and attributed them to Isaiah. If Jesus had made a mistake, then he could not be equal with God, or be God, because God is onmiscient (all-knowing), incapable of making a mistake.

Further, when Isaiah describes vegetation and geography, he is describing Palestine in both sections, not Babylon, where the liberals say the second part of Isaiah was written. Finally, when the Dead Sea Scrolls were discovered, there was no break in the book of Isaiah between the first and second half; if anything, the break occurred in the middle of a line in the middle of the page. There wasn't even a paragraph break. Hence, those who study Isaiah carefully treat it as one book by one author.

How was Isaiah called?

In Isaiah 6, Isaiah saw the Lord "high and lifted up" (v. 1), probably while mourning the death of King Uzziah. Uzziah had been a good king until the very last when he committed an act of defiance against God and was judged with leprosy. However, King Uzziah had been a strong king who built forts and walls, established a great army, and increased national pride. The nation prospered under Uzziah. Apparently Isaiah was looking to a human leader for deliverance and protection of the nation of Israel, but God wanted Isaiah to see that the Lord was the Deliverer and Protector of Israel. God instructed Isaiah to warn the nation that they would be destroyed and taken into captivity because of their sin, though his message would be rejected, even when he warned the people of the future (Isa. 6).

What archaeological verification is there for the events of Isaiah?

Sennacherib, king of Assyria (705–681 B.C.), captured all of the surrounding nations, plus forty-six cities in Judah. He surrounded the city of Jerusalem and demanded its surrender. Archaeologists have found the chronicle of Sennacherib, which says, "I shut up [King] Hezekiah like a caged bird within his royal capital." This story is found in Isaiah 36–37. As God predicted, Sennacherib fled Judah upon report of an impending invasion from a Thirhakah Ethiopian ruling pharaoh of Egypt's twenty-fifth dynasty.

Why is Hezekiah's sickness out of chronological order?

The sickness of Hezekiah (chapters 38–39) was deliberately out of chronological order because it was the introduction of Babylon, which is the theme of the last part of the book (chapters 40–66). Before Assyria invaded Judah,

Hezekiah was sick, but God gave him an additional fifteen years to live. Why? Because in that additional fifteen years, God used Hezekiah to deliver Israel from Assyria and to have a son. If Hezekiah had died without a physical son, the physical line to the Messiah—Jesus Christ—would have been cut off.

Why did God miraculously extend Hezekiah's life?
First, because Hezekiah became the human instrument to deliver Israel from Assyria. Second, because he did not yet have a male heir. Without a male heir, the physical line to Messiah would have been cut off.

What happened when Hezekiah's life was extended?
The Bible describes the "shadow on the sundial" (Isa. 38:8), the steps of the sundial reversing ten degrees. Some believe God reversed the spin of the earth on its axis to give him additional time. Others believe God caused the earth to stop spinning on its axis, or that He did it another way that we don't understand. Still others believe that "the sundial going backwards" was only symbolic language that meant that God was going to give him an additional fifteen years of life, as if the sundial went backwards.

What was Hezekiah's great sin?
After Hezekiah was healed of his sickness, the king of Babylon sent him a letter (a "get-well card") to congratulate his recovery. Hezekiah then showed the Babylonians who brought the message to him his entire treasure house. Because of his bragging and pride (Isa. 39:2), God sent Hezekiah a message, saying, "All [Israel] shall be carried to Babylon" (Isa. 39:6–7).

What are some of the prophecies about Jesus Christ in Isaiah?
Isaiah predicted that:
- Jesus would be born of a virgin (Isa. 7:14)
- a Child-King would come to rule over Israel (Isa. 9:6)
- a "Rod" (this phrase is translated "Branch," which is a sprig that grows on a cut-down tree stump) would come forth from the stem of Jesse (Isa. 11:1)
- after the nation was chopped down (became the tree stump), a Sprig, or Branch, (the Messiah) would grow out of the roots (Isa. 11:1)
- the Branch would be God (Isa. 4:2)

- Jesus would be an ensign to the Gentiles (Isa. 11:10)
- Christ would have victory at Armageddon (Isa. 34:2–6)
- a forerunner would come to prepare the way of Messiah (Isa. 40:3)
- Jesus would be the Servant of the Lord (Isa. 42:1–4), the Redeemer of Israel (Isa. 44:6), the Light to the Gentiles (Isa. 49:6), and the suffering Servant (Isa. 52:13–53:12)
- Messiah would be a preacher (Isa. 61:1–2) and the coming King (Isa. 65:15–18)

QUESTIONS ABOUT THE BOOK OF JEREMIAH

Who wrote the book of Jeremiah?

Jeremiah authored the book. He is called the "weeping prophet" because he weeps over the message of judgment that he wrote in this book.

When did Jeremiah minister?

Jeremiah ministered during the reigns of the last four kings of Judah (626–586 B.C.).

What are the key words in Jeremiah?

The key words are *the word of the Lord*, which constantly came to Jeremiah.

What are the key verses in Jeremiah?

"But this is what I commanded them, saying, 'Obey My voice, and I will be your God, and you shall be My people. And walk in all the ways that I have commanded you, that it may be well with you.' Yet they did not obey or incline their ear, but followed the counsels and the dictates of their evil hearts, and went backward and not forward" (Jer. 7:23–24).

What was the message of Jeremiah?

He gave the final warning of the coming captivity by Babylon, even though the people to whom he spoke were still fearful of Egypt or Assyria. Israel couldn't believe God meant that Babylon (a small nation at the time) could capture Israel.

What was happening in the world when Jeremiah ministered?

Judah had been captured by Egypt and paid taxes to Pharaoh-Necho. When Egypt attacked Babylon, Nebuchadnezzar defeated Necho at the battle of Carchemis in 605 B.C., in one of the great battles that became a turning point of history. Almost immediately, Nebuchadnezzar invaded Judah, received "spoils" from Jerusalem, and took the first captives of God's people from Judah back to Babylon. Daniel went to Babylon at this time.

What did Jeremiah predict?

Jeremiah said that Israel would spend seventy years in captivity in Babylon, and at the end of that time, the nation of Israel would return to the land and reestablish the kingdom. But the Jewish people did not believe Jeremiah or his predictions that Babylon would capture them because they thought Jerusalem was invincible.

What was the reaction of Judah's kings to Jeremiah's preaching?

King Jehoiakim branded Jeremiah a traitor. Later, King Zedekiah, an evil king, privately consulted with Jeremiah, then put him in prison, keeping him in a slime pit.

How accurate were Jeremiah's prophecies?

Nebuchadnezzar encamped about Jerusalem and destroyed the city in 586 B.C., demolishing the walls, the temple, and the entire city. The book of Lamentations was an eyewitness account by Jeremiah as he lamented the destructive siege that lasted almost ten months.

What happened to Jeremiah after the destruction of Jerusalem?

Nebuchadnezzar told his army to release Jeremiah and take him back to Babylon and to freedom because of his positive prophecies about Babylon. Jeremiah refused to go because he wanted to remain with the Jewish remnant in Jerusalem. But the Jewish remnant forced Jeremiah to go with them to Egypt. At Tahpanhes (a fortress city in the Nile River delta) the Jews built "another temple" that included animal sacrifices. Jeremiah died in Egypt.

How authentic is the book of Jeremiah?

Archaeologists have found the Lachish letters written on ostraca (broken pottery) in 588–586 B.C. that accurately reflect the events and culture that Jeremiah describes in his book. Also, Jesus quoted Jeremiah, treating him as an author and a historical person. Finally, other New Testament writers quoted Jeremiah as an authority.

QUESTIONS ABOUT
THE BOOK OF LAMENTATIONS

Who wrote Lamentations?
Jeremiah wrote the Lamentations as an eyewitness account of the city of Jerusalem being destroyed by Nebuchadnezzar in 586 B.C. This book is a *lament* over the destruction of Jerusalem.

What is the key word in Lamentations?
The key word is *weep(ing)*, because this is how Jeremiah and the people expressed their lament for Jerusalem.

What are the key verses in Lamentations?
The Lord was like an enemy.
He has swallowed up Israel,
He has swallowed up all her palaces;
He has destroyed her strongholds,
And has increased mourning and lamentation
In the daughter of Judah.
He has done violence to His tabernacle,
As if it were a garden;
He has destroyed His place of assembly;
The LORD has caused
The appointed feasts and Sabbaths to be forgotten in Zion.
In His burning indignation He has spurned the king and the priest.
(Lam 2:5–6)

What is the significance of Lamentations?
Even though it is an eyewitness account of Jeremiah, it shows the love that God has for the city of Jerusalem, and His sorrow at its destruction.

Why did God destroy the city?
"Jerusalem has sinned gravely" (Lam. 1:8). God chastened His people because of their transgressions, and each of the five chapters is a different "lament" over Israel's fall.

QUESTIONS ABOUT
THE BOOK OF EZEKIEL

Who wrote Ezekiel?
Ezekiel was a priest who was called to be a prophet (Ezek. 1:1ff). He was taken into Babylonian captivity in 597 B.C. (the second wave of captivities by Nebuchadnezzar), where he wrote to explain why Israel was in captivity and what future plans God had for the nation.

Where did Ezekiel write his book?
He wrote his book from Babylon after he arrived in captivity. It is highly autobiographical, referring to himself as "son of man" approximately eighty times. This title suggests Ezekiel is the "representative man." It was a title used by Jesus to identify Himself with humanity.

What are the key issues in Ezekiel?
Ezekiel emphasizes the temple and the Shekinah-glory cloud that rested upon the temple, which was God's presence. Ezekiel describes the departure of God's glory because of Israel's sin, and the return of God's glory in the future kingdom.

What is the key word in Ezekiel?
The key word is *restoration*. God will restore Israel to her promised land.

What are the key verses in Ezekiel?
"For I will take you from among the nations, gather you out of all countries, and bring you into your own land. Then I will sprinkle clean water on you, and you shall be clean; I will cleanse you from all your filthiness and from all your idols. I will give you a new heart and put a new spirit within you; I will take the heart of stone out of your flesh and give you a heart of flesh" (Ezek 36:24–26).

How did Ezekiel see the temple of God while he was still in Babylon?

Some teach that Ezekiel wrote while in a prophetic trance because he had a vision of what was happening in the house of God (Ezek. 8:1). Others teach that he was taken physically by the Spirit to Jerusalem where he witnessed the sins in the temple as they were being committed.

What did Ezekiel see in the temple?

He saw an idol of jealousy (Babylonian) in the temple (Ezek. 8:5). He also saw figures of Canaanite idols drawn on the temple walls (Ezek. 8:10). He saw women weeping for the Assyrian God, Tammuz (Ezek. 8:14), and he saw twenty-five men worshiping the Egyptian sun God, Re (Ezek. 8:16).

What was God's response to the idolatry in the temple?

Ezekiel saw the Shekinah-glory cloud lift up from above the ark of the covenant (Ezek. 9:3). The cloud lifted above the Holy of Holies (Ezek. 10:4). It then lifted higher above the temple (Ezek. 10:18), and finally it tarried momentarily over the Mount of Olives (Ezek. 11:23). Eventually God's glory left, and it will not return until the future kingdom is established.

What were Ezekiel's main prophetic predictions?

Ezekiel predicted the coming millennial kingdom, the return of Israel to the land, and the rebuilding of the millennial temple.

Why will God have the temple rebuilt in the coming Millennium?

The millennial temple will demonstrate God's holiness, provide a dwelling place for His divine glory, and perpetuate the animal sacrifices, which will be memorials in nature. The temple will be the center of divine government, and water will flow out of the temple that will heal the land (Ezek. 47:1–12).

Since Christ has done away with sacrifices, why will there be animal sacrifices in the future?

The sacrifices will have nothing to do with forgiveness of sin, but will be memorial in nature, such as the memorial nature of the Lord's Table that is celebrated today.

QUESTIONS ABOUT
THE BOOK OF DANIEL

Who wrote the book of Daniel?

A young man named Daniel was carried into captivity in Babylon at age fifteen (605 B.C.) and lived there the entire time Israel was in captivity. He had an extended ministry late in life under the Medo-Persian Empire.

What are the key words in Daniel?

The key words are *Most High,* the name for God used by Gentiles to designate His rulership over the world. God's program no longer focuses on Israel in the promised land, but with "the Gentiles," until a future date when the Davidic kingdom will be established.

What are the key verses in Daniel?

Daniel answered and said:
"Blessed be the name of God forever and ever,
For wisdom and might are His.
And He changes the times and the seasons;
He removes kings and raises up kings;
He gives wisdom to the wise
And knowledge to those who have understanding.
He reveals deep and secret things;
He knows what is in the darkness,
And light dwells with Him." (Dan 2:20–22)

Why are some scholars critical of the book of Daniel?

Daniel predicted the coming four world empires that conquered the known Western world: (1) Babylon, (2) Media-Persia, (3) Greece, and (4) Rome. The accuracy of these supernatural prophecies demands that readers accept the Scriptures as a revelation from God. Since God demands all people to repent and believe, many would rather deny the supernatural nature of the Bible because it demands they change their lifestyles.

How have critics tried to deny the book of Daniel?

Some say it is only literary fiction. Others say it is written by an unknown author and has no reliability. Still others say it was written in the first century A.D., and is therefore not prophetic in nature, but only an historical account of the past four world empires. Some critics reject the book of Daniel because the Old Testament Jews did not place the book with the prophets, but included it in the scroll with the historical section. Finally, some rejected it because the book of Daniel was written in both Chaldean and Hebrew. Many zealous Jews reject anything other than the Hebrew language.

What arguments prove the historical Daniel?

First, the Dead Sea Scrolls demonstrate that the book was written before the second, third, and fourth world empires ruled the known world. (Some Dead Sea scrolls were written during the Media-Persian rule of the world, and they included the book of Daniel.) Also, Jesus recognized Daniel as both a prophet and an author. But primarily, the early Jewish writers placed Daniel in the Hebrew Canon, as did both Josephus and the Septuagint.

How was Daniel's life parallel to Joseph's?

Both Daniel and Joseph had no recorded sin, both ministered to Gentile nations, both influenced political leaders of their day, and both were faithful to moral purity. Both interpreted dreams for Gentile rulers. Both arose from obscurity to national recognition.

Why did Daniel refuse to eat from the king's table? (Dan. 1:8)

Perhaps the meat was unclean according to Old Testament law, or perhaps the meat had been offered to idols and Daniel didn't want to eat anything offered to idols. Some even feel that the wine was intoxicating, and Daniel wasn't going to stupefy his mind.

Who was Nebuchadnezzar?

Nebuchadnezzar was the son and successor of King Nabopolassar of Babylon, who delivered his nation from its dependence on Assyria. He was the greatest and most powerful of all the Babylonian kings. He married the daughter of Cyaxares, and thus, the Median and Babylonian empires were united.

Nebuchadnezzar defeated Pharaoh Necho, the Egyptian king, at Carchemish during the fourth year of Jehoiakim's reign in 605 B.C. (Jer. 46:2). This battle forever tilted the balance of power in the Near East world. Egypt never again became a world power. Out of the victory, Nebuchadnezzar became the first world ruler (Daniel 1–4). After the victory at Carchemish, Nebuchadnezzar besieged Jerusalem, eventually carrying off many choice Jewish citizens to Babylon, including Ezekiel and the prophet Daniel (2 Kings 24:10–16). Judea's last three kings, Jehoiakim, Jehoiachin, and Zedekiah, were severely dealt with by Nebuchadnezzar. Finally, in 586 B.C., Jerusalem itself was destroyed by him (2 Kings 25). Nebuchadnezzar reigned as king of Babylon from 605 B.C. to 562 B.C., a period of forty-three years.

What was Nebuchadnezzar's dream?

He saw an image that was extremely tall. Its head was gold, arms and breast silver, thighs brass, legs iron, and feet were iron mixed with clay. The dream involved "latter days," a prediction of coming kingdoms (Dan. 2:28).

What was the interpretation of the dream?

The gold head stood for Nebuchadnezzar and the kingdom of Babylon, the silver arms and breast stood for the kingdom of Medo-Persia, the hips of brass stood for Greece, and the legs of iron stood for Rome.

What was so remarkable about Daniel's interpretation?

Daniel not only told the contents of the dream to Nebuchadnezzar, miraculous since its contents were a secret, but was faithful to also tell Nebuchadnezzar the meaning of his dream. As a result, Daniel and his three friends were promoted to greater offices in Babylon (Dan. 2:46–49).

What was the idol in chapter three?

The idol was an image that was ninety feet tall, made entirely of gold. Perhaps since Nebuchadnezzar didn't want his kingdom to come to an end, this was signifying his defiance and perpetuity. All who refused to worship the idol, a tribute to Nebuchadnezzar, were cast into a furnace of fire. Daniel's three friends, Shadrach, Meshach, and Abednego, were faced with a decision that involved life and death. His friends refused to worship the image and were cast into the fire but were delivered by God. Nebuchadnezzar saw a fourth person, a Christophany (Jesus Christ) in the fire.

How was Nebuchadnezzar converted in chapter four?

Nebuchadnezzar's pride was his downfall (Dan. 4:28–37). God judged him with a disease similar to modern-day lycanthropy, a psychiatric disorder that made him think and act like an animal. When Nebuchadnezzar came to his senses, he recognized the lordship of God over all and was converted (Dan. 4:1–3, 37).

Is there any historical evidence to substantiate this event?

In 576 B.C. Nebuchadnezzar had a mental breakdown, and his wife, Amyti, accompanied by the priest, kept Nebuchadnezzar's illness a secret, and hence, kept the kingdom intact. They ruled (secretly) in his place, even though certain military men tried to conquer the kingdom. After seven years of insanity in 569, Nebuchadnezzar was healed and the rule was returned to him. He died in 562 B.C.

How can we answer the critics' claim that there was no such person as Belshazzar?

Archaeologists have uncovered the Nadunidus Chronicle that included the name of a leader of Babylon named Belshazzar.

How did Belshazzar become king?

History says that Nebuchadnezzar married Amyti and had a daughter, Nitoeris, who married Nabonius, who became Nebuchadnezzar's son-in-law and ruler of the kingdom after Nebuchadnezzar. Nebuchadnezzar's own son, Belshazzar, was coregent with Nabonius, and technically the second ruler in the kingdom.

How could Medo-Persia defeat Babylon in one night?

Because of the immense fortifications around cities, it usually took several months or years to defeat a city, especially one as fortified as Babylon. However, the Medes and the Persians dug canals and diverted the water of the Euphrates River into the desert. Suddenly, when the river went dry during the night, soldiers from Media-Persia came under the wall in the riverbed into the heart of the city and captured it just as God predicted.

Who was Darius the Mede?

The critics claim there is no record of Darius the Mede, who ruled the city of Babylon after the collapse of the nation. However, this ruler was Gubaru, a man who had many names and titles. He was governor of Babylon under Cyrus.

Why was Daniel thrown to the lions? (Daniel 6)

A man was thrown into the lion's den to determine if he was guilty or innocent of an accused crime. It was trial by ordeal. God vindicated Daniel, because the lions didn't touch him. Those who accused Daniel were thrown in the pit and were immediately eaten by the lions, determining their guilt.

Why did Daniel not mention the Chinese, Aztecs, and so forth in his prediction of world empires?

Daniel did not mention these because God's key to world history is the Jews. Those nations that related to the Jews are mentioned in Daniel: Babylon, Media-Persia, Greece, and Rome.

Who was the nation depicted as the feet of iron and clay? (Dan. 2:33, 41–43)

This was probably the nation of Rome that will be revived in the end times.

Who are the ten nations symbolized by the ten toes? (Dan. 2:41–43)

Some feel they are the actual ten nations that originally made up Rome. Others feel they are European nations who have been transplanted around the world. Still others believe they are only a symbolic picture and could mean any nation existing at the time of the end.

Who are the four wild beasts prophesied in chapter seven?

The lion is Babylon, symbolic of royalty and great strength. The bear with its two sides is symbolic of the dual kingdoms of Media and Persia. The leopard with four heads is Greece. The four heads probably depicted the four sections of the Greek empire, which divided after the death of Alexander the Great (Antigonus ruled Syria, Ptolemy ruled Egypt, Lysimacus ruled Greece, and Cassander ruled Macedonia). The fourth beast is Rome with its ten horns, i.e., its ten nations.

Who are the two nations in chapter eight?

The ram with two horns pushing west is the empire of Medo-Persia trying to cross over to conquer Europe (Dan 8:1–4). The male goat from the west that won the battle was Alexander and the Greeks (Dan. 8:5–10).

What is Daniel's prophecy of seventy weeks?

Daniel realized the return of the Jews to the promised land was near when he read Jeremiah (Jer. 9:8–11). Jeremiah had predicted that the captivity would last seventy years. So Daniel began praying and getting ready for the return of God's people to the land of Israel when the seventy years were up. God told Daniel there would be seventy "weeks," or periods of time (Dan. 9:24) until Israel returned to the promised land. The Hebrew word for "week," is a period of time that could be longer than seven days; it could be seven years. Seventy weeks, when translated in seven-year periods of time, means that 490 years of Jewish history remained on the prophetic calendar before Israel would return to again live safely in the land.

Daniel predicted that there would be sixty-nine weeks, a total of 483 years, until Messiah would be "cut off" (the death of Jesus). The prophetic calendar would begin with "the decree to rebuild Jerusalem" (Dan. 9:25), the time when Artaxerxes allowed Nehemiah to rebuild the city walls in 454 B.C. Add 483 years to that date and the result is A.D. 29, the time when Jesus Christ died on Calvary.

A gap between the sixty-ninth and seventieth weeks starts with the death of Jesus, which is an unknown length of time. At the end of this gap, the "time of the Gentiles," God will finish the prophetic calendar by reintroducing the Seventieth Week (this is the seven years of the coming Tribulation).

QUESTIONS ABOUT THE MINOR PROPHETS

HOSEA, JOEL, AMOS, OBADIAH,

JONAH, MICAH, NAHUM, HABAKKUK,

ZEPHANIAH, HAGGAI, ZECHARIAH, MALACHI

QUESTIONS ABOUT
THE BOOK OF HOSEA

Who was Hosea?
He was a prophet, the son of Deeri, who ministered in the northern Kingdom of Israel during the reign of Jeroboam II.

What was the unique message of Hosea?
Hosea warned against the coming Assyrian invasion of the northern Kingdom of Israel.

What are key words in Hosea?
The key words are *faithless adultery.* Just as Gomer—Hosea's wife—commits faithless adultery, so the prophet accuses God's people of being faithless to God by committing adultery with idols.

What are the key verses in Hosea?
"For the children of Israel shall abide many days without king or prince, without sacrifice or sacred pillar, without ephod or teraphim. Afterward the children of Israel shall return and seek the LORD their God and David their king. They shall fear the LORD and His goodness in the latter days" (Hos. 3:4–5).

Why does Hosea call the Northern Kingdom "Ephraim"?
Because the Northern Kingdom had ten tribes and Ephraim was the strongest of the ten tribes.

What is known about Hosea's family?
Hosea's ministry centers largely on a divinely inspired parallel between his love for his unfaithful wife, Gomer, and the Lord's love for unfaithful Israel.

Many question why the book of Hosea includes the unfaithful sexual exploits of his wife and the apparent recognition of her prostitution. Don't look at the obvious sin of Gomer; look at the parallel of how God's people flirt with sexual sins and are unfaithful by spurning God's love.

What is Hosea's nickname?

He has been called the "brokenhearted prophet" because of his unfaithful wife.

What was the expressed sin of the Northern Tribe of Israel?

They were guilty of idolatry, specifically, the worship of Baal and its golden calves (chapter 13).

What is unique about Hosea's position in the Bible?

The book of Hosea is the first of the "Minor Prophets." The last twelve books of the Old Testament are called "minor" because they are shorter than the "Major Prophets." However, Hosea is placed first in the Minor Prophets because it is the longest book of the Minor Prophets.

QUESTIONS ABOUT THE BOOK OF JOEL

Who was Joel?

Very little is known about the personal life of Joel, except that he lived in Jerusalem and his father's name was Pethuel (Joel 1:1). His date is uncertain since there are no contemporary kings or other chronological data given in the book, nor warning of impending invasions by either Assyria or Babylon.

What are the key words in Joel?

The key words are *the day of the Lord.*

What are the key verses in Joel?

"Alas for the day! For the day of the LORD is at hand; it shall come as destruction from the Almighty" (Joel 1:15). "And it shall come to pass afterward that I will pour out My Spirit on all flesh; your sons and your daughters shall prophesy, your old men shall dream dreams, your young men shall see visions. And also on My menservants and on My maidservants I will pour out My Spirit in those days" (Joel 2:28–29).

What is Joel's motive for writing?

Joel probably wrote during a time of famine, as he describes devouring locusts, and the fields and vegetation being burned up because of lack of water.

What is Joel's message?

Joel describes the coming "day of the LORD" (Joel 1:15), comparing God's coming judgment to a plague of locusts.

What gives the book of Joel credibility?

Peter quotes from Joel (2:28–32) on the day of pentecost, describing the coming revival when God will pour out His spirit upon on all flesh (Acts 2:16–21).

What does Joel call on the nation to do?

He wants them to mourn over and repent of their sins, fast, and pray for deliverance.

QUESTIONS ABOUT
THE BOOK OF AMOS

Who was Amos?

Amos described himself simply as a shepherd (rather than a priest or a prophet) and as one called to prophetic ministry: "The words of Amos, who was among the sheepbreeders of Tekoa, which he saw concerning Israel in the days of Uzziah king of Judah, and in the days of Jeroboam the son of Joash, king of Israel, two years before the earthquake" (Amos 1:1).

What is the key word in Amos?

The key word in Amos is *judgment*.

What are the key verses in Amos?

"Hear this word that the LORD has spoken against you, O children of Israel, against the whole family which I brought up from the land of Egypt, saying:

'You only have I known of all the families of the earth; therefore I will punish you for all your iniquities'" (Amos 3:1–2).

When did Amos minister?
Amos wrote during the time of Uzziah, king of southern Judah, and Jeroboam II of Israel (776–760 B.C.). He begins two years before the earthquake, apparently one known to his listeners and readers.

How was the message of Amos received?
When he spoke, the Northern Kingdom was at its zenith of power under Jeroboam II, and the fulfillment of his message of judgment seemed improbable. Therefore, the people were doubtful of Amos.

How is Amos quoted in the New Testament?
James the elder cited the prophecies of Amos in Acts 15:15–18, and Stephen, in his sermon of Acts 7, quoted from Amos 5:25–27 (Acts 7:42–43). These New Testament citations give credibility to the Old Testament book of Amos.

QUESTIONS ABOUT
THE BOOK OF OBADIAH

Who was Obadiah?
Obadiah was an obscure prophet. Nothing is known about his hometown or his family, nor do we know where he lived and ministered. He probably lived in southern Judea, because he wrote of nearby Edom. His one-chapter message is a warning that the small nation of Edom will be destroyed. However, he does have a secondary theme: the future restoration of Israel because of the Lord's faithfulness to His covenant promises.

There are thirteen men who have the name Obadiah in the Old Testament. The minor prophet Obadiah is probably not one of the other twelve, but is a different person altogether. Some scholars think that the prophet Obadiah might be (1) "the minister in Ahab's time who hid God's prophets in a cave" (1 Kings 18:3); (2) the official, or priest, sent out by Jehoshaphat to teach the Law in Judea (2 Chron. 17:7); (3) the manager who repaired the temple under Josiah (2 Chron. 34:12); or (4) a priest during the time of Nehemiah (Neh. 10:5). However, he was probably none of these.

Who wrote the book of Obadiah?

Obviously from verse 1, Obadiah wrote the book: "The vision of Obadiah. Thus says the Lord GOD concerning Edom."

When was Obadiah written?

Scholars are not sure when Obadiah was written because he does not associate his message with a particular king. Obadiah describes the invasion of Judah and condemns Edom for not coming to help Judah. Because the Edomites will not help Judah, they are sentenced by God. By determining which invasion Obadiah refers to, the time of writing can be established.

There are four major invasions of Judah when enemies attacked Jerusalem: first, when Pharaoh Shishak of Egypt plundered the temple during the reign of Rehoboam (1 Kings 14:25–26); second, during the reign of Jehoram (848–841 B.C.), when the Philistines and Arabians plundered the palace in Jerusalem (2 Chron. 21:16–17); third, when the ten northern tribes of Israel invaded Judah (2 Kings 14; 2 Chron. 25); and fourth, when Nebuchadnezzar destroyed Jerusalem and the temple in 585 B.C. In studying all of these, most scholars feel Obadiah was writing of the second invasion, when the Philistines and Arabians invaded Israel, and Edom did not come to their aid. This invasion happened somewhere between 848 and 841 B.C. Therefore, the book of Obadiah is one of the earliest of the Minor Prophets. He was probably a contemporary of Elisha.

Who was Edom?

Edom is a nation that came from Esau, the twin brother of Jacob (Obad. 1:10, 21). Esau was also called Edom (the original word suggests "red"), because he was covered with red hair when he was born. The struggle between Jacob and Esau began in the womb of their mother, continued while they were young men, and even when they parted peacefully as old men, they still did not stop hating each other.

When Israel returned from Egypt, Edom did not help the Israelites return to the land, but instead hindered them and fought against them (Num. 20:14–21). Therefore, Obadiah declared judgment against Edom by

(1) describing their crime, (2) pronouncing their guilt, and (3) announcing how God would judge them—His total destruction of the nation.

What is the key word in Obadiah?

The key word is *judgment*; God will judge Edom for her crime.

What is the key verse in Obadiah?

"For violence against your brother Jacob, shame shall cover you, and you shall be cut off forever" (Obad. 1:10).

QUESTIONS ABOUT
THE BOOK OF JONAH

Who was Jonah?

Jonah (his name means "dove") was a prophet to the northern kingdom of Israel, living in the land of Zebulon from the city of Gath Hepher (2 Kings 14:25) near the Sea of Galilee (during the reign of Jeroboam II, 2 Kings 14:23–25).

What are the key words in Jonah?

The Lord prepared. God prepared several things in Jonah's life: a storm, a fish, a vine, a worm, and so forth.

What is the key verse in Jonah?

"And he said: 'I cried out to the LORD because of my affliction, and He answered me. Out of the belly of Sheol I cried, and You heard my voice'" (Jonah 2:2).

Why is Jonah so famous?

Jonah is perhaps the most familiar of all the Minor Prophets because of the well-known story of Jonah being swallowed by a whale (actually a fish). The story includes the miracle of being swallowed by the fish, being deposited on the land, the powerful preaching that brought the capital city of Nineveh to repentance, and the account of how God prepared a vine to protect Jonah from the searing sun, then allowing a worm to destroy the vine to teach him God's sovereignty.

Is the book of Jonah credible?

The fact that Jonah is identified by the Lord Jesus Christ (Matt. 12:40) gives it credibility. If there had not been a historical person named Jonah, and if he had not been swallowed by a great fish, then the credibility of Jesus could be called into question. If Jesus is not a credible witness, then everyone can doubt the credibility of the substitutionary death—the sinless One dying for the sinful.

Where was the city of Nineveh?

Nineveh was the capital of the ancient nation of Assyria, located on the banks of the Tigris River. The Bible describes it as an "exceedingly great city," a three-days' journey around it (sixty miles). The vast ruins discovered confirm the immense size of Nineveh.

Why did Jonah run away from his commission to preach to Nineveh?

Perhaps Jonah was afraid of being persecuted in Nineveh, or he had a false concept of the separation of Jews from Gentiles, or he didn't understand God's love and commission for the world. Whatever the reason, Jonah did not want to preach to the heathen nation of Assyria and its capital, Nineveh. So Jonah ran toward Spain, in the opposite direction.

How did Jonah manifest his rebellion to God?

He got on a ship to go to Tarshish (probably Tartessus, Spain), but God sent a storm to threaten the boat that he had taken. The sailors tried to preserve the ship; they called on their heathen gods, but finally decided Jonah was the cause of the storm, and that it was a judgment from God. When they threw Jonah overboard, the storm subsided. But a great fish had been prepared by God to swallow Jonah.

What was the result of Jonah's preaching to Nineveh?

The king and the people of the city believed Jonah; they repented of their sin and turned from their evil ways.

What was the response of Jonah when he saw the revival?

Jonah was angry that the city had repented and that the Lord did not judge Nineveh. As he sat on a hill overlooking Nineveh to wait for God's judgment on the city, the Lord sent a vine to cover him from the fierce noonday heat. Obviously Jonah enjoyed the vine. Then God sent a worm to destroy the vine. The message was that God could sovereignly send either protection or judgment. This was a rebuke to Jonah's anger.

What does the Bible teach about Jonah's "whale"?

There seems to be some controversy surrounding whether or not Jonah was swallowed by an actual whale. The Bible says, "The LORD had prepared a great fish" (Jonah 1:17). The King James version of the Bible translates it "whale" from the Greek *ketos*, but this word actually means "a great fish." Jewish tradition felt that the word *prepared* (Hebrew *manah*) meant that God created this particular fish that could swallow a man. But the word *prepare* means "to appoint, ordain, or order," so the idea probably is one of commission rather than creation: God guided this especially large fish to swallow Jonah, and God "commissioned," not created, this fish. The Hebrew text merely says that it was a "great fish" (Hebrew *dag gadol*). There are excellent commentaries that present in-depth study on the subject of the fish of Jonah referred to in Jonah 1:17 and Matthew 12:40. Other commentators have suggested that the fish was a dogfish, which has a stomach so large that the body of a man in armor was once found in it. Still others suggest that the fish was a shark, some of which grow to a weight of ten thousand pounds and a length of thirty to forty feet, and in whose stomachs full-grown horses have been found.

QUESTIONS ABOUT
THE BOOK OF MICAH

Who was Micah?

Micah was a prophet from the Southern Kingdom of Judah, whose message dealt with the Northern Kingdom of Israel. Some feel he was a disciple of Isaiah. Micah warned that the Northern Kingdom, still in the land, would shortly be invaded by Assyria and destroyed (Mic. 1:1–6). Micah also prophesied the eventual Babylonian captivity of the Southern Kingdom of Judah (Mic. 4:10), but he also included the wonderful prophecy that Messiah would be born in Bethlehem. In this prophecy, he recognized the eternal deity of Messiah (Mic. 5:2).

What is the key word in Micah?

The key word is *judgment*.

What are the key verses in Micah?

"He has shown you, O man, what is good; and what does the LORD require of you but to do justly, to love mercy, and to walk humbly with your God?" (Mic. 6:8). "Who is a God like You, pardoning iniquity and passing over the transgression of the remnant of His heritage? He does not retain His anger forever, because He delights in mercy" (Mic. 7:18).

What evidence is there that Micah wrote the book?

Approximately a century after Micah wrote, Jeremiah quoted Micah 3:12, saying, "Micah of Moresheth prophesied in the days of Hezekiah . . ." (Jer. 26:18).

What is Micah's promise concerning the latter days?

Micah says that Zion will be restored to the land, there will be a reign of peace, the Gentiles will come to the knowledge of the true God, and Messiah will reign (Mic. 4:1–4).

When did Micah minister?

Micah lived during the reigns of Jotham, Ahaz, and Hezekiah, kings of Judah.

QUESTIONS ABOUT
THE BOOK OF NAHUM

Who was Nahum?

Very little is known about Nahum, but his name means "comfort." Nahum had a message of comfort to Israel, but a message of judgment for Nineveh. His message outlined the destruction of Assyria, the constant enemy of Israel.

When did Nahum write?

Most Bible scholars believe that he wrote between 664 and 606 B.C. He speaks of the destruction of No-Amon (Nah. 3:8), which took place in 664 B.C. The fact that Nineveh was still a powerful nation when he wrote meant that he wrote before the destruction of Nineveh.

What is the key word in Nahum?

Nineveh. Nahum predicted the destruction of Nineveh.

What are the key verses in Nahum?

"Behold, I am against you," says the LORD of hosts; "I will lift your skirts over your face, I will show the nations your nakedness, and the kingdoms your shame. I will cast abominable filth upon you, make you vile, and make you a spectacle. It shall come to pass that all who look upon you will flee from you, and say, 'Nineveh is laid waste! Who will bemoan her?' Where shall I seek comforters for you?" (Nah. 3:5–7)

What is known about "Elkoshite?"

Nahum is called an Elkoshite, but nothing is known about the site. Most Bible scholars think that this was the city known as Kathar-Nahem, the village named in honor of Nahum and later known as Capernaum, which was Jesus' base of ministry on Lake Galilee.

What is the message of Nahum?

Nahum predicted the defeat and destruction of Nineveh, the capital city of Assyria.

QUESTIONS ABOUT THE BOOK OF HABAKKUK

Who was Habakkuk?

Little is known about the life of Habakkuk, other than he was a contemporary of Jeremiah the prophet and ministered in the closing years of the Southern Kingdom of Judah before Babylon destroyed the nation. Habakkuk ministered during the turbulent years following the death of King Josiah, one of the revival kings.

What was the message of Habakkuk?

He warned that the Babylonians were going to come and judge the nation of Judah.

What is the key word in Habakkuk?

The key word is *faith*. Habakkuk questions why God is doing the things he cannot understand. God gives him an answer that he should live by faith and trust his God: "But the just shall live by his faith" (Hab. 2:4).

What are the key verses in Habakkuk?

"I will stand my watch and set myself on the rampart, and watch to see what He will say to me, and what I will answer when I am corrected. Then the LORD answered me and said: 'Write the vision and make it plain on tablets, that he may run who reads it. For the vision is yet for an appointed time; but at the end it will speak, and it will not lie. Though it tarries, wait for it; because it will surely come, it will not tarry. Behold the proud, his soul is not upright in him; but the just shall live by his faith.'" (Hab. 2:1–4)

What do we know about the personal life of Habakkuk from this book?

Because the author reflects deep spirituality in chapter 3, as well as deep concern about the holiness of God, many see him as a very sensitive prophet. He has a very eloquent but deep prayer expressing great faith in the Lord.

What is most remembered about Habakkuk?

Habakkuk used the phrase, "The just shall live by his faith" (Hab. 2:4). This phrase was repeated three times in the New Testament (Rom. 1:17; Gal. 3:11; Heb. 10:38).

How did the commission come to Habakkuk for ministry?

"I will stand upon my watch, and set me upon the tower, and will watch to see what he will say unto me, and what I shall answer when I am reproved. And the LORD answered me, and said, Write the vision, and make it plain upon tables, that he may run that readeth it. For the vision is yet for an appointed time, but at the end it shall speak, and not lie: though it tarry, wait for it; because it will surely come, it will not tarry. Behold, his soul which is lifted up is not upright in him: but the just shall live by his faith." (Hab. 2:1–4 KJV)

QUESTIONS ABOUT
THE BOOK OF ZEPHANIAH

Who was Zephaniah?

The first verse identifies Zephaniah as the son Cushi, and the great-great-grandson of the godly King Hezekiah, suggesting he was the only prophet of royal descent. His writings suggest he had free access to the court of King

Josiah (the revival king), and was quite familiar with the city of Jerusalem (1:9–10; 3:1–7). The name Zephaniah means "Jehovah has hidden." Apparently he was born during the reign of evil King Manassas and was "hidden" as a young child from Manassas' atrocities.

When did Zephaniah write?

He wrote his book "in the days of Josiah the son of Amon, king of Judah" (1:1). This means he wrote during Josiah's reign, 640–409 B.C., during the time that included the destruction of Nineveh (612 B.C.).

What was Zephaniah's message?

Zephaniah warned Israel of a coming day of judgment from God. His ministry played a significant role in preparing Judah for the revival that took place under the revival king, Josiah, the last godly king of Judah.

What are the key words in Zephaniah?

The key words are *the day of the LORD.*

What are the key verses in Zephaniah?

"The great day of the LORD is near; it is near and hastens quickly. The noise of the day of the LORD is bitter; there the mighty men shall cry out. That day is a day of wrath, a day of trouble and distress, a day of devastation and desolation, a day of darkness and gloominess, a day of clouds and thick darkness" (Zeph. 1:14–15).

QUESTIONS ABOUT
THE BOOK OF HAGGAI

Who was Haggai?

Haggai was a minor prophet and the writer of the book bearing his name (Hag. 1:1). Many think he was born in Israel before the 586 B.C. captivity and was taken to live in Babylon for the seventy years of captivity. King Cyrus, the Persian king, had issued a decree in 538 B.C. that allowed the Jews to return to their land and rebuild the temple. Haggai returned from Babylon with the remnant under Zerubbabel in 536 B.C., and the people began work on the temple (Ezra 4–6), but stopped shortly thereafter. The

Samaritans hindered the work of the temple and wrote a letter to the Persian king, adding to the delay of the work. The remnant that returned found the land desolate, the crops failed, and hostility from their neighbors. They faced hard work, not to mention the enemies who attacked them.

In this context God called Haggai to preach to the people, encouraging them to complete the temple. Perhaps of all the prophets, Haggai and Zechariah might be considered the most successful prophets, because the temple was completed under their ministries.

Haggai preached his first message on September 1, 520 B.C. (Hag. 1:15). The prophet Zechariah, who also preached with him, began preaching between Haggai's second and third messages. The last message of Haggai was December 4, 518 B.C. The people responded and began work immediately on the temple, and completed it in four years, in 516 B.C. (Ezra 6:16). However, when the temple was rebuilt, it did not contain the ark of the covenant, so the Shekinah-glory cloud did not fill the Holy of Holies, nor were the Urim and Thummin present to supernaturally determine the will of God for the people.

What does the name *Haggai* mean?

His name in Hebrew (*Haggay*) is probably derived from "festival" which suggests his name means "festival of Jehovah." Most people think that he was born on a festival day, perhaps on one of the feast days. Inasmuch as the Feast of Tabernacles is emphasized, Haggai 2:1 suggests that he was born on this day.

What is the key word in Haggai?

The key word is *consider*. Haggai told the people to consider or think about what they were doing and what they could accomplish for God by rebuilding the temple. The word *consider* appears six times in Haggai (1:5–7; 2:15, 18).

What name of the Lord does Haggai emphasize?

Throughout the book Haggai refers to the Lord of Hosts, *Jehovah-Sabaoth*, a name that gives emphasis to God's power and glory. The name emphasizes an army that belongs to the Lord, and refers to either the Lord's army or the heavenly bodies of angels (Gen. 2:1; Josh. 5:15; Judg. 4:2). In the vernacular this name could be called "God of the fighting angels." It is significant that when Israel does not have an army, and is powerless to defend itself, God is depicted as *Jehovah-Sabaoth*, the One who will fight for the nation.

What are the key verses in Haggai?

"Thus says the LORD of hosts: 'Consider your ways! Go up to the mountains and bring wood and build the temple, that I may take pleasure in it and be glorified,' says the LORD" (Hag. 1:7–8).

What is the focus of Haggai?

The focus of Haggai is the "unfinished temple." The people had begun rebuilding the temple, but had stopped. The prophet reminded them that, "the glory of this latter house shall be greater than of the former" (Hag. 2:9 KJV). By that he meant that the former house, Solomon's temple, had contained the Shekinah-glory cloud, but the house that they were building, Zerubbabel's temple, would experience a far greater glory when the Lord Jesus Christ visited it during His earthly ministry.

QUESTIONS ABOUT THE BOOK OF ZECHARIAH

Who was Zechariah?

The name *Zechariah* means "God remembers," and Zechariah shares his name with twenty-nine other Old Testament characters. Most of the time the name Zechariah was given out of gratitude for God's gift of a baby boy, usually when people had been praying for a child. Zechariah was of the priestly line, the son of Berechiah, and the grandson of Iddo (1:1, 7). He was born in Babylon and was brought to Palestine by his grandfather when the Jewish exiles returned under Zerubbabel in 536 B.C. He was called as a young man (2:4), perhaps as early as 520 B.C., and eventually became a member of the Great Synagogue that collected and preserved the Old Testament Canon. Many people believe he was "murdered between the temple and the altar," the same way that an earlier Zechariah was martyred (2 Chron. 24:20–21).

What is the significance of Zechariah?

For a dozen or more years the Jewish community had not completed the temple. Rather than rebuking them, Zechariah encouraged them to action by reminding them of the future importance of the temple. He indicated that the temple must be built because Messiah's glory would one day fill the temple. He indicated that future blessing was contingent upon their present obedience.

What is the key word in Zechariah?

Messiah. While the exact word is not used, the coming Messiah is the dominant thrust of Zechariah (3:1, 8; 6:12–13; 9:9–10; 11:4–13; 12:10; 13:1, 7).

What is the key verse in Zechariah?

"Rejoice greatly, O daughter of Zion! Shout, O daughter of Jerusalem! Behold, your King is coming to you; He is just and having salvation, lowly and riding on a donkey, a colt, the foal of a donkey" (Zech. 9:9).

How is Christ seen in the book of Zechariah?

Jesus Christ is seen in both His two advents: first as Servant and then as King; first as man and then as God. Zechariah calls Christ the "Angel of the LORD" (3:1–2), the "BRANCH" (3:8; 6:12–13), "the stone" (3:9), a "priest on His throne" (6:13), the "King" (9:9–10), the "cornerstone" (10:4), the One "whom they pierced" (12:10), a cleansing "fountain" (13:1), and the smitten "Shepherd" (13:7). He is also the Shepherd depicted in Zechariah 11:4–13. In chapter 14 He is depicted as the coming Judge.

QUESTIONS ABOUT
THE BOOK OF MALACHI

Who was Malachi?

Very little is known about Malachi because he never introduces himself other than by his name. *Malachi* means "my messenger." Someone has said that when asked who he was, Malachi answered, "I am no one but God's messenger." Some believe Malachi is not his name, but is only a description of a prophet who wanted to be known as a messenger of the Lord.

What is the key word in Malachi?

The key word is *curse.* Malachi warned the people that God would curse them for their rebellion (Mal. 2:2; 3:9), and the last word in the book, and in the Old Testament, is *curse* (Mal. 4:6).

What is the key verse in Malachi?

"You have wearied the LORD with your words; yet you say, 'In what way have we wearied Him?' In that you say, 'Everyone who does evil is good in the sight of the LORD, and He delights in them,' or, 'Where is the God of justice?'" (Mal. 2:17).

How is the book unified?

Malachi uses a series of questions and answers to develop the message of the book. He asks questions that people might be asking of God and answers for God with condemnation and a message of judgment.

How effective was the ministry of Malachi?

Malachi reveals Israel's hypocrisy, infidelity, mixed marriages, false worship, arrogance, and nonpayment of the tithe. Malachi is so stinging in his condemnation that God remained silent for four hundred years after he spoke, until the coming of John the Baptist (Mal. 3:1).

How does Malachi end?

The last book in the Old Testament concluded with the announcement of the coming of John the Baptist, who would proclaim the coming of the Lord. The Lord promised, "I will send my messenger, and he will prepare the way before me" (Mal. 3:1). When John the Baptist came announcing the arrival of Messiah, he quoted Malachi and Isaiah, saying, "Prepare the way of the Lord" (Matt. 3:3). Then before Malachi ended the book, he added the promise, "Behold I will send you Elijah the prophet before the coming of the great and dreadful day of the LORD. And he will turn the hearts of the fathers to the children, and the hearts of the children to their fathers, lest I come and strike the earth with a curse" (Mal. 4:5–6).

QUESTIONS ABOUT THE GOSPEL ACCORDING TO MATTHEW

Who wrote the Gospel according to Matthew?

Almost all Christians have accepted the authorship of Matthew, and no one has seriously questioned that he wrote the book that bears his name. Matthew was an early disciple, leaving his post as tax collector in Capernaum to follow Jesus Christ. Later he was chosen as one of the twelve apostles. Many think that as tax collector, he was compulsive in taking notes as he surveyed the caravans and travelers who passed through his tax table. They suggest his compulsive note taking carried over as he followed Jesus' ministry on earth. Matthew took notes on Jesus' sermons, and wrote down the miracles that He performed. Then very early after Jesus died, Matthew transferred his notes into the book we know as the Gospel of Matthew.

When did Matthew write?

Many feel that Matthew was the first of the books written in the New Testament, and was therefore placed first in order. If this is so, then he wrote within ten years of Jesus' death. Only a few people think that he wrote at a later date, between A.D. 58–68 It is obvious that Matthew did write before the destruction of the Jewish temple, because his writing included the prediction that the temple would be destroyed (Matt. 24–25). Apparently, the temple was still standing when he wrote. Two expressions, "to this day" (27:8) and "until this day" (28:15), suggest that he wrote fairly soon after the events occurred because things he described had not changed when he was writing.

Who was Matthew?

Matthew was the son of Alphaeus (Mark 2:14), a Jew who had become a tax collector in Capernaum for the Roman government. Because tax collectors were hated by all people, perhaps his alienation from his people and society motivated him to follow Jesus Christ. Matthew responded quickly to Jesus (Matt. 9:9–13, Mark 2:14, Luke 5:27–28), indicating that he had been listening to His sermons and was ready to make a commitment to discipleship. Immediately he gave a large banquet for Jesus, where the Lord preached to publicans and sinners. Many think that Zacchaeus, a chief tax collector, came to faith because of Matthew's conversion. Zacchaeus would have been stationed in Jericho, and would have supervised all of the tax collectors in the Jordan River area from Capernaum and Galilee, including where Matthew was located. The last time Matthew's name occurs in Scripture is when he is mentioned with the eleven disciples praying in the Upper Room (Acts 1:13).

What is the theme of Matthew?

Matthew presents Jesus Christ as the promised messianic King (1:23; 2:2; 3:17; 4:15–17; 21:5–9; 22:44–45; 26:64; 27:11, 27–37). Because of this, the key word is *king*, and the key phrase is "the kingdom of heaven." This phrase occurs thirty-two times in Matthew (but nowhere else in the New Testament), strongly identifying Jesus with messianic fulfillment. Matthew also includes more Old Testament quotations and references than any other book in the New Testament (almost 130). Therefore, one of his characteristic statements is, "that which was spoken through the prophets might be fulfilled" (occurring nine times). Matthew begins his book, "The genealogy of Jesus Christ, the Son of David"—hence, identified strongly with the prophetic kingdom (1:1). The phrase "Son of David" occurs nine times in Matthew.

What is the key word in Matthew?

The key word is *king*, and Matthew attempts to demonstrate that Jesus fulfills the prophecies of Messiah, the coming King.

What is the key verse in Matthew?

The key verse includes the question that gives direction to the entire book: "Where is He who has been born King of the Jews? For we have seen His star in the East and have come to worship Him" (Matt. 2:2).

What is the turning point in the book of Matthew?

Jesus comes to offer Himself as the King of Israel, but Israel rejects His offer. The Pharisees, acting as the spokesman for the nation, formally reject Jesus as their King and Messiah in Matthew 12. The Pharisees claim that Jesus heals by the power of Satan, (Beelzebub), not by the power of God. The focus of Jesus' ministry shifts to the church (Matt. 16:18), and immediately Jesus speaks in parables about the coming kingdom of heaven. Jesus also makes repeated references to His coming death.

Who are the three kings referred to in Matthew?

Ever since the hymn "We Three Kings" was written, people refer to the visiting wise men who came from the east as "kings" when, in fact, they were "wise men from the East" (2:1). They probably came from the nation of Persia, while some believe they might have come from as far east as India. They were the equivalent of scholars in our university, and they had wealth so they could devote themselves to study. They also probably held high positions in their government. Because they studied astronomy, they were "captivated" by the appearance of a supernatural star that they called "His star" (2:2). Because they represented heads of state, they presented themselves as an official delegation to King Herod in Jerusalem. It was from there that King Herod sent them to Bethlehem based upon the priests' and scribes' knowledge of Micah (2:4). The star was not a comet, like Halley's comet, nor was it a transposition of several stars in the sky, but was a supernatural phenomenon that moved in the atmosphere and stood over the place where the baby was lying.

What does tradition say about the three wise men?

Tradition has it that there were three kings or wise men, because they brought three types of gifts. Tradition also tells us their names were Balthazar, Caspar, and Melchior, and that their gifts were gold, frankincense, and myrrh.

What was the star that guided the wise men to the home of the baby Jesus in Jerusalem?

"Now after Jesus was born in Bethlehem of Judea in the days of Herod the king, behold, wise men from the East came to Jerusalem, saying, 'Where is He who has been born King of the Jews? For we have seen His star in the East and have come to worship Him'" (Matt. 2:1–2).

The first view is that the star that guided the Magi (wise men) was a supernatural phenomenon, a starlike object that appeared in their eastern sky, and afterwards reappeared to guide them as they journeyed from Jerusalem to Bethlehem to the house where Jesus was located. It was more than a comet or a meteor; rather, it appeared in the lower regions of the air. This star differed so much from anything that was common that they concluded that it signified something uncommon.

The second view is that the star was a natural phenomenon (a comet) passing over the earth at the time of Christ's birth. One such explanation comes from the astronomer Kepler, who noted a conjunction of Jupiter and Saturn, joined in March 1604 by Mars, becoming a brilliant new star in October 1604, and gradually fading and vanishing in February 1606. Kepler calculated that the planets were in conjunction in 7 and 6 B.C. (about the time of Jesus' birth), as they were in 1604.

What does it mean when God spoke from Heaven, "this is My beloved Son in whom I am well pleased"? (Matt. 3:17)

You must recognize that the title "beloved Son" does not speak of physical relationship, for God is Spirit. Jesus was "the only begotten Son" (John 3:16) and the second person of the Godhead. The phrase "only begotten" means He was uniquely related to God the Father, and of the same essence as God the Father. This has been called by scholars "eternal generation," indicating that Jesus is eternal (He was never born or "started") and in a timeless relationship with God as His Father. Remember, the Trinity is equal in nature, separate in person, but submissive in duties.

Who were the scribes?

The word *scribe* comes from *granmateisie*, meaning "the writers." These scribes were men in the temple who were assigned the task of making copies of the Scriptures. Because they learned the Scriptures by copying them, they were qualified to teach the Law. These scribes usually kept very careful count of every letter in the Old Testament pages they were writing. Because of their knowledge, they were asked many questions about their religion. This is why Herod asked for their opinion on where the Messiah was to be born when the wise men came from the East looking for Messiah.

Why did Joseph take Mary and the baby Jesus to Egypt?

Because an angel had warned him that there was danger to the baby Jesus, they went and lived in Egypt for two to three years.

How did they end up in Egypt?

Apparently the gifts that were brought by the wise men supplied enough money to make the trip there and back and to support them while they were there. Tradition tells us that Joseph got a job as a carpenter while in Egypt.

If Herod slaughtered all of the children, why is it not recorded in Roman history?

Technically, Herod did not slaughter all of the babies in all of the promised land. He only killed the babies in Bethlehem, where Jesus was living. This would have probably amounted to less than twenty babies, which would not have been a crisis large enough to catch the attention of Roman historians.

What does the phrase "the kingdom of heaven" mean?

The phrase literally means "the kingdom of heavens," and only Matthew uses this phrase in Scripture. Jesus is referring to a time when the rule of heaven over the earth will take place (Matt. 6:10). The phrase comes from Daniel 2:37, which mentions "the God of heaven," who will rule in His theocratic kingdom.

Who were the Pharisees?

The word *Pharisee* means "separate," and describes a group of legalistic leaders who zealously kept the Law in its smallest detail. The Pharisees formed a self-righteous, self-denying Jewish sect that was very vindictive of those who didn't teach the Law.

Who were the Sadducees?

These were a different group of Jews, who were more liberal in their orientation than the Pharisees. They denied the existence of the supernatural, angels, spirits, miracles, and especially the Resurrection. They were religious rationalists, and many of the priests, as well as laypersons in the Sanhedrin (the religious ruling body over Jerusalem) followed their interpretation.

Why was Jesus tempted at the beginning of His ministry?

Just as the first Adam was tempted in the Garden of Eden, where he demonstrated his disobedience to God, the "last Adam," Jesus Christ, was tempted so that He might demonstrate His obedience to God. And as Adam lost everything in *dis*obedience, Jesus gained everything in obedience. Because Jesus didn't sin, He was able to redeem a race that had fallen under the curse (Rom. 8:19–23).

What does Jesus mean when He says to pluck out your eye and cut off your hand? (Matt. 5:29–30)

"If your right eye causes you to sin, pluck it out and cast it from you; for it is more profitable for you that one of your members perish, than for your whole body to be cast into hell. And if your right hand causes you to sin, cut it off and cast it from you; for it is more profitable for you that one of your members perish, than for your whole body to be cast into hell" (Matt. 5:29–30).

Passages such as Matthew 5:29–30, Matthew 18:8–9, and Mark 9:42–48 are examples of a type of figure of speech known as a *hyperbole* (a metaphorical exaggeration), illustrating the harm associated with adultery and lustful thoughts. Thus, the suggestion of cutting off one's hand or plucking out one's eye is definitely not to be taken literally. What Jesus implied in these passages is that if "thy right eye offend thee," then the logical thing to do would be to do something about it (the cause of offense) and bring the passions of the heart under the control of the Spirit of God. It would be far better to sever a member of the body than to keep it and go to hell. It is obvious, however, that the real problem lies in the heart and mind of sinful man.

Why is there inconsistency between the two renderings of the Lord's Prayer?

In Matthew 6:10 (KJV), Jesus said, "in earth, as it is in heaven," yet in Luke 11 (KJV), He says, "as in heaven, so in earth." This inconsistency appears only in the original King James Version, not in some of the newer translations.

Jesus related the Lord's Prayer twice in His ministry. In His first year, He included it in the Sermon on the Mount (Matthew 6). In His last year, His disciples said, "Teach us to pray." In response Jesus told them to pray the Lord's Prayer. The phrase in question appears in two different sequences because the Bible records it the way Jesus said it on each occurrence. Since the Bible is word-for-word accurate, each writer (Matthew and Luke) recorded exactly what Jesus said. The newer revisions have changed the order for modern readers.

Why did Jesus not say the Lord's Prayer the same way each time?

Because when Jesus said, "after this manner," the word *manner* simply meant a "pattern" that He wants us to follow when we pray, not an exact formula to be used.

How could Jesus say the kingdom of heaven was "at hand" when it didn't appear? (Matt. 4:17)

When Jesus said the kingdom was "at hand," He was affirming that it could come immediately if the people would repent and receive it. However, the Jewish leaders rejected the message of Jesus, and the predicted kingdom did not come during the time of Jesus' life. The kingdom will not come until after the Tribulation, when the Davidic Kingdom will be set up at the return of Jesus Christ to earth.

How could Jesus say that He came to "fulfill" the Law? (Matt. 5:17)

Jesus fulfilled the Law in that He was born under the Law (Gal. 4:4), and then perfectly kept the Law (John 8:46; Matt. 7:5; 1 Peter 2:21–23). Jesus was the fulfillment of the Old Testament types (Heb. 9:11–26) and fulfilled the Law when He became the substitute for sin on the cross (Gal. 3:13–14). In his death Jesus was the Mediator by His blood of a new covenant that surpassed the old covenant (Rom. 5:2; Heb. 8:6–13).

Did Jesus believe there was a hell or lake of fire?

Jesus warned that certain people would be "in danger of hell fire" (5:22). The word here is *gehenna*, which was a reference to the valley of Hinnon, outside the city of Jerusalem, where garbage was burned. It was also the place where human sacrifices were made (2 Chron. 33:6; Jer. 7:31). Jesus used *gehenna* to warn of the eternal consequences of sin. It is a place where "their worm does not die, and the fire is not quenched." *Gehenna* is translated "lake of fire" (Matt. 5:29–30; 10:28; 18:9; 23:13, 15; Mark 9:43, 45, 47; Luke 12:5; James 3:6).

What is the difference between the "kingdom of God" and the "kingdom of heaven"?

The kingdom of God seems to be universal and refers to God's reign over all people, including angels, the church, and those in the Old and New Testaments, while the kingdom of heaven seems to be a messianic term that refers to the coming kingdom. The kingdom of God can only be entered by the new birth (John 3:3, 5–7), while the kingdom of heaven is entered by the coming rule of Jesus Christ on earth. Therefore, the kingdom of heaven is primarily an earthly rule, while the kingdom of God includes both earth and heaven. The kingdom of God does not "come outwardly" (Luke 17:20), but is an inward and spiritual rule (Rom. 14:17), while the kingdom of heaven is an outward rule whereby Jesus Christ will put "all things under His feet" and shall "deliver the kingdom to God the Father" (1 Cor. 15:24–28).

What is the difference between a disciple and an apostle? (Matt. 10:1–2)

Jesus originally called *disciples*. The meaning of the word *disciple* is "a follower." Hence, these people followed Jesus and learned from Him. Then Jesus chose out of all of His disciples (more than twelve) certain ones who were to be apostles. The word *apostle* means "sent one." In Acts 1:16–26, Peter said the criteria for being an apostle is that he must have followed Jesus Christ in His earthly ministry and been a witness of the Resurrection.

Why is John the Baptist the greatest man to ever live? (Matt. 11:11)

John the Baptist was given a position greater than anyone else because he announced the coming of Jesus Christ to the earth. Jesus said of John the Baptist, "There has not risen one greater than John the Baptist" (Matt. 11:11). Surely Abraham was greater in faith; and Moses, the servant of the Lord, was great as a lawgiver and a miracle worker; and we cannot rule out the greatness of David as a man after God's own heart. Some have said the greatness of John the Baptist is in his announcement of the kingdom, not necessarily in who he was. Jesus went on to say, "But he who is least in the kingdom of heaven is greater than he [John]" (11:11). This means the greatness of John extends only to the kingdom he announced, but that anyone could be greater than John the Baptist by completely yielding to God.

What does the Bible teach about the "mysteries"? (Matt. 13:11)

The Bible does not use the word "mysteries" to mean something mysterious, ethereal, or unknown, as in Eastern religions. Rather, a mystery refers to previously hidden truth in the Old Testament that is revealed in the New Testament. A mystery is supernatural because God is the One who declares its truth. There are many mysteries spoken of in the Bible: (1) the mysteries of the kingdom of heaven (Matt. 13:3–50); (2) the mysteries of Israel being blinded during this church age (Rom. 9:25); (3) the mystery of the rapture, when living saints will be resurrected at the return of Jesus (1 Cor. 15:51–52; 1 Thess. 4:14–17); (4) the mystery of Jews and Gentiles being one body (the church) in Jesus Christ (Eph. 3:1–11); (5) the mystery of the church as a bride (Eph. 5:28–32); (6) the mystery of Christ living in each believer (Col. 1:26–27); (7) the mystery of Christ, the incarnate fullness of the Godhead (Col. 2:2, 9; 1 Cor. 2:7); (8) the mystery of God restoring godlikeness to men in the future (1 Tim. 3:16); (9) the mystery of iniquity of Antichrist in the future (2 Thess. 2:7); (10) the mystery of the seven stars (Rev. 1:20); and (11) the mystery of Babylon (Rev. 17:5–7).

Why did Jesus originally ignore the Syrophenician woman's request for her daughter to be healed? (Matt. 15:21–28)

The Gentile woman addressed Jesus and, up to that time, His ministry was not to Gentiles. But Jesus recognized the faith of the woman. Notice she called Him "Lord," and even requested "the crumbs which fall from [their] masters' table" (Matt. 15:27). By this title she was prefiguring that when the Jews did not take the bread of God, the Gentiles would get the crumbs that fell from their table, i.e., the Gentiles would receive the grace of God.

Did Jesus say that Peter would be the foundation of the Church? (Matt. 16:18)

Jesus said to Peter, "You are Peter, and on this rock I will build My church, and the gates of Hades shall not prevail against it" (Matt. 16:18). By this Jesus did not mean that He would build a church on Peter. This statement by Jesus is a play on Greek words. When Jesus said, "You are Peter," He was literally using the word *petros*, that is, "a little rock." Then He said, "on this rock," or *petra*, which was a large shelf rock or foundation rock. Jesus was saying that Peter's statement of faith, "You are the Christ, the Son of the living God" (Matt. 16:16), was a rock, and that He would build a church upon this great statement of faith that acknowledged the deity of Christ.

What did Jesus mean, "the gates of Hell shall not prevail against it?" (Matt. 16:18)

Jesus is stating that the church will be primarily attacking, that is, going into hell to rescue those who are lost, bringing them out for salvation. This is not a picture of the defensive church as a fortified castle trying to keep Satan out. Rather, the picture is reversed. The church is on the offensive to defeat Satan.

What is meant by the statement, "I will give unto thee the keys of the kingdom of heaven"? (Matt. 16:19 KJV)

Some mistakenly think that Peter was given the keys to heaven, and therefore by apostolic authority could determine who would enter or not enter.

However, the overwhelming teaching of Scripture is that any person who believes in Jesus Christ can enter heaven. So this statement by Jesus meant that Peter would open the door of Christian opportunity to Israel on the day of Pentecost by his preaching (Acts 2:38–42). Peter would again open the door to Gentiles when he preached in the house of Cornelius (Acts 10:34–46). Peter did not have authority over the church. Even in the first church council that Peter attended, James was the moderator who became its spokesman (Acts 15:13).

What does the Bible mean when it says, "whatsoever thou shalt bind on earth, shall be bound in heaven"? (Matt. 16:19 KJV)

This does not mean that Peter has apostolic authority to bind up people in heaven, or to determine those who go to hell. This did not give him the right to determine the eternal destiny of anyone (Rev. 1:18). Jesus has these keys. This determination was given to all of the disciples (Matt. 28:19–20). When any Christian goes soul-winning and leads someone to Christ, that person is "loosed," and when the gospel is presented but people reject it, that person is "bound."

What happened to Jesus when He was transfigured? (Matt. 17:1–13)

The Bible says that Peter, James, and John saw Jesus transfigured, and that "His face did shine as the sun, and his raiment was white as the light" (Matt. 17:2 KJV). This is what Jesus would look like after His humiliation was over. When Jesus returned to heaven, He returned to His formal glory (John 17:5).

Why did Moses and Elijah appear with Jesus on the Mount of Transfiguration?

There have been many reasons suggested why these two were chosen to come back with Jesus. First of all, Moses is probably a representative of those redeemed who passed through death (Deut. 34), yet shall live again in the future resurrection. Elijah is here because he represents those who will enter heaven through translation, as he did in the Old Testament. Christians in this generation will do so by the rapture.

Why is there an inconsistency regarding "the Mountain"?

In Matthew 17:20, Jesus said, "Move from here to there, and it will move; and nothing will be impossible for you." This was a reference to Mt.

Hermon, close to where He spoke. However, in Mark 11:23 Jesus said, "Whoever says to this mountain, 'Be removed and be cast into the sea,' . . . he will have whatever he says." This was a reference to the Mount of Olives where He spoke.

There is no inconsistency. Jesus used the phrase about "removing mountains" on several occasions. Once He refers to Mount Hermon in the north (Matt. 17), and He repeated the statement about Mount Tabor in Galilee, and again about the Mount of Olives (Mark 11). The context and background of each statement tells you where Jesus made this statement. There is nothing wrong with Jesus repeating Himself to different audiences to get the same point across.

In what sense shall the twelve apostles judge for Jesus Christ in the coming Millennium? (Matt. 19:28)

Jesus will administer the kingdom over all the earth in the coming thousand-year reign through the apostles. They will manage the affairs on this earth for Him.

Is there a discrepancy involving the healing of the blind men in Jericho?

A discrepancy has been imagined because Jesus is said to have healed the blind men as He departed from Jericho (Matt. 20:29). However, in Luke 18:35, Jesus healed as He entered Jericho. In Bible times, as today, there are two cities of Jericho. There was the old city that is today covered by a heap of gravel (technically this is a *tell*, a city covered by a man-made mountain), and there is a new, modern city of Jericho. Therefore, Jesus could have been leaving the old city and entering a new city, healing the blind men at that time. A few others explain the apparent discrepancy by saying that the blind men asked for healing when Jesus entered the city, but Jesus waited to heal until He left the city.

Is there a discrepancy in the number of blind men healed at Jericho? (Matt. 20:29–34; Luke 18:35–43)

Matthew was written to the Jews, and the Jews always wanted to verify any activity "at the mouth of two witnesses." Since there were two healed, Matthew includes a record that both were healed. However, one blind man,

Bartimaeus, was more prominent than the other (Mark 10:46). He was also more persistent in begging Jesus for healing. That's why Mark and Luke indicated that he was healed and gave him prominence in their narrative.

What did Jesus mean when He said, "this generation shall not pass, till all these things be fulfilled"? (Matt. 24:34 KJV)

Some people teach that the signs and destructions that Jesus taught about in the Olivet Discourse happened to the generation of Jews who were listening to Him on that day, to those in that generation when Titus destroyed Jerusalem in A.D. 70. The word *generation* is a reference to race or family, and is not used here to speak of that specific generation (those born in a twenty-year period) but of the larger Jewish people. In other words, the nation of Israel will be preserved until the future tribulation time when "all these things be fulfilled" (Matt. 24:34).

Are there contradictions involving the anointing of Jesus at the feast during His final week of life?

In Matthew 26:6–13, a woman came to Jesus during the feast and poured precious ointment "on His head as He sat at the table" (Matt. 26:7). In the John 12:1–11 account, Mary came and poured the ointment on His feet (v. 3). This apparent contradiction is explained in two ways. Some say that the ointment was put both on His head and feet, the two different gospel writers recording what they observed. Others say that it was two different feasts. The feast in the house of Simon the leper (Matt. 26:6) was celebrated on Wednesday evening of the final week, while the feast in Bethany at the home of Mary, Martha, and Lazarus, was celebrated on Saturday evening, six days before the feast (John 12:1).

What was the order of events at the Last Supper? (Matt. 26:20–35)

Apparently when they entered the room, Jesus and His disciples all took their places at the table. Then they began to argue about who should be the greatest, apparently because some felt they didn't get the proper place next to the Lord. Jesus washed their feet as a sign of humility and then identified Judas as the traitor. Jesus instituted the Communion (the bread and the cup), then gave the Upper Room Discourse (John 14 and 15).

Why is there a question whether the bread or the cup should be served first at the Lord's Supper?

Matthew suggests that Jesus served the bread first (Matt. 26:26), while Luke suggests He served the cup first (Luke 22:17). The majority of Christians have always celebrated the Lord's Table first taking the bread, then taking the juice or the cup. The account in Luke says that they took the cup first; however, Luke also mentions that they took the cup later (22:17, 20). Apparently the first cup in Luke is a reference to the first cup of the Jewish Passover meal, not a reference to the institution of the Lord's Supper, the Communion. The second cup mentioned by Luke is a reference to the Lord's Supper.

Is there a contradiction between the intercessory prayer of Jesus (John 17), and His prayer in the Garden of Gethsemane? (Matt. 26:36–46)

No, these are two distinct times when Jesus prayed on the night before He died. The high priestly prayer of Jesus in John 17 was offered before He went across the Brook Kidron (John 18:1). This high priestly prayer might have been prayed somewhere in the city of Jerusalem, a garden, a small room off of the Upper Room, etc. However, I believe Jesus went into the Holy of Holies in the temple and made His prayer there (John 17), a view supported by many deeper life Bible teachers such as J. C. Ryle and Arthur Pink. The Holy of Holies is the place where the high priest carried blood annually for the remission of sin for the nation of Israel on the Day of Atonement. It is only natural to think that Jesus found His way into that place for His High Priestly prayer. After praying in the city of Jerusalem, Jesus crossed the Brook Kidron (John 18:1) into the Garden of Gethsemane (a garden toured by visitors to Jerusalem today). There He prayed three different times, asking His disciples to pray with Him, but they fell asleep and He exhorted them, "What? Could you not watch with Me one hour?" (Matt. 26:40).

Did Judas repent and get saved? (Matt. 27:3)

"Then Judas, His betrayer, seeing that [Jesus] had been condemned, was remorseful" (Matt. 27:3). This word *remorseful,* from the Greek word *metameleoma,* which means "to regret," is different from the term for repentance to salvation (Greek *metanoia*). Because Judas saw Jesus being taken to Pilate, he regretted what he did to Jesus, but he did not repent.

"Then Judas . . . brought back the thirty pieces of silver to the chief priests and elders, saying, 'I have sinned by betraying innocent blood.' And they said, 'What is that to us? You see to it!' Then he threw down the pieces of silver in the temple and departed, and went and hanged himself" (Matt. 27:3–5). Judas shows every indication of still being unsaved: He betrays innocent blood for money, feels guilty, returns the money, and commits suicide. These are the actions of a guilty conscience, not a forgiven and regenerate one. His admission "I have sinned" is not necessarily a true confession to faith.

Are there contradictions surrounding Judas's death? (Matt. 27:5)

There are two descriptions of Judas's death. First, he hanged himself (Matt. 27:5). Second, he fell from a cliff or high place, and his intestines spilled as he died. The reference to Judas's "falling headlong" (Acts 1:18–19) is generally thought to have happened while he was attempting to commit suicide. Perhaps Judas hanged himself over a ledge or cliff, when the rope broke, he then fell into the valley below.

Is there an inconsistency concerning the "field" after Judas's death?

"But the chief priests took the silver pieces and said, 'It is not lawful to put them into the treasury, because they are the price of blood.' And they consulted together and bought with them the potter's field, to bury strangers in. Therefore that field has been called the Field of Blood to this day" (Matt. 27:6–8). The potter's field was probably bought by the legally minded priests in Judas's name. The priests took the thirty pieces of silver returned by Judas and purchased it to bury people who couldn't afford a burial place. The Bible does not say Judas was buried here.

While traveling with Jesus, Judas was the treasurer. He was stealing money that was given to Jesus. "Now this man purchased a field" (Acts 1:18–19). He committed suicide in this place and was buried there.

The account of Judas's death (Acts 1:18–19) is not inconsistent with that set forth by Matthew (27:3–8).

What is the order of the trials of Jesus?

The four Gospels give us different accounts of different trials of Jesus. Actually, there were six trials, or if not technically called "trials," some would have been like our grand jury investigation.

1. Jesus was first brought before Annas, the former high priest (John 18:12–14). Apparently, they were here going to determine what charges to bring against Jesus.

2. Jesus was next brought before Caiaphas, the ruling high priest, to get his approval and to determine Jesus' guilt.

3. Jesus was led to the Sanhedrin, seventy men who ruled Israel, again to verify the charges brought against Jesus (Matt. 27:1–2; 11–14).

4. Jesus was brought before Pilate, the ruling Roman officer.

5. Pilate didn't want to try Jesus because he didn't see clearly the charges or the indictment, so he sent Jesus to Herod (Luke 23:6–12). Because Jerusalem was not in Herod's jurisdiction, Herod sent Jesus back to Pilate.

6. Jesus was finally tried before Pilate, then led out to be crucified.

Is there a discrepancy regarding where Peter was questioned about being a follower of Jesus?

Peter was questioned at different places. First, he was "with the servants" (Matt. 26:58). Second, he was on "the porch" where a great number of people were. He was then questioned by a maid, but the whole crowd was involved (Matt. 26:71–75 KJV). Remember, Peter denied the Lord three times.

What is the order of events at the Crucifixion?

First Jesus arrived at Golgotha (Matt. 27:33), then He was offered a stupefying drink but refused it (v. 34). He was actually crucified between two thieves (27:35–38). He uttered His first cry from the cross: "Father, forgive them" (Luke 23:34). The soldiers divided His garments (Matt. 27:35), then the Jews began to mock Him (27:39–44). The thieves began to criticize Jesus, but one repented and believed in Him (Luke 23:42). Jesus answered, "Today you will be with Me in Paradise" (Luke 23:43, second cry). Then Jesus turned the care of His mother over to John: "Woman, behold your son!" (John 19:26–27, third cry). Total darkness fell over the earth (Matt. 27:45). Jesus then cries, "My God, My God, why have You forsaken Me?" (Matt. 27:46–47, fourth cry), followed by His fifth cry, "I thirst." The sixth cry was, "It is finished" (John 19:30), and the seventh and last cry was, "Father, into Your hands I commend My spirit" (Luke 23:46). The Lord dismissed His spirit (Matt. 27:50), and died.

Are the four different Gospel accounts of the inscription on the cross contradictory?

There is no contradiction involved. All four authors have written, "THE KING OF THE JEWS." Luke adds, "THIS IS" (Luke 23:38). Matthew quotes the name "JESUS," while John gives the additional words to identify his address "OF NAZARETH." From each author's individual recollection, we have the various renderings of the inscription. The unsaved human instruments put an inscription above the cross in the first place to mock Jesus. We see the inscription as a divine guide of humans that best describes Jesus, i.e., "This is Jesus of Nazareth, the King of the Jews."

How did Jesus "dismiss His Spirit"? (Matt. 27:50)

By an act of His own will, Jesus volitionally terminated His life. Jesus had earlier said, "No one takes it from Me, but I lay it down of Myself" (John 10:18). The physical death of Christ is different from all others, because He died for all men.

Why was the veil in the temple ripped from top to bottom at the time Jesus died? (Matt. 27:51)

The veil divided the Holy of Holies from the rest of the temple. No priest could go into the Holy of Holies except the high priest, once a year on the day of atonement (Lev. 16:1–30). The veil was ripped to signify that all people now had access to God through the sacrificial blood of Jesus Christ (Heb. 10:20). All people can now come into the very presence of God by "a new living way" (Heb. 9:1–8; 10:19–22). The fact that it was ripped from top to bottom signifies this was the work of God. If it had been ripped from bottom to top, that would have implied the work of men ripping it apart, which would have been difficult. (According to Jewish tradition, the veil was a series of "matted" veils, approximately twelve inches thick.)

When Jesus died, what bodies were was resurrected in the cemetery?

At the moment Jesus died, the Bible says, "The graves were opened; and many bodies of the saints who had fallen asleep were raised; and coming out of the graves after His resurrection, they went into the holy city and appeared to many" (Matt. 27:51–53). Some feel that an actual resurrection, or resuscitation, took place in a cemetery near Golgotha, and that some who had physically died came back to life and returned to their families in the city. This was a symbolic picture of Old Testament saints being released from sheol, so they might enter into heaven (Eph. 4:8–10).

What does the Bible teach about Joseph of Arimathaea burying the body of Jesus?

Joseph of Arimathaea was a member of the Sanhedrin, the seventy ruling men of Israel. Apparently he was not present early on Friday morning when they voted against Jesus. After the death of Jesus, he begged Pilate for the body (Matt. 27:58) and then buried the body of Jesus in his own grave. The Bible identifies him as a secret believer (John 19:38).

What does the Bible teach about Nicodemus's role in burying Jesus?

Nicodemus was a member of the Sanhedrin, but like Joseph of Arimathaea, he was probably not present when the council met early on Friday morning to vote on an indictment against Jesus. After the death of Jesus, Nicodemus brought an expensive mixture of spices, about one hundred pounds weight, to anoint the body of Jesus (John 19:39–40). He was a secret believer until this event.

How was the body of Jesus prepared?

The Bible says it was wrapped in a linen cloth (John 19:40) and anointed with a mixture of spices and oil. The Jewish pound only had twelve ounces, so when the Bible says one hundred pounds of oil and spices were used (John 19:39), it was actually seventy-five pounds.

Technically the body of Jesus was mummified with a large cast, similar to a plaster-of-paris cast used to mend a broken bone today. However, the cast would not have been hardened, but would have been more like a "soft cast." When Peter and John examined the linen cloths, they found that they were not unwrapped, but the body was gone. This is an indication of the miracle of the Resurrection—Jesus' body passed right through the "soft cast."

What does the Bible teach about the order of events at the tomb on Easter Sunday morning?

It seems there might be a contradiction, because Matthew said that Mary Magdalene and another Mary came to the tomb (Matt. 28:1). Mark indicates that there were three ladies (Mark 16:1), but John says there was only one, Mary (John 20:1). Apparently at least four women came together to the tomb, but

Mary Magdalene went ahead of the other women to check on the soldiers and the encampment around the tomb. They all thought the tomb was sealed and guarded. When Mary saw that the soldiers were gone and the stone was rolled away from the tomb, she left by another way—forgetting the other women— and ran into the city to tell Peter and John. After a period of waiting, the other women came to the tomb and found out from the angel that the Lord was risen, so they departed quickly to Jerusalem. In their haste they met Jesus and worshiped Him (Matt. 28:9). When Mary Magdalene got to town, she told Peter and John. The two disciples ran to the tomb; John, the younger of the two, out-ran Peter. They examined the tomb and determined that the Lord was not there. John believed Jesus was resurrected (John 20:2–10). After a while Mary Magdalene returned to the tomb. It was here that she met the Lord, and when she touched Him, He told her, "Do not cling to Me" (John 20:17).

Later that day, perhaps in the early afternoon, the Lord appeared to Peter (Luke 24:34; 1 Cor. 15:5), then to two disciples on their way to Emmaus (Luke 24:13–31). Finally, in the evening the Lord appeared to ten apostles in the Upper Room (John 20:19–24).

Why does Jesus give different commands in the Great Commission, and why is each command recorded differently in each Gospel?

These are not conflicting commands, but the Great Commission was given five times in five locations. Each time, Jesus adds more to the Great Commission. In essence, it becomes one command in our thinking, but each of the four Gospel writers adds a different facet. Technically, each Gospel writer gives a different command that is given at a different place and a different time. All five commands make up one Great Commission.

The first has to do with just "Go" (John 20:21); the second tells them to preach to everyone, everywhere (Mark 12:15); the third relates to their strategy (Matt. 18:19–20); the fourth regards content (Luke 24:46-48); and the fifth has to do with geographical tactic (Acts 1:8).

The first giving of the Great Commission was in the Upper Room on Easter Sunday when Jesus appeared to ten disciples. He told them, "As the Father has sent me, I also send you" (John 20:21). In His first command, Jesus only told them to go; He didn't tell them where to go, or to what group to preach, or even what to do.

The second command was given seven days later, again in the Upper

Room, but this time there were eleven disciples present (Mark 16:14). Jesus said, "Go into all the world and preach the gospel to every creature" (v. 15). Now He was telling them to go everywhere and to preach to everyone, but He still didn't tell them the strategy by which they were to preach.

The third command was given at a different place, on a mountain in Galilee, and was probably at least one week later (Matt. 28:16). On this occasion Jesus sharpened their understanding of the Great Commission: "Go therefore, and make disciples of all the nations, baptizing them in the name of the Father and of the Son and of the Holy Spirit, teaching them to observe all things that I have commanded you; and lo, I am with you always, even to the end of the age" (Matt. 28:19–20). Here Jesus told them that their strategy was to make disciples of each ethnic group, to baptize them, and then to teach them His words.

The fourth command was given in Jerusalem on the fortieth day before Jesus was taken up into heaven. This command involved the content of their preaching. "Thus it is written, and thus it was necessary for the Christ to suffer and to rise from the dead the third day, and that repentance and remission of sins should be preached in His name to all nations, beginning at Jerusalem. And you are witnesses of these things" (Luke 24:46–48).

A few hours later, Jesus took the disciples out to the Mount of Olives. Before He ascended into heaven, He gave them the last aspect of the Great Commission, which involved geography. He commanded, "But you shall receive power when the Holy Spirit has come upon you; and you shall be witnesses to Me in Jerusalem, and in all Judea and Samaria, and to the end of the earth" (Acts. 1:8). Therefore, what seems like a contradiction in the commands of the Great Commission is actually a continuous development of the one command, so that when we understand the Great Commission, we understand the full aspect of how we are to carry out His commission: where to go, to whom to preach, how to get it done, what to preach, and what geographical path we should follow.

QUESTIONS ABOUT THE GOSPEL ACCORDING TO MARK

Who was Mark?

Many think that Mark was the young man who was accosted during the arrest of Jesus but ran away into the night (Mark 14:51, 52). He was very involved and associated with many other believers in the early-church days.

His mother had a large house that was used for the meeting of believers in Jerusalem (Acts 12:12). Peter apparently visited his house often, because Rhoda, the girl who kept the gate, recognized his voice (12:13–16). Mark was related to Barnabas (Col. 4:10 KJV), and because of Barnabas, Mark accompanied Paul and Barnabas on the first missionary tour. When it came to the second tour, Barnabas decided to take Mark, but Paul resisted because Mark had "run away" and left them in the middle of the first tour. The contention became so great between Barnabas and Paul that they split company, and Mark went with Barnabas to evangelize Cyprus. However, Peter is the one who probably led him to Christ, because Peter calls him, "Mark my son" (1 Peter 5:13). Many feel that Mark's close association with Peter resulted in information and interviews that led to Mark's writing of this Gospel. Even though Paul refused to take Mark with him on the second journey, at the end of Paul's life he wrote that Mark was important to him, and that he wanted Mark to come to him in prison (Col. 4:10; Philem. 23). Paul said, "He is useful to me for ministry" (2 Tim. 4:11).

Who wrote the Gospel according to Mark?

The early church declared that Mark was the writer of this Gospel. Such church fathers as, Clement of Alexander, Origen, and others affirm Mark's authorship.

When did Mark write the Gospel?

Most scholars believe that he wrote before the destruction of the temple in A.D. 70 (Mark 13:2), so perhaps it was written about the time that Peter, Mark's source, was martyred, around A.D. 65.

What is the theme of Mark?

Mark directs his book toward a Roman readership because he pictures Jesus as a Man of action, showing what Jesus did. When you compare the stories of Mark with the stories in the other Gospels, they are shorter and more action-packed. Mark is a book of deeds, and there are more recorded miracles performed by Jesus in Mark than in the other Gospels. Mark contains a total of twenty-seven of the thirty-seven recorded miracles performed by Jesus in His lifetime. Mark also omitted a number of items that Romans would not have cared about, such as the genealogy of Christ, fulfilled prophecies, references to the Jewish law and customs, and so on. Mark also interpreted Aramaic words, because they would have been unfamiliar to Romans.

What is the key word in Mark?

The key word in Mark is *immediately*. This word is translated "anon" and "straightway" in the King James Bible. Because Mark shows Jesus as a servant, he shows that Jesus is obedient to the Father, instantly carrying out the duties assigned to Him.

What is the key verse in Mark?

"For even the Son of Man did not come to be served, but to serve, and to give His life a ransom for many" (Mark 10:45). This verse shows Jesus as a servant, and how He went about doing good in service to people.

How is Jesus presented in the Gospel of Mark?

Jesus is presented as a servant (Mark 10:45). There is no genealogy, because a servant does not have a genealogy. Mark presents Jesus as the Branch; He is "My servant the branch" (Zech. 3:8).

What does Mark tell about the "long day?"

Because Jesus is a servant, Mark describes the events of one extremely long, involved day of ministry. In the summer of A.D. 29, Jesus began the morning in Capernaum ministering in the house of Peter. When he cast out a devil, the Jewish leaders accused Him of casting out demons by the power of Satan. Here is where Jesus dealt with the topic of the unpardonable sin. Shortly thereafter, His mother, Mary, and some of His brothers came to call Him away from ministry. It is here that Jesus said that His "family" is made up of those who do the will of God (Mark 3:31–35). Jesus then went to the seaside where He gave the sermon that included the parables of the mysteries of the kingdom of God (Mark 4:1–34). After preaching this long sermon, Jesus departed to cross the Sea of Galilee, and fell asleep because He was weary from the continuous pressure of ministry. A storm developed that threatened the disciples, and Jesus miraculously calmed the waves. The disciples were amazed that even the winds and the sea obeyed the Lord.

On the other side of the sea, Jesus met the demon-possessed man in

Gadara. After casting the demon out of the man, the people forced Jesus to leave the area, and He returned to Capernaum. Immediately upon arrival, Jairus asked Jesus to come to his house to heal his little girl, who was at the point of death. But in the interim, a woman touched the hem of Jesus' garment and was healed. Jesus paused to establish the faith of the woman. Meanwhile, Jairus's little girl died. But Jesus went to the home of Jairus and raised the little girl from the dead. This long, involved day is reflective of Jesus the Servant, who was also the Son of God.

QUESTIONS ABOUT THE GOSPEL ACCORDING TO LUKE

Who was Luke?

Luke was a Gentile (Col. 4:10–14), who was also a doctor, called by Paul, "Luke the beloved physician" (Col. 4:14). Little is known about Luke before he joined Paul on the second missionary journey. Some think he was a Greek physician who attended to a Roman family but was set free and given

Roman citizenship. Many think he was from Antioch, where Paul and Barnabas established the church. Others think that Luke was from Tarshish, and that Paul met Luke and won him to Christ while Luke was a medical student at the medical school in Tarshish. Luke joined Paul in Asia Minor, as evidenced by the use of the pronoun *we* in Acts (16:1–17; 20:5–21:18; 27:1–28:16). That made Luke a close friend and traveling companion with Paul on the missionary journeys. We don't know what Paul's "thorn in the flesh" was, but he had some serious illness that necessitated constant medical attention. Luke was with Paul during his arrest and first Roman imprisonment, and many think Luke wrote the books of Luke and Acts during this time. He was also with Paul in his second Roman imprisonment: "Only Luke is with me" (2 Tim. 4:11). Therefore, Luke was a man who was loyal to Paul during profound danger. However, when Paul was martyred, Luke was apparently released. Tradition says he remained unmarried and died at age eighty-four.

How did Luke write the Gospel?

We know that Luke was not an eyewitness of the things he wrote in the Gospel, but he relied heavily on the testimony of eyewitnesses and other short biographical sketches that had been written about Jesus Christ. He carefully examined all of his sources and put his material in chronological order, obviously rejecting some of the information that he did not include.

He wrote to "set in order a narrative of those things which have been fulfilled among us" (Luke 1:1). Of all of the Gospels, Luke is the most chronologically correct. He tells us that he got his material from "eyewitnesses and ministers of the word" (Luke 1:2). However, Luke did not rely only on his own ingenuity or insight. He relied on God. He testified that he "had perfect understanding," meaning that he studied many sources and interviewed many people, but that he wrote "from the very first" (Luke 1:3), which is the Greek word *anothen*, meaning "from above." This word tells us that he was relying on the Holy Spirit's inspiration to write this text.

Why did Luke write this book?

Apparently he was writing a twin volume to Theophilus, a rich or influential Christian, who in turn would distribute the books among others. This two-volume set, Luke and Acts, constitutes what Jesus began (the Gospel of Luke), and what He continued to do through the church (Acts). Some have felt that Theophilus may have been the wealthy family that first paid for Luke's medical training and later gave him his freedom and Roman citizenship. Other people think Theophilus was an affluent Christian who would make sure that the gospel was published broadly so that many could read it. This would have meant that Theophilus had slaves who were scribes. They would copy the book and send it out to many New Testament churches.

When was the book of Luke written?

Luke was with Paul for two years when Paul was in prison in Caesarea. During that time, Luke probably traveled throughout the Holy Land to interview eyewitnesses, gather documents, and study the life and ministry of Jesus Christ. It is probably here that Luke wrote the gospel of Luke while in his early sixties. Luke may have sent it to Theophilus by courier or Roman mail, which was secure and trustworthy. Remember, all of the possessions of Paul and Luke would have been lost during the shipwreck (Acts 27) on their trip to Rome. When they arrived in Rome, it was probably there that Luke began writing his second volume, the book of Acts.

What are the key words in Luke?

The key words are *the son of man,* which occur approximately eighty times. Because Luke wanted to create a record of the earthly life of Jesus that was chronological, accurate, and complete, he wrote about Jesus the Son of Man, emphasizing the humanity of Jesus Christ. A doctor would obviously know more about humanity than any other person.

What is the key verse in Luke?

"For the Son of Man has come to seek and to save that which was lost" (Luke 19:10).

To whom was the book of Luke written?

Luke wrote to Gentiles, specifically to Greeks. He translates Aramaic words into Greek words, and always explains the Jewish customs and geography for the Greek reader. Because the Greeks would have been interested in stories, Luke includes more parables than do the other Gospels. He was the only non-Jew to write Scripture, and he writes to his own people, telling of Jesus Christ—the perfect man.

What does the Bible teach about the taxation when Jesus was born?

Caesar Augustus sent out a decree that everyone in the Roman Empire had to return to their hometowns to be registered for a census. The Bible uses the phrase "all the world," from *oikounene*, which is "inhabited earth." This does not mean all of humanity and tribes unknown, but the entire sphere where Roman rule extended.

What does the Bible teach about the dedication of the infant Jesus in the temple?

The baby Jesus was taken to the temple for dedication and circumcision (Luke 2:21–24). There a man named Simeon met the young couple and apparently was the human instrument to dedicate the baby Jesus. Simeon is described as "just and devout, waiting for the Consolation of Israel: and the Holy Ghost was upon him" (Luke 2:25 KJV). Simeon "took Him [Jesus] up in his arms and blessed God" (Luke 2:28). This is the technical blessing of the infant Jesus. Because the corrupt priest who would later be responsible for crucifying Jesus was not spiritually able to dedicate the baby Jesus, God had prepared a spiritual man named Simeon to dedicate Jesus. Simeon met the young couple out in the crowd among the people where Jesus was dedicated; the baby was not dedicated in the temple under the influence of the priest.

What did the baby Jesus know?

The Bible says, "And the Child grew and became strong in spirit, filled with wisdom; and the grace of God was upon Him" (Luke 2:40). While this verse does not say Jesus *grew* in wisdom, apparently He was *filled* with wisdom, getting something He had not previously had. Later the Bible says, "Jesus increased in wisdom and stature, and in favor with God and men" (Luke 2:52). This means that Jesus grew in wisdom, spiritual discernment, and social understanding as He grew physically. While Jesus was God, and His birth was a supernatural incarnation, He grew normally as other boys would grow. That means that as a small child playing in the yard of Mary and Joseph, Jesus wouldn't have known everything that was going on in the village of Nazareth.

However, He knew all that He needed to know, and God the Father in heaven clearly protected, guided, and gave Jesus all the knowledge He needed at every moment of His earthly life.

Why is the genealogy in Luke different from the genealogy in Matthew? (Luke 3:23–38)

The Matthew genealogy traces the line from David to the father, Joseph (Matt. 1:16), giving Jesus the family title of Messiah. In Luke we have Mary's genealogy. Note that the genealogy of Mary is through Nathan, son of David. Joseph's genealogy is through Solomon, son of David.

How can both Joseph and Mary be the descendants of Heli? (Matt. 1:16; Luke 3:23)

When Joseph is called "the son of Heli," remember that the word *son* does not occur in the Greek language. It is italicized, meaning it is not there. Joseph is the son-in-law of Heli, not the biological son.

What do we know about Jesus' ministry from the Scriptures He read in Nazareth? (Luke 4:17–20)

When Jesus returned to Nazareth, He read from Isaiah 61:1–2, but He stopped in the middle of the passage at the phrase "the acceptable year of the Lord." Jesus read the events associated with His first advent: preaching, healing, delivering captives, and giving sight to the blind. Jesus did not include the next portion of Isaiah 61, which refers to His second advent, that is, His return in glory.

Why is the statement "on Earth as it is in Heaven" from Matthew reversed in Luke to read, "in Heaven, so in Earth" (the Lord's Prayer)?

The Lord's Prayer was orated by Jesus twice during His earthly ministry. The first time was in the Sermon on the Mount, and it occurs in the middle of His sermon, which was delivered in His first year of ministry. The next time Jesus recites the Lord's Prayer was in His third year of ministry. After Jesus had been praying all night, the disciples asked Him to teach them to pray, and He gave them the Lord's Prayer as an example of how to pray. The Lord never intended for us to repeat the Lord's Prayer repetitiously as formula. He said that we should pray the Lord's Prayer "after this manner" (Matt. 6:9 KJV). The word *manner* is "pattern," so the Lord's Prayer is a pattern for us to pray, not an exact formula. So it's not required that we repeat every word in its exact order. However, the first time Jesus gave the Lord's Prayer, He used one order of words, the next time He gave the Lord's Prayer, He reversed the order of words. Since the Bible is an accurate translation of the events and speech of Scripture, Matthew wrote exactly what Jesus said in His sermon, and Luke wrote exactly what Jesus said after He had prayed all night.

Should the Lord's Prayer be prayed today?

Some think the Lord's Prayer should not be prayed today because it involves kingdom or millennium truth. (Note the words *thy kingdom come,* which refer to the coming millennial kingdom.) Also, they say the concept of "forgive us our sins as we forgive those who sin against us" is law, and not the basis of grace. Today God forgives our sins on the basis of the blood of Jesus Christ (1 John 1:7). They further say that the reference to "kingdom" in the conclusion is again a reference to the future kingdom.

It is the dispensationalists of today who do not pray the Lord's Prayer, teaching that it only applies to the future kingdom. However, church history teaches that Christians have used the Lord's Prayer since it was first given. The first historical and archaeological reference we have to the Lord's Prayer was found in Pompeii, Italy, where Mount Vesuvius overflowed the city with lava. Two homes in the city had the phrase *patra nostra* ("our Father") chiseled on the stone walls. Whereas today we call it the Lord's Prayer, it was originally called by its first two words, the "Our Father." The reference to "king" and "kingdom" is an application of God's broader rule in the "kingdom of God." Just as you must be born again to enter His kingdom, so all Christians put themselves under the rule and reign of King Jesus (see *Praying the Lord's Prayer* by Elmer Towns, Regal Books, 1997).

What does the Bible teach about "importunity" in prayer?

The word *importunity* means "persistence" or "diligence" and suggests that we should pray consistently and continually as Paul prescribed when he said to "pray without ceasing" (1 Thess. 5:17). The lesson is that we should not be discouraged when God delays the answers, but should continue praying.

What did Jesus mean when He said that we should ask for the Holy Spirit? (Luke 11:13)

In this reference, Jesus was referring to the church age, also called the age of the Holy Spirit. The Bible teaches that when you are saved, the Holy Spirit comes to dwell in you (Rom. 8:9; John 7:37–39). But there is also a filling of the Holy Spirit whereby the third person of the Trinity will come into the Christian to lead, use, empower, and enlighten. Paul said we are to be continually filled with the Holy Spirit (Eph. 5:18). This is the ministry of the Holy Spirit that Jesus promised right before He returned to heaven (Acts 1:4–5). Jesus was saying to "ask" for the Holy Spirit to help us, to be filled with the Holy Spirit.

Was the story of the rich man in hell and Lazarus in heaven a parable? (Luke 16:19–31)

Some claim that this story is a parable, and as such, the flames of hell are not real, but only a figure of speech to describe future punishment for unbelievers. Those who deny the existence of hell say that the flames are only allegorical, and that hell does not last forever. However, a parable was a teaching device that Jesus used to tell an earthly story with a heavenly meaning. A parable never identifies people by name, but Lazarus was identified by name in this story, indicating he was a real person. Also, when Jesus gave a parable, He interpreted it either at the beginning or end, but the story of Lazarus and the rich man does not have an interpretation. Parables are stories of natural people and natural situations. None of the parables include miracles or the supernatural. Since the characteristics of a parable are not found in the story of the rich man and Lazarus, this is not a parable.

What do we know about hell from this story that Jesus told about the rich man who went there? (Luke 16:19–31)

First of all, hell is an unseen world of the departed human spirit. Those in hell have a conscious existence. They are tormented, and they suffer thirst, fire, and separation from their loved ones and other people. But perhaps the greatest characteristic of hell is the constant awareness of *lost opportunity*. Jesus gave the story of the rich man in hell to tell us that those who die have full exercise of their mental faculties (memories, emotions, and so forth).

What did Jesus mean when He asked, "When the Son of Man comes, will He really find faith on the Earth?" (Luke 18:8)

This is not a reference to one's personal faith. There will be a remnant of believers when the Lord Jesus Christ returns, and individuals will have faith in Him. This reference to "faith" is to corporate faith, or to doctrinal faith. Jesus is saying that when He comes, people will have compromised the truth, and corrupted the Word of God (2 Tim. 3:1ff).

What did Jesus mean when He said that Jerusalem will be under siege by armies? (Luke 21:20)

When Jesus gave the Olivet Discourse, He predicted that Jerusalem would be seized by an army that would bring desolation to the city. This prophecy was literally fulfilled when the Roman general Titus destroyed Jerusalem in A.D. 70. However, this is also a future reference to the attack on Jerusalem during the Great Tribulation (Matt. 24:15–28; Mark 13:14–16; Rev. 19:11–21).

What does the phrase "the times of the Gentiles" mean? (Luke 21:24)

God's program was with the seed of Abraham, Israel (Gen. 12:1–3). God sealed His commitment to Abraham when His presence filled the tabernacle, and later, the temple in Jerusalem. However, when Jerusalem was captured by Nebuchadnezzar in 586 B.C. (2 Chron. 31:1–21), it began a time when Gentiles would rule the Jews, God's people.

Since that time, a seed of David has not sat upon the throne, the Shekinah-glory cloud has not rested on the ark of the covenant, and Gentile nations have been in rulership over Israel.

QUESTIONS ABOUT THE GOSPEL ACCORDING TO JOHN

Who was John?

John was apparently the youngest of the twelve disciples. Originally he had a hot temper, because Jesus called John and his brother James "Sons of Thunder" (Mark 3:17). Their father was Zebedee, a fisherman, and their mother was Salome, who later followed Jesus (presumably after Zebedee died), and was present at the crucifixion (Mark 15:40–41). John first became a follower of John the Baptist, until he was called to follow Jesus at the beginning of His ministry (John 1:19–51). John was one of the main disciples to later become one of the twelve apostles (Luke 6:12–16). He was one of the three "inner-circle" disciples who were close to Jesus, along with Peter and James. At the foot of the cross, Jesus committed Mary to John's care. Tradition tells us that Mary stayed with John the apostle, even living to a ripe old age. When John pastored the church in Ephesus, tradition points to a small house outside the city where Mary lived.

Who wrote the Gospel according to John?

Conservatives have unanimously said John the apostle wrote the book, even though a few liberals have said there was an elder in Ephesus that wrote the book in the second century. Recent discoveries have discounted that theory. The John Rylands papyrus found in Egypt contains portions of John. This papyrus, dated A.D. 135, proves the book of John would have been written before the presumed elder lived. Also, many copies of John were circulated throughout the Mediterranean world, thus, necessitating its early date. The book of John was written approximately A.D. 90.

How do we know John wrote this Gospel?

The author is identified as the disciple "whom Jesus loved" (John 13:23; 19:26; 20:2; 21:7, 20). John was a meticulous eyewitness of numbers, names, and events (John 1:34; 1:45; 3:1; 11:1; 18:10).

What is the key word in John?

The key word is *believe*. John uses the word approximately ninety-eight times to tell that the central core of Christianity is simply believing in Jesus Christ. "For God so loved the world that He gave His only begotten Son, that whoever believes in Him should not perish but have everlasting life" (John 3:16).

What is the key verse in John?

The key verse is John's stated purpose for writing the book: "But these are written that you may believe that Jesus is the Christ, the Son of God, and that believing you may have life in His name" (John 20:31).

What was the purpose for the gospel of John?

John stated his purpose was twofold: First, "that you may believe that Jesus is the Christ, the Son of God" (John 20:31). He wanted to demonstrate the deity of Jesus Christ. He was writing late in the first century, around A.D. 90, when people were beginning to question whether Jesus was truly or fully God. John heard these questions, along with the questions of gnosticism, and wrote a strong declaration of Christ's deity, declaring that Jesus was who He said He was, the Son of God.

But there was a second purpose: "that believing you may have life in His name" (John 20:31). John wanted people to experience eternal life that comes through belief. The word *life* is the second key word in the gospel of John and occurs thirty-six times.

Why was John so focused on unbelief?

The opposite of belief is unbelief. "Men loved darkness rather than light, because their deeds were evil" (John 3:19). Those who put their faith in the Son of God have eternal life, but those who reject Him will suffer the wrath of God (John 3:36; 5:24–29). John presents the fact that Jesus came to His own, but His own received Him not (John 1:11). John shows the greatest opposition of Jesus was from "the Jews," a phrase symbolizing the Jewish establishment of Jerusalem. They rejected Him early during the first Passover in the first year of Jesus' ministry when Jesus cleansed the temple (John 2:13–22). They rejected Jesus again during the second Passover (John 5:16, 17). They planned to kill Him at least one year before He died (John 7). The Jews were in open debate and opposition to Jesus (John 8). They were the antithesis of John's thesis of belief.

How is Jesus "the Word"? (John 1:1)

John called Jesus the *Logos*, that is, "the Word," which is not a term John picked up from the philosophies of Greece. Some believe John got the term "the Word" from the use of "wisdom" as seen in the book of Proverbs.

However, *word* is constantly repeated in the Old Testament in the phrase "the word of the LORD," a reference to the authority of God communicated in words. As the Word, Jesus is the concept of God Himself and the expression of God Himself. John teaches, "No one has seen God at any time. The only begotten Son, who is in the bosom of the Father, He has declared Him" (John 1:18). The phrase "has declared" means to "demonstrate." As the Word, Jesus demonstrates to us what God really is like.

Why is there no genealogy in John?

Both Matthew and Luke contain a genealogy of Jesus; Matthew because he is demonstrating that Jesus is the rightful heir to the throne of David, and Luke because he is demonstrating that Jesus is true humanity. However, John shows the Incarnation—that is, that Jesus is God—and God doesn't have a genealogy.

What does the phrase mean, "The law was given by Moses, but grace and truth came by Jesus Christ"? (John 1:17 KJV)

The Law demonstrates that man is evil; grace demonstrates God's desire to save man. The Law shows how far man has fallen into wickedness; grace saves the bad. The Law demonstrates that blessings can be earned; grace is a free gift. Grace is God's love demonstrated in Jesus Christ (John 3:16).

Why does Jesus do an "insignificant" miracle to begin His ministry?

The first miracle of Jesus was changing water into wine (John 2:11). The only persons present were family members and His disciples. Jesus could have demonstrated His power before a great crowd somewhere else, but He began manifesting Himself to family because He wanted the endorsement of family. Also, just as God created at the beginning of the Old Testament, so Jesus, the Son of God, created wine out of water at the beginning of the New Testament. Since water was the fulfillment of the Law for the purifying of the Jews (John 2:6), Jesus was demonstrating that His message of grace is greater than the Old Testament message of judgment. Jesus began declaring Himself to those closest to Him, knowing they would take the message to the multitude. Wine, a symbol of joy, demonstrated that Jesus came to bring joy into the world.

Did Jesus use a whip to drive people out of the temple?

Some see Jesus only as a "meek and mild" man who came to be a moral example to all. But when Jesus entered the temple, He saw corruption and greed in His Father's house. So He displayed judgment: "When He had made a whip of cords, He drove them all out of the temple, with the sheep and the oxen, and poured out the changers' money, and overturned the tables" (John 2:15). God has two sides. God is at the same time both holiness and love. While God loves people at all times, He must always judge them for their sin. Jesus is God, who always loves people, but when He saw sin, especially in the religious establishment, He judged them by cleansing the temple.

Who was Nicodemus? (John 3:1–10)

Nicodemus was a ruler of the Jews who sat on the Sanhedrin. This meant he was numbered with the seventy religious rulers who had oversight of the religious, social, and financial matters of Jerusalem (the political oversight was in the hands of Rome). Nicodemus was considered one of the wealthiest men in Jerusalem, as well as one of the most pious (John 3:1–10). After talking with him Jesus said, "Art thou a master of Israel, and knowest not these things?" (John 3:10 KJV). The phrase "a master" in the Greek is *ho didaskolos,* which means "the teacher of Israel." Perhaps he was the most respected of all the religious teachers in Israel.

What must religious teachers do?

When Nicodemus came to Jesus, he tried to compliment Jesus by saying, "You are a teacher come from God; for no one can do these signs that You do, unless God is with him" (John 3:2). But Jesus told him, "Unless one is born again, he cannot see the kingdom of God" (John 3:3). All religious teachers, like all people, must be born again. "Do not marvel that I said to you, 'You must be born again'" (John 3:7).

What is the meaning of the phrase "born again"? (John 3:3, 7)

When one is born again, he (or she) is made to live spiritually again, which means the individual is regenerated. When a person is regenerated, he is given a new nature that desires righteousness; he has eternal life and is made a member of God's family. Regeneration is not reformation, because it means "to make new." The condition of the new birth is believing and receiving Jesus Christ (John 1:12–13).

What does the phrase "believeth not" mean? (John 3:18 KJV)

Every person has an awareness of God, including a knowledge of what is right and of his or her obligation to God. Those who "believe not" have simply rejected or refused to believe in Jesus Christ. John says, "He who believes in Him is not condemned; but he who does not believe is condemned already, because he has not believed in the name of the only begotten Son of God" (John 3:18). If a person does nothing about salvation, he or she has "believed not," and will be condemned.

Why does the Bible say that Jesus "needed to go through Samaria"? (John 4:4)

Jesus was leaving Jerusalem, and the shortest route from Jerusalem to His home in Galilee was through Samaria. However, most Jews would not go through Samaria because of ethnic segregation. They took the longer route through the Jordan River valley. Jesus went through Samaria and overcame segregation because a woman needed His message. By taking this route He laid the foundation for a future church in Samaria.

What did Jesus offer the woman at the well?

"But whoever drinks of the water that I shall give him will never thirst. But the water that I shall give him will become in him a fountain of water springing up into everlasting life" (John 4:14).

What did Jesus mean, "God is a Spirit"? (John 4:24 KJV)

The article *a* is not in the original language. God is not one spirit among many. Rather, God is spirit in nature. This means God is an incorporeal being; He does not have physical being. When you ask the question, "Why can't I see God?" you cannot see God because there is nothing to see. God is spirit. Yet God is a person, with intellect, emotion, and will.

What does "this is again the second miracle" mean? (John 4:54 KJV)

This reference to a "second miracle" seems to contradict a previous statement: "When He [Jesus] was in Jerusalem at the Passover, in the feast day, many believed in His name, when they saw the miracles which He did" (John 2:23 KJV). Obviously, we know that Jesus had done many miracles because Nicodemus said as much (John 3:2). If Jesus did many miracles in Jerusalem, what does "second miracle" suggest—"This again is the second sign that Jesus did when He had come out of Judea into Galilee" (John 4:54)? This could be the second miracle He did when He reentered Galilee, a miracle quite different from the many miracles He did in Jerusalem. Or it could be only the second miracle that He had ever done in Galilee (the first miracle was changing water into wine).

Why do some leave out part of John 5:3 and all of verse 4?

Certain translations of the Bible leave out John 5:3–4, while others only place it as a footnote. The portion in question is "waiting for the moving of the water. For an angel went down at a certain time into the pool and stirred up the water; then whoever stepped in first, after the stirring of the water, was made well of whatever disease he had" (John 5:3–4).

There are three reasons why some leave it out of the text. First, it is not found in all of the ancient texts. Some of the copies have left this portion out. However, the majority of the texts have listed this passage. A second reason it is left out is because God does not usually perform miracles through an angel. And the third reason is that the miracle is on a "first come, first served" basis, meaning that whoever was first in the water got healed. God doesn't heal the fastest or the quickest. God always relies on faith on the part of the person for healing. Nonetheless, even though a few of the early texts leave out this portion of Scripture, there is enough evidence to prove that this section should not be left out.

Note: The Bible does not say that an angel actually healed the person who got into the water first. Those around the pool of Bethesda were "waiting." Many believe the story about the angel was a tradition, but not a fact. However, denying the angel tradition does not deny the healing power of God. While God may not heal on a basis of "first come, first served," God surely healed the man who had been lame for thirty-eight years. He picked up his bed and walked.

Why did the Jews want to kill Jesus three years before they actually did it?

At the pool of Bethesda Jesus said, "My Father has been working until now, and I have been working" (John 5:17). Jesus was not just calling God His

Father as we might do it today. Jesus used a unique Greek word to say that He was just like the Father. The Jews understood what Jesus meant. "Therefore the Jews sought all the more to kill Him, because He not only broke the Sabbath, but also said that God was His Father, making Himself equal with God" (John 5:18).

How did Jesus claim to be God?

First, Jesus claimed to be equal with God in nature (John 5:17–18). Second, Jesus claimed to do the same works that the Father did (John 5:20), and third, Jesus claimed to have the same task of judging people as does the Father (John 5:21–22).

What is the difference between everlasting life and eternal life?

The New King James Version renders John 5:24, "He who hears my word and believes in Him who sent me has everlasting life." The King James Version also uses the phrase "everlasting life." But the New American Standard Version (NASB) reads, "He who hears My word, and believes Him who sent Me, has *eternal* life" (italics mine). Technically, the words *everlasting* and *eternal* come from the same Greek word, *ainois*. Both *everlasting* and *eternal* mean "life without end." However, when the King James Version was being translated, the translators chose to use two English words based on the contexts of their translations. When God saves you, you have everlasting life from that moment on. The word *everlasting* means life begins and never ends. However, *eternal* life means life that never began *and* life that will never end. Only God has eternal life. Technically, when you get the life of God— eternal life—you get the life of God that has always been in existence. When you are saved, you have both everlasting and eternal life.

What did Jesus mean, "If I bear witness of Myself, My witness is not true"? (John 5:31)

Jesus was not saying that His words were not true. He was defending His Messianic claims based on two or more witnessing. The Jews taught that the biblical rule of evidence required "two witnesses" (John 8:17; Num. 35:30; Deut. 17:6). Jesus gave not just two witnesses, but four that testify He is Messiah: (1) John the Baptist, (2) His miracles, (3) the Father, and (4) the Scriptures (John 5:33–39).

Why have some called the feeding of the five thousand the most popular of all of Jesus' miracles?

This miracle has been called the most popular for two reasons: first, because it affected the largest number of people, about five thousand men (John 6:10), and second, because it's the only miracle to occur in all four of the Gospels.

What did the crowd mean when they called Jesus the "Prophet"? (John 6:14)

There are two references to the prophet. First, some feel this is a reference to the prophet that God will raise up, who is likened unto Moses—that is, the Messiah (Deut. 18:15–18). Others believed that the prophet would be Jeremiah. The rabbis taught that before Messiah would come, Jeremiah would return with the pot of manna that was in the ark of the covenant, that had been originally hidden by Jeremiah. He would take that bread and feed the entire multitude, just as the manna fed the entire nation of Israel. Since Jesus fed the entire multitude with five loaves and two fishes, the people were wondering if Jesus was Jeremiah who would come to feed the multitude. But Jesus was greater than Jeremiah. He answered, "I am the bread of life: he that cometh to me shall never hunger; and he that believeth on Me shall never thirst" (John 6:35 KJV). Jesus was saying He was more than one like Moses or Jeremiah; Jesus was saying He was life. Just as the people in the wilderness had physical life from manna, He would give them spiritual life when they believed on Him.

What did Jesus mean, "Except ye eat the flesh of the Son of Man, and drink His blood, ye have no life in you"? (John 6:53 KJV)

Some have accused the church of cannibalism, that the Christians hid the body of Jesus Christ and ate it. This is not true. Others have said that the communion bread and wine turns to the actual body and blood of Jesus Christ. This is also not true. Jesus was using a metaphor to say that we must take Him into our lives, almost like eating or drinking; He must become a part of us, and we a part of Him (John 14:20).

What did Jesus mean about going to the Feast of Tabernacles, "I go not up yet unto this feast"? (John 7:8 KJV)

Some believe that Jesus was misleading His brothers. His brothers asked Jesus to go up to the Feast of Tabernacles and "show [Himself] to the world"

(John 7:4). Jesus told His brothers He was not going then, but two days later He decided to go. When He told His brothers He was not going, it was in reference to "revealing Himself." Jesus would not reveal Himself as the true Messiah of the world until later when He died for the sins of the world. Notice He said to His brothers, "For My time has not yet fully come" (John 7:8). This meant His time to declare Himself as Messiah and die for the sins of the world had not yet come.

Why is John 8:1–11 not found in some of the Bible translations?

"But Jesus went to the Mount of Olives. Now early in the morning He came again into the temple, and all the people came to Him; and He sat down and taught them. Then the scribes and Pharisees brought to Him a woman caught in adultery. And when they had set her in the midst, they said to Him, 'Teacher, this woman was caught in adultery, in the very act. Now Moses, in the law, commanded us that such should be stoned. But what do You say?' This they said, testing Him, that they might have something of which to accuse Him. But Jesus stooped down and wrote on the ground with His finger, as though He did not hear. So when they continued asking Him, He raised Himself up and said to them, 'He who is without sin among you, let him throw a stone at her first.' And again He stooped down and wrote on the ground. Then those who heard it, being convicted by their conscience, went out one by one, beginning with the oldest even to the last. And Jesus was left alone, and the woman standing in the midst. When Jesus had raised Himself up and saw no one but the woman, He said to her, 'Woman, where are those accusers of yours? Has no one condemned you?' She said, 'No one, Lord.' And Jesus said to her, 'Neither do I condemn you; go and sin no more.'" (John 8:1–11)

This passage was not found in all of the ancient manuscripts; however, it was found in enough ancient manuscripts to give evidence that it should be included. Augustine declared that it was stricken from many copies because a few people thought it taught immorality. They thought that Jesus was condoning the woman's immorality, and Augustine said people didn't want to read or teach it because they might see that as a "loophole" for committing adultery. However, this passage teaches the "blackened" understanding of the Jewish leaders who rejected Jesus Christ. Against that backdrop He said, "I am the light of the world" (John 8:12).

What did Jesus mean when He said, "Your father Abraham rejoiced to see My day, and he saw it and was glad"? (John 8:56)

Jesus might have been referring to several occasions where Abraham saw God, that is, a physical appearance of Jesus Christ. He might have referred to when Abraham saw the smoking oven and burning torch (Gen. 15:17), or to the time when the Lord appeared to Abraham (Gen. 17:1). He could also have been referring to the time Abraham interceded to God to save Sodom and Gomorrah (Gen. 18:23–33). I think Jesus refers to the last reference, when Abraham presented himself before God to pray.

What did Jesus mean, "Verily, verily, I say unto you, Before Abraham was, I am"? (John 8:58 KJV)

Jesus was claiming deity in this statement. The statement "I am," *Ego amimni*, is a unique expression whereby Jesus identifies with the Lord (Jehovah) of the Old Testament. Just as the root meaning of Lord is "I am, I am," Jesus came identifying Himself with God when He said, "I am light, I am bread, I am vine . . ." When Jesus said, "Before Abraham was, I am," He was equating Himself with deity. His opponents picking up stones to kill Him for blasphemy demonstrates they understood what Jesus meant.

How did Jesus pass through the crowd without being stoned? (John 8:59–9:1)

The Jews hated Jesus Christ, and were so agitated that they were ready to kill Him, but didn't. Jesus could have passed through them by any of the following means: (1) He could have become invisible, but that probably didn't happen. (2) He could have blinded their eyes so they didn't see Him passing by. (3) His disciples could have surrounded Him, as the secret service surrounds the president to protect him from harm. (4) God could have imposed an internal constraint on each of the men so that they were not able to cast the stones in their hands. While we don't know how it happened, we do know that Jesus walked through an angry mob without being hurt.

Why did Jesus make clay from spit on the ground to heal the blind man? (John 9:6)

Jesus knew that man's law said they could not make clay on the Sabbath. He was breaking man's sabbatical law, but not God's law. In this endeavor

Jesus was freeing the people from man's law. Also, since man was originally created from dust, Jesus used dust in the form of clay to heal the man. Finally, rather than putting water on his eyes to cleanse them and effect healing (if He had used water, people might have said He was not really a healer), Jesus used clay, which would destroy sight, to give the man healing. This way Jesus demonstrated the credibility of His healing, and that He was God.

Why did the disciples think that the man was born blind because of his or his parents' sin?

The Old Testament Law said that the sins of the parents passed to the children of the third and fourth generations (Ex. 20:5). Therefore, people in Jesus' day tended to interpret any birth defect as an evidence of sin in parents or grandparents. In addition to healing the man, Jesus corrected the misunderstanding that birth defects come from the sin of the parents or grandparents.

Why did Jesus say of Lazarus's sickness, "this sickness is not unto death"? (John 11:4)

When Jesus was told that Lazarus was sick, He knew that Lazarus was already dead. When He said that the sickness was not unto death, He meant not unto death *at that time.* Jesus knew He would raise Lazarus from the dead, and that Lazarus would live a normal life and die at a later time.

What did Jesus mean when He referred to Mary's ointment, and said, "Against the day of my burying hath she kept this"? (John 12:7)

Mary seemed to understand the coming death of Jesus Christ more than others. Jesus was saying that Mary had loved Him so much that she kept this ointment to anoint His body when He died.

Was Jesus being callous to poor people when He said, "The poor you have with you always, but Me you do not have always"? (John 12:8)

Jesus was putting priority on His death and resurrection, and the fact that Mary's anointing His body right before He actually died was an act of faith to her. But it was also an act of testimony to those who observed it. Jesus was not putting down the poor, but indicating that Judas, who had the bag, was only using "the poor" as an excuse to get more money. Judas wanted money from the ointment in the bag so that he might steal it.

What did Jesus mean when He said, "He that is washed needeth not save to wash his feet, but is clean every whit: and ye are clean, but not all"? (John 13:10 KJV)

Jesus was using Far Eastern symbolism to portray salvation. People would go to the public bath to clean their whole bodies. On the way home their feet would get dirty, so when they entered the house they had to wash their feet. Jesus was saying that when we are saved, we are cleansed from every sin. But in our daily walks during this life, we become contaminated and influenced by sin. So we need to daily ask for God's forgiveness of our sin (1 John 1:8–10).

Should Christians wash feet today as part of the Lord's Table?

Some believe that "footwashing" is a required ordinance along with the broken bread and the cup. They do so because Jesus said, "If I then, your Lord and Teacher, have washed your feet, you also ought to wash one another's feet" (John 13:14). However, most Christians do not believe that "footwashing" is a required church ordinance. They say that because there is no command repeated to the New Testament church to wash feet, as there is to baptize and serve Communion, footwashing is not required. They also believe that since there is no illustration of washing feet in the book of Acts, it is not a requirement. Finally, they see that the symbolism of footwashing is weak when compared to the symbolism of the Lord's Table. Washing feet is symbolic of humility—a wonderful symbolism. Everyone needs humility, but it is not as imperative as the broken body symbolized in the bread, and the spilled blood symbolized in the cup. We must celebrate the Lord's Table, but we are not required to wash feet as a church ordinance.

Why didn't all of the disciples know Judas would betray Christ when Jesus said, "It is he to whom I shall give a piece of bread when I have dipped it"? (John 13:26)

In biblical times, the father of the family—or in this case, Jesus—would have been the first to dip a morsel of bread into the lamb stew and then pass it to the honored guest, the person sitting next to him. On this evening Judas was the honored guest, even though Jesus knew Judas would betray Him. So when Jesus gave him the morsel of bread dipped in lamb stew, he was doing what everyone expected. But as the master of ceremonies, Jesus would have given a morsel of bread to everyone there. Therefore, no one knew who the betrayer was except Judas; he knew what he was going to do.

What did Jesus mean when He said, "If I go and prepare a place for you, I will come again, and receive you to Myself; that where I am, there you may be also"? (John 14:3)

Some feel this passage teaches that Jesus would come into our hearts to save us after He went to heaven. Some teach that Jesus will come at death to receive us to Himself. Others teach that Jesus will come at the rapture to join our bodies and souls together, then take us to heaven.

What is Jesus' favorite name for the Holy Spirit?

Jesus' favorite name for the Holy Spirit is "Comforter" (KJV). The Holy Spirit is also called "Helper" in other translations. The Greek word *paraklete* has the concept of *para* ("beside") and *kaleo* ("to call"). This is a person who is called alongside to help us. The Holy Spirit is called to help us find salvation, to help us live for God, and to help us glorify and worship God. The Helper is the third person of the Trinity, the Holy Spirit (John 14:17).

Why did Jesus liken Himself unto a vine when He said, "I am the true vine"? (John 15:1)

After Jesus instituted the Communion service in the Upper Room, He made the statement, "I am the true vine" (John 15:1). He may have been walking through the city of Jerusalem, and a vine that grew over a wall may have brushed Him. Jesus may have passed the large gate to Herod's temple and saw the vine there that symbolized Israel. Whatever the case, Jesus wanted His disciples to know that He was the True Vine and Life of Israel. Some say He saw the fires burning in the distance of the "smudge pots" to keep away the late winter frost. Then He made an analogy: "He is cast out as a branch, and is withered; and they gather them and throw them into the fire, and they are burned" (John 15:6). Jesus may have been reminded of the vine when He saw the fires on the distant hills. Still others think that the cup of His spilled blood was fresh in His mind, and He wanted them to know that just as the life-giving grape comes from the vine, He is the True Vine that gives life.

What did Jesus mean when He said, "the prince of this world is judged"? (John 16:11 KJV)

This is a reference to the judgment of Satan at the cross that happened within a few hours after Jesus made this prediction. Because of Satan's sin, he would receive the "cross-judgment." This is the fulfillment of what God told the serpent in the garden, "And He shall bruise your head" (Gen. 3:15). When a judge passes down a death sentence, he might say, "You shall be hanged by the neck until you are dead." Just as the judgment sentence takes sometimes weeks or years to carry out, Satan was judged at the Cross; but not until the Second Coming of Jesus Christ will he finally be judged in the lake of fire.

What did Jesus mean, "Hitherto have ye asked nothing in my name: ask, and ye shall receive, that your joy may be full"? (John 16:24 KJV)

The word *hitherto* means "up to now," and Jesus was reminding them that up until that time they had prayed to God in heaven, following the example of the Psalms. But once Jesus died and became the Mediator between God and man, they would have to pray "in His name." This means they would come through the blood of Jesus Christ and through His intercessory work at the right hand of God the Father.

When the soldiers came to arrest Jesus, why did they "fall to the ground"? (John 18:6)

Many feel that when they asked Jesus who He was, He answered them, "I am He." That was a statement of deity, and for just a moment, Jesus drew back the veil of his humanity, allowing the soldiers to see His deity. Just as no man can stand in the presence of God, they fell to the ground when they were confronted with the full glory of Jesus Christ.

What did Jesus mean, "Shall I not drink the cup which My Father has given Me?" (John 18:11)

The cup is the "cup of vengeance," which God the Father had promised to pour out on sin. Jesus knew He was going to become the Sin-Bearer of the world on the cross, and that He needed to drink the cup of vengeance of God the Father. This is when the Old Testament was fulfilled: "It pleased the Lord to bruise Him" (Isa. 53:10).

What was the meaning of the crown of thorns put upon the head of Jesus? (John 19:2)

Jesus is the King of those who follow Him, and in the future He will be the recognized King of Israel. Because of this, Jesus said to Pilate, "I am a king. For this cause I was born, and for this cause I have come into the world" (John 18:37). Because He was King, the world (soldiers) put a crown of thorns upon Him to mock Him. However, the crown of thorns has become our symbol of love and adoration. He wore the crown of thorns for you and for me.

Why did Mary Magdalene not recognize Jesus when He met her at the tomb? (John 20:11–17)

First of all, His face might have been so deformed by the suffering and punishment that He endured that He was not recognizable. Second, the Bible says she was weeping (John 20:13), so she might not have been able to see clearly through her tears. Third, it might have been spiritual blindness because of her unbelief (2 Cor. 4:3–4). She did not recognize Him until she heard Him speak.

Why did Jesus tell Mary, "Touch me not; for I am not yet ascended to my Father"? (John 20:17 KJV)

Apparently it was all right to touch Jesus after He was raised from the dead. The women who met Him leaving the tomb held Him by the feet (Matt. 28:9). And Jesus said on other occasions "Touch me" (John 20:27). However, Mary Magdalene apparently was holding on to His feet, as though she were trying to restrain Him and not let Him out of her sight. Jesus was saying that He would not have a physical relationship with His people in the future, but rather, it would be a spiritual relationship. He said, "I am ascending to My Father and your Father, and to My God and your God" (John 20:17).

How did Jesus appear to the disciples in the Upper Room on Easter Sunday afternoon?

The Bible says the doors and windows were shut, then "Jesus came and stood in the midst, and said to them 'Peace be with you'" (John 20:19). Apparently the resurrected body of Jesus Christ walked right through the walls, but they could not see Him until He appeared to them. Some have said He "materialized," but that doesn't seem to be the case as though He was not there and suddenly was there. Rather, He stood in their midst, but they could not see Him until He appeared to them.

Why was Thomas given the opportunity to put his finger in the wounds of the Lord? (John 20:24–29)

Thomas was the only one absent on the first Easter Sunday when Jesus appeared to them. The following Sunday Jesus appeared to them again when Thomas was present. Jesus knew the statements of unbelief that Thomas "the doubter" had said. "The other disciples therefore said to him, 'We have seen the Lord.' So he said to them, 'Unless I see in His hands the print of the nails, and put my finger into the print of the nails, and put my hand into His side, I will not believe'" (John 20:25). Jesus invited Thomas, "Reach your finger here, and look at My hands; and reach your hand here, and put it into My side. Do not be unbelieving, but believing" (John 20:27).

How many miracles did Jesus perform?

No one really knows how many miracles Jesus performed. The book of John ends Jesus' conversation with Thomas by saying, "And truly Jesus did many other signs in the presence of His disciples, which are not written in this book" (John 20:30). So we really don't know. In another place John tells us, "And there are also many other things that Jesus did, which if they were written one by one, I suppose that even the world itself could not contain the books that would be written. Amen" (John 21:25). Some have speculated that Jesus performed two to three thousand miracles. Others have speculated just a few more than those recorded, around fifty. There are thirty-seven recorded miracles in the four Gospels. Mark records twenty-seven miracles, more than any other Gospel. John has the fewest, recording eight miracles.

Why does the number seven occur so often in the gospel of John?

Many have said that John is the most Jewish of all of the Gospel writers, and that because of his Jewish background, he understood that seven was God's favorite number. So John includes seven miracles in his book, but chapter 21 seems to be an addendum or postscript, obviously added by the inspiration of the Spirit of God, but nevertheless an addition. Chapter 21 records an additional miracle. Therefore, John has seven plus one miracles. Seven is the number of perfection; eight is the number of the Holy Spirit.

John also includes the seven "I Ams": I am Bread; Light; the Shepherd; the Door; the Resurrection; the Way, the Truth, and the Life; and the Vine. For more study on John and the number seven, see *The Gospel of John: Believe and Live* by Elmer Towns (Chattanooga, Tenn.: AMG Publishers, 2002).

QUESTIONS ABOUT THE ACTS OF THE APOSTLES

Why is it called "the Acts of the Apostles"?

The Greek manuscripts designated it simply as *Praxeis*, that is, "Acts." Many of the books in Greek literature summarize great men with the phrase *praxeis*. Thus, this could be called the acts of Peter (Acts 1–12) and the acts of Paul (Acts 13–28). However, others have called it "the acts of the Holy Spirit" because He is evident in the expansion of the church. Some have called it "the acts of the church" as believers carried the message around the world. Still others have called it "the acts of prayer" because of the devotion to prayer by the church throughout the book of Acts.

Who wrote Acts?

The book is dedicated to Theophilus, the same one to whom the book of Luke was dedicated. Hence, Acts is the second of a two-volume work; therefore, you would expect that the author is Luke, who wrote the Gospel. The book of Acts includes the "we" sections that show Luke's authorship (Acts 16:10–17; 20:5–21; 27:1–28:16). The "we" indicates the times when Luke was traveling and ministering with Paul. Therefore, Luke wrote much of the book from an eyewitness point of view. At other times he interviewed people who were on the missionary journeys, Paul and/or others. Also, when Luke spent time in Jerusalem during Paul's trips there, he could have interviewed other "eyewitnesses" (Luke 1:1–4) to write the material for chapters 1–12. Luke included written documents in Acts 15:23–29 and 23:26–30 that he may also have studied.

When was Acts written?

The book of Acts ends abruptly with Paul waiting in Rome for his trial before Caesar. What was Paul doing? "Preaching the kingdom of God and teaching the things which concern the Lord Jesus Christ with all confidence, no one forbidding him" (Acts 28:31). Therefore, Luke completed the book about A.D. 62, before Paul was tried before Caesar, before the persecution of Nero (A.D. 64), before Paul's death (A.D. 68), and before the destruction of Jerusalem (A.D. 70).

Why did Acts have such an abrupt ending?

The book of Acts does not have a logical conclusion whereby the author draws all things into a summary and completes all details. Rather, the book of Acts stops with Paul preaching and teaching, with no one stopping his ministry (Acts 28:31). Some have suggested that Luke needed to get the manuscript to Theophilus so that it could be published. Others suggest that the Holy Spirit intended that the book of Acts not be concluded, to show that the Holy Spirit is still doing ministry today of preaching and teaching, as was done in Paul's day.

What are the key words in Acts?

The key words for Acts are *church growth*. These words do not appear in the book of Acts, but Luke demonstrated that, like a seed, when the gospel is planted, the church grows to full bloom and brings forth fruit.

What is the key verse in Acts?

"But you shall receive power when the Holy Spirit has come upon you; and you shall be witnesses to Me in Jerusalem, and in all Judea and Samaria, and to the end of the earth" (Acts 1:8).

How does the book of Acts show church growth?

The book of Acts puts great emphasis on numbers and arithmetic. First, it mentions that there were approximately 120 in the Upper Room praying (Acts 1:15). Then to that number were added three thousand souls who were converted and baptized on the day of pentecost (Acts 2:41). Next, it mentions that "the Lord added to the church daily those who were being saved" (Acts 2:47).

"However, many of those who heard the word believed; and the number of the men came to be about five thousand" (Acts 4:4). Here we see another number. This represents men, not women and children. Probably the early church would have numbered approximately twenty-five thousand at this time, including men, women, and children.

Next, "Believers were increasingly added to the Lord, multitudes of both men and women" (Acts 5:14). The number had become so large that Luke only described it as being "multitudes." But the church continued growing. The next word used was *multiplied*, not just "added" to the church. The number increased exponentially: "The number of the disciples multiplied greatly in Jerusalem" (Acts 6:7).

Next, Luke described a number of churches growing, not just individual believers: "Then the churches throughout all Judea, Galilee, and Samaria had peace and were edified. And walking in the fear of the Lord and in the comfort of the Holy Spirit, they were multiplied" (Acts 9:31). Notice that believers are now counted by churches, and the number of the churches was multiplying. When the Gospel reached Antioch, "a great number believed and turned to the Lord" (Acts 11:21), and because of the ministry of Barnabas and Paul, "many people were added to the Lord" (Acts 11:24). This was external growth, but the church also grew internally: "The word of God grew and multiplied" (Acts 12:24).

As the Gospel grew throughout the Mediterranean world, again it is said, "So the word of the Lord grew mightily and prevailed" (Acts 19:20).

Why were the disciples still interested in the Jewish kingdom right before Jesus ascended to heaven?

Jesus spent forty days of Postresurrection ministry teaching His disciples "things pertaining to the kingdom of God" (Acts 1:3). It is only natural that before He went back to heaven they asked, "Lord, will You at this time restore the kingdom to Israel?" (Acts 1:6). Jesus said it was not for them to know the "time" when this would happen (Acts 1:7). Jesus gave them the promise of the Great Commission in place of a promise of a restored kingdom: "But you shall receive power when the Holy Spirit has come upon you; and you shall be witnesses to Me in Jerusalem, and in all Judea and Samaria, and to the end of the earth" (Acts 1:8).

Where were the disciples praying after Jesus ascended to heaven?

"They went up into the upper room" (Acts 1:13). This was probably the home of Mary, the mother of John Mark. The church on another occasion prayed in "the house of Mary, the mother of John whose surname was Mark, where many were gathered together praying" (Acts 12:12). She would have been a wealthy Christian with room enough in her house for a large crowd.

Were the apostles correct in adding Matthias to their ranks?

The disciples only numbered eleven before Matthias took the place of Judas (Acts 1:26). Since the Jews thought that twelve was a complete number, the apostles felt they needed a twelfth person to complete their ranks. Also, until the place of Judas was filled, perhaps the disciples suffered guilt over what Judas had done.

Many believe that the disciples acted prematurely, and should have waited for the appointment of Paul as an apostle. "Born out of due time" (1 Cor. 15:8), Paul constantly defended his apostleship throughout his life (2 Cor. 12:1–21). Also, many feel that the church should no longer have resorted to "casting lots," which was an Old Testament method that implied "luck." God's choice was Judas, but since they used "luck" to appoint Matthias, they didn't get God's choice to replace Judas. Since the twelve apostles were going to sit on twelve thrones in the coming kingdom (Matt. 19:28), both Matthias and Paul obviously couldn't sit on the twelfth throne. Since Matthias is never heard of again, perhaps he should not have been chosen, and the church should have waited for Paul.

Was Judas buried in the potter's field? (Acts 1:18–19)

The potter's field was probably a plot of ground in Jerusalem bought by the legally minded priests in Judas's name. The priests took the thirty pieces of silver returned by Judas and purchased a field to bury people who couldn't afford a burial place. The Bible does not say Judas was buried here. "But the chief priests took the silver pieces and said, 'It is not lawful to put them into the treasury, because they are the price of blood.' And they consulted together and bought with them the potter's field, to bury strangers in. Therefore that field has been called the Field of Blood to this day" (Matt. 27:6–8).

While traveling with Jesus, Judas was the treasurer. He was stealing money that was given to Jesus. "Now this man purchased a field" (Acts 1:18–19). He committed suicide in this place and was buried there. This field is different from the potter's field.

What does the Bible teach about the mighty wind on the day of pentecost?

This was probably not a hurricane blowing in their faces, but rather, it was "a sound from heaven as a rushing mighty wind." Wind is the symbol of the new birth and represents the movement of the Spirit of God; therefore this sound of a mighty wind shows the might of the Holy Spirit in this new dispensation.

What does the Bible teach about the tongues of fire that sat upon the believers on the day of pentecost?

This was not literal fire, because it said it was "divided tongues, as of fire" (Acts 2:3). Because it was "as of fire," it looked like fire, but it wasn't actual fire that would have burned. It was a symbol of fire that would cleanse or consume, a sign of judgment and purification. God was purifying the church, and when they went preaching the Word of God, the power of God flowed through them to judge and convict of sin.

What does the Bible teach about tongues on the day of pentecost?

When the 120 in the Upper Room were filled with the Holy Spirit, they began to speak with "other tongues," which means they were speaking the languages of those who were observing and listening to the leaders of the early church. "We hear, each in our own language" (Acts 2:8, 11). The Bible indicates what languages they were speaking (Acts. 2:7–11). The foreigners were saying, "We hear them speaking in our own tongues the wonderful works of God" (Acts 2:11).

Why did Peter quote from the book of Joel when he preached on the day of pentecost?

Perhaps there were two things he wanted to convey to the people. First, he wanted them to know the essence of revival, which is God's presence among His people. Peter quoted from Joel, "I will pour out of My Spirit on all flesh" (Joel 2:28), which is a biblical definition of revival. Second, he wanted them to know why both men and women were speaking in tongues that day. Joel said, "Your sons and your daughters shall prophesy" (Acts 2:17, from Joel 2:28). Again Peter quoted, saying, "And on My menservants and on My maidservants I will pour out My Spirit in those days; and they shall prophesy" (Acts 2:18, Joel 2:29). But finally, Peter quoted from Joel to offer salvation to all: "Whoever calls on the name of the LORD shall be saved" (Acts 2:21, from Joel 2:32).

Is salvation only to those who are baptized in the name of Jesus Christ?
On the day of pentecost Peter preached, "Repent, and let every one of you be baptized in the name of Jesus Christ for the remission of sins; and you shall receive the gift of the Holy Spirit" (Acts 2:38). Some have interpreted this command to mean you have to be baptized in the name of Jesus Christ to be saved. However, in this reference, Peter is preaching to Jews who rejected Jesus Christ. The historical Jesus had preached, had performed miracles, and had been crucified in their city. Therefore, they must repent by acknowledging Jesus and what He had done for them. They had to repent and believe, then testify to their salvation by "being baptized in the name of Jesus Christ." However, this is not the only formula to be used for baptism. Later Jesus said, "baptizing them in the name of the Father and of the Son and of the Holy Spirit" (Matt. 28:19). Those who rejected Jesus had to be baptized in "Jesus name." Those who rejected the Trinity had to be baptized in the name of the Father, Son, and Holy Spirit. You must be baptized according to God's formula, not your own.

There is a second problem: Some people think you must be baptized to be saved. They point out that baptism is the only way to get remission of sins. However, a careful reading of the Greek text shows that they were not being baptized *to be* saved, but they were being baptized because they had received the remission of sins.

How long was the sermon on the day of pentecost?
The sermon that is recorded in Scripture (Acts 2:15–39) is not the complete sermon. Actually the sermon was probably a much longer discourse, but Luke included the essence of the sermon to help understand what God was saying to Israel. The sermon ends with the statement, "And with many other words he testified and exhorted them, saying, 'Be saved from this perverse generation'" (Acts 2:40).

Was Peter giving a reoffer of the Jewish kingdom in Acts 3:19?
In Acts 3:19–21 Peter said, "Repent therefore and be converted, that your sins may be blotted out, so that times of refreshing may come from the presence

of the Lord, and that He may send Jesus Christ, who was preached to you before, whom heaven must receive until the times of restoration of all things, which God has spoken by the mouth of all His holy prophets since the world began."

The phrase "times of refreshing" may be a reference to future millennial blessing, but it is also a reference to the revivals that come upon the church from time to time. When God's presence is "poured out on the church" that is a description of revival—that is, atmospheric revival. The phrase "He may send Jesus" is not a reference to the Second Coming, but of God's offer of salvation to all. The phrase "restitution of all things" is both a reference to the coming future kingdom and to how God wants to give us all things in Jesus Christ.

Was the house literally shaken when the early church prayed?

The Bible states, "When they had prayed, the place where they were assembled together was shaken" (Acts 4:31). Some believe that a localized earthquake shook the house and surrounding areas. Others believe it was the supernatural power of God that shook just the house where they were praying. Still others believe that the word *shaken* refers to a manifestation of the Holy Spirit (there is a sect known as the "shakers," who shake uncontrollably when they are filled with the Holy Spirit and speak with other tongues).

Did the early church practice "common ownership"?

There are two verses that seem to imply that the early church practiced a form of Christian communism, having common ownership of all things. On the day of pentecost it is described: "And all that believed were together, and had all things common; and sold their possessions and goods, and parted them to all men, as every man had need" (Acts 2:44–45 KJV). Later the Christians are described: "Nor was there anyone among them who lacked; for all who were possessors of lands or houses sold them, and brought the proceeds of the things that were sold, and laid them at the apostles' feet; and they distributed to each as anyone had need" (Acts 4:34–35). While these seem to suggest common ownership of all things, notice that the believers were selling and giving to *other believers* according to the needs that people had. It was not a "board" or "association" that was the recipient of the things, nor one entity owning all things for the multitude. Many in the early church had come from all parts of the known world. Because of pentecost and evidence of the Holy Spirit, they did not return home. Soon their money ran out, and Christians shared what they had with those who were away from home. By chapter 4 the process had become sophisticated, and many were selling all that they had, giving it at "the apostles' feet" which was to the church. The church was distributing to the needs of the individuals.

Notice two things: First, there was not a common ownership of all property. Instead, everything that was owned was sold and distributed. These people were practicing what Jesus said: "If anyone desires to come after Me, let him deny himself, and take up his cross daily, and follow Me" (Luke 9:23). They were sacrificing everything. Second, the church was not holding ownership of anything but was distributing everything as it received the money.

How did Peter know that Ananias and Sapphira were keeping back part of the money they brought to the church?

Some have suggested that there were people in the city of Jerusalem who knew the price Ananias and Sapphira got for selling their property, and when they saw that only part of the money was given to the church, they told Peter. Others believe the Holy Spirit by direct revelation gave Peter this information. Peter implies this when he said, "Why has Satan filled your heart to lie to the Holy Spirit?" (Acts 5:3).

How did Ananias and Sapphira die?

Notice what the Bible says: "Ananias, hearing these words, fell down and breathed his last. So great fear came upon all those who heard these things" (Acts 5:5). "Then immediately [Sapphira] fell down at [Peter's] feet and breathed her last" (Acts 5:10). It seems that they could have died of a stroke or heart attack or some other physical reason. Or God could have just stopped their internal life processes. Whatever the cause, it doesn't seem that they died as a result of circumstances but died by the hand of God.

What does the Bible teach about healing by the shadow of a godly man?

After the deaths of Ananias and Sapphira, the unsaved were greatly convicted of God's work in the church (Acts 5:13). "So that they brought the sick out into the streets and laid them on beds and couches, that at least the shadow of Peter passing by might fall on some of them" (Acts 5:15). This does not say that the people were saved because of Peter's shadow. It doesn't even say they were healed. God heals through faith. A woman came to Jesus and touched just the hem of his garment, and might have gone away to tell everyone that she was healed by touching Jesus, but Jesus called her forth and reminded her, "Your faith has made you well" (Mark 5:34). So even if they were healed when the shadow passed over them, it was faith, and not the shadow, that effected healing.

How did the church handle its first segregation or ethnic problem?

"In those days, when the number of the disciples was multiplying, there arose a complaint against the Hebrews by the Hellenists, because their widows were neglected in the daily distribution" (Acts 6:1). The apostles determined to handle the matter correctly, and they chose seven godly men who fit the criteria of spiritual leadership and ordained them (praying with their hands on the men's heads, setting them apart) for this ministry. It is noteworthy that the seven men all had Greek names (Acts 6:5), thus they represented the Greeks who were being discriminated against.

What supernatural event occurred at the death of Stephen?

As Stephen—the first martyr—died, God gave him a revelation of heaven. "But he, being full of the Holy Spirit, gazed into heaven and saw the glory of God, and Jesus standing at the right hand of God" (Acts 7:55).

Was Simon the sorcerer saved? (Acts 8:9–25)

Some say Simon the sorcerer was saved because he believed, was baptized, and "he continued" (Acts 8:13). However, others believe he was not saved because he wanted to buy the power of God with money. Peter suggests he was lost: "Your money perish with you" (Acts 8:20). Also Simon had no "portion in this matter" (Acts 8:21), and Peter told him, "Repent therefore of this your wickedness, and pray God if perhaps the thought of your heart may be forgiven you. For I see that you are poisoned by bitterness and bound by iniquity" (Acts 8:22–23). It seems as if both arguments are strong, so we will not know whether Simon was saved until we get to heaven.

Who was the Ethiopian eunuch?

The Ethiopian eunuch was the treasurer of Ethiopia, and served under Queen Candace. He was a "proselyte of the gate," which meant he could enjoy salvation, could bring a sacrificial lamb to the gate of the temple, but was not allowed to go in to fellowship with the priest in the temple.

Jesus said there were three ways by which a man became a eunuch. First, some eunuchs "were born thus from their mother's womb" (Matt. 19:12). Second, there were some who "were made eunuchs by men" (Matt. 19:12), meaning they were castrated or had some other procedure so they could not have children. Those who worked in the king's harem were such eunuchs. Third, there were those "who have made themselves eunuchs for the kingdom of heaven's sake" (Matt. 19:12). These chose not to marry or have children because they made a spiritual vow of chastity. The Ethiopian eunuch was probably of the second type. If he had had physical deformities, he would not have been allowed into the temple, therefore, he would have been a "proselyte of the gate."

How did Philip leave the Ethiopian eunuch? (Acts 8:39)

The Bible says, "When they came up out of the water, the Spirit of the Lord caught Philip away, so that the eunuch saw him no more; and he went on his way rejoicing" (Acts 8:39). Apparently Philip was supposed to lead the eunuch to full understanding of Jesus Christ and baptize him. After Philip had completed this task, the Spirit led him away. Some say that when Philip finished his task of teaching and baptizing, he made a normal departure, meaning he said good-bye and exhorted the eunuch to faith in Jesus Christ. Others say the Spirit caught him away in a manner similar to the rapture of the Christians—he actually disappeared. Still others say the Spirit led him to walk away after he baptized the eunuch. This suggests an abrupt departure.

What authority did Saul have to arrest Christians in the city of Damascus?

Some have questioned whether Saul had the authority as a Jew serving in Jerusalem to go to Damascus, a Syrian city, and there compel the Syrian government to arrest Christians so he could bring them back to Jerusalem. When Caesar was dealing with insurrection and rebellion, the high priest in Jerusalem backed Caesar and in return was given spiritual authority over all

Jews throughout the Roman world. Therefore Saul had a letter from the high priest in Jerusalem to exercise that authority, which the Roman authorities in Damascus would have honored.

What did Paul see when he fell to the Earth?

Paul did not see just a vision of Jesus Christ, nor did he have a hallucination from a heat stroke; Paul saw the actual Postresurrection appearance of Jesus Christ to him on the road to Damascus. Paul saw and heard Jesus Christ. When Paul asked, "Who are You, Lord?" he got the answer, "I am Jesus, whom you are persecuting" (Acts 9:5).

Is there a contradiction as to whether those with Paul actually heard the voice of Jesus?

The contradiction is only perception. The account reads in Acts 9:7, "And the men who journeyed with him stood speechless, hearing a voice but seeing no one." The Greek word is *phone*, which means they heard a sound, but did not understand the articulated words. In Acts 22:9, the text reads, "They did not hear the voice of Him who spoke to me." This means they did not understand the words that Jesus was saying to him, though they did hear an indistinguishable voice talking.

What fell from Paul's eyes when he was converted?

The Scriptures say, "Immediately there fell from his eyes something like scales, and he received his sight at once; and he arose and was baptized" (Acts 9:18). Luke, the medical doctor, is describing scales, suggesting they were something like scabs. Perhaps when Paul saw Jesus, the Lord was transformed into the brightness of the sun, and as result, Paul fell to the ground and dug at his eyes with sandy hands, creating scratches, bruises, and abrasions both on the skin and cornea, resulting in scabs around the eyes. When God healed him, the scabs fell off and he was able to see.

How long was Paul in Arabia after he was converted?

The Bible says that after he was converted, "Saul spent some days with the disciples at Damascus" (Acts 9:19). In another place Paul said that he did not get his teaching from Jerusalem, "nor did I go up to Jerusalem to those who were apostles before me; but I went to Arabia, and returned again to

Damascus. Then after three years I went up to Jerusalem to see Peter, and remained with him fifteen days" (Gal. 1:17–18). Some suggest that Paul went to Arabia for three years (probably not Saudi Arabia as we know today; the word *Arabia* means "desert"). Others suggest a shorter time. But Paul had a desert experience. Tradition tells us he was forty days in the wilderness, as was Jesus. While he was there God taught him the truth of grace, the mysteries of the kingdom of heaven, and the truths of the church, the body of Christ. The text suggests Paul returned to Damascus and stayed there three years preaching "Christ in the synagogues, that He is the Son of God" (Acts 9:20). Then after three years, Paul went to Jerusalem. He stayed in Jerusalem fifteen days.

Why was an attempt made to kill Paul in Damascus?

Because Paul was effective in preaching Jesus Christ to the Jews, they tried to kill him.

Why was an attempt made to kill Paul in Jerusalem?

Paul only stayed fifteen days in Jerusalem, but again, the Jews wanted to kill him because of his effectiveness in preaching that Jesus was the Messiah.

Why did the angel give a vision to Cornelius, and not preach the gospel to him?

Cornelius was a godly man that gave alms and prayed, but he was not yet converted. Since it is not the job of angels to preach the gospel (because the Great Commission was given to believers), the angel told him to go find Peter, who preached the gospel to him: "Now send men to Joppa, and send for Simon whose surname is Peter . . . He will tell you what you must do" (Acts 10:5–6).

Why did God show Peter a sheet filled with unclean animals?

There are perhaps two reasons why Peter saw the sheet filled with unclean animals. First of all, God was preparing him to go to a Gentile (Cornelius) and preach to him. Jew considered Gentiles unclean. Second, the ceremonial law concerning what a Jew could not eat was done away with in the death of Christ (Col. 2:14–17), the Law now being fulfilled. Therefore, God used the occasion of the sheet to tell Peter, "What God has cleansed you must not call common" (Acts 10:15).

What happened when Peter preached the gospel to Cornelius?
The Bible says, "The Holy Spirit fell upon all those who heard the word" (Acts 10:44). "They heard them speak with tongues and magnify God" (Acts 10:46). As a result, Peter baptized them in water (Acts 10:48).

Why did the church at Antioch get so much attention in Scripture?
This was the church where Gentiles first responded to the gospel in a significant way (Acts 11:19–20). It became a great missionary church for the spreading of the gospel throughout the Mediterranean world (Acts 13:1–5). It was also the church where Paul received his internship, demonstrating the power of God upon him, equipping him for missionary duty (Acts 11:25–26).

Why did Herod turn against the church and kill James?
When Caligula was Caesar, he took emperor worship seriously, putting a statue of himself in the Jewish temple. This resulted in Jewish struggles with Rome, and persecution of the Jews. When Claudius became Caesar in A.D. 41, he backed down on emperor worship and made peace with the Jews. Then the Jews turned their hatred against the church and caused Rome to persecute Christians. "Now about that time Herod the king stretched out his hand to harass some from the church" (Acts 12:1).

How did God judge Herod?
God judges people in various ways. Sometimes God judges people directly, as when He directly struck Ananias and Sapphira dead (Acts 5). At other times God uses intermediate means, such as this judgment on Herod: "Then immediately an angel of the Lord struck him, because he did not give glory to God. And he was eaten by worms and died" (Acts 12:23).

Where was the prayer meeting held for Peter's release?
The prayer meeting was held in the Upper Room, in "the house of Mary, the mother of John whose surname was Mark, where many were gathered together praying" (Acts 12:12).

What does the phrase "his angel" mean?
When Rhoda went to tell the people in the prayer meeting that Peter was at the gate, they said she was mistaken, and that it was "his angel" (Acts 12:15).

They believed that every person had a guardian angel, one sent by God to protect them. When talking about children, Jesus said, "In heaven their angels always see the face of My Father who is in heaven" (Matt. 18:10). From this suggestion, Christians believe everyone has a guardian angel.

Was Paul unmarried or a widower?

There is no clear Scripture reference to Paul ever having been married. We know that Paul was born at Tarsus of Cilicia (Acts 9:11; 21:39; 22:3) of the tribe of Benjamin (Phil. 3:5). In Romans 16:7–11 Paul salutes three persons as his (physical) kinsmen, two of whom were "of note among the apostles," and had become Christians before him. Acts 23:16 refers to "Paul's sister's son." It seems that if Paul had been married, there would have been some mention of his wife in the Scriptures.

Most Bible scholars believe Paul was single. However, some feel he was widowed. Paul says, "I wish that all men were even as I myself" (1 Cor. 7:7). For the gospel's sake he chose to remain unmarried, and in his ministry, it was best for him to be single. Others say that since Paul had probably been a member of the Sanhedrin, which demanded a man be married to qualify for membership, he was probably a widower who never remarried.

What was the judgment on Elymas the sorcerer? (Acts 13:6–12)

Elymas, a Jewish sorcerer and false prophet, opposed Paul when the gospel was preached to Sergius Paulus, the Roman ruler of Cyprus. Paul prayed for God to judge Elymus. He said, "'And you shall be blind, not seeing the sun for a time.' And immediately a dark mist fell on him, and he went around seeking someone to lead him by the hand" (Acts 13:11).

Why did John Mark leave Barnabas and Paul?

John Mark was never called of God, as were Barnabas and Paul, so he probably thought that since he had decided to come with them, he could decide to leave. Also, as long as they were in Cyprus, they were in familiar territory, the country of his relative Barnabas. But when they left to go to Asia Minor, this was not only unfamiliar territory, but also Mark, being a Jew, might have sensed persecution against the Jews in Asia Minor. To this add the fact that a transfer of leadership took place at this time. Paul became the leader, and Barnabas the follower. Since Mark was a relative of

Barnabas, and the leadership changed, Mark felt he could leave and go home.

Why did the leadership pass from Barnabas to Paul? (Acts 13:2–13)

When the missionary tour began, Barnabas's name was mentioned first, but as they left Cyprus, Paul's name was mentioned first. This might be because they were going into Gentile territory, and Paul was the apostle to the Jews. Also, Paul had prayed for the miracle of blinding Elymas, and was effective in getting the Roman ruler of Cyprus saved. As the change in leadership was being made, Saul's name was changed to Paul. He gave up his Jewish name for a Gentile name to remove barriers when he preached to Gentiles.

Did Mark sin by leaving Paul and Barnabas?

Jesus had encouraged His followers to not give up after beginning a task (Luke 9:57–62). Paul felt Mark had given up, and when Barnabas wanted to take him on the next missionary journey, Paul objected (Acts 15:37–39). Since Paul was the leader who was pushing the Great Commission into all the known Mediterranean world, Mark apparently had let him down, and "Paul insisted that they should not take with them the one who had departed from them in Pamphylia, and had not gone with them to the work" (Acts 15:38). Barnabas disagreed and "took Mark and sailed to Cyprus" (Acts 15:39).

Why was Saul's name changed to Paul?

Saul was his Jewish name, and while he ministered primarily among the Jews his name opened up doors of opportunity for ministry. However, when Paul ministered to Sergius Paulus (a Roman official) on Cyprus, Paul probably saw the wisdom of using a Gentile name to effectively reach Gentiles. Also notice that when Paul did his first miracle of blinding Bar-Jesus, it was in the presence of Sergius Paulus (a person named Paul).

Did Paul die when he was stoned at Lystra? (Acts 14:19–20)

There are many reasons to think that Paul died under the stoning. First, stoning is a brutal form of punishment that usually leads to death. Second, the Jewish enemies hated Paul so intensely that they would not knowingly leave him with a shred of life left. Third, the text says that they left him "supposing him to be dead" (Acts 14:19), and fourth, when Paul gave an account of being caught up into the third heaven (2 Cor. 12:1), he indicated that it was approximately fourteen years earlier, the approximate time when Paul was stoned at Lystra. This suggests Paul died under the stoning and went to heaven.

Some feel he was not stoned, but was only severely beaten. They point to the fact that "supposing him to be dead" (Acts 14:19) suggests that the crowd only "supposed" he was dead, but he really wasn't. To support this argument, they suggest the nature of Gentile stoning was humiliation and punishment, not death. The author believes it was the Jews who came to Lystra that actually stoned Paul, leading to his death. Paul was immediately raised up and the next day continued his travels, suggesting he was raised from the dead. To support this view, see 2 Corinthians 12:2–4 that gives the approximate time of the stoning, fourteen years before Paul wrote the book of Second Corinthians: "I know a man in Christ who fourteen years ago— whether in the body I do not know, or whether out of the body I do not know, God knows—such a one was caught up to the third heaven. And I know such a man—whether in the body or out of the body I do not know, God knows—how he was caught up into Paradise and heard inexpressible words, which it is not lawful for a man to utter" (2 Cor. 12:2–4).

What was the cause for the first church council?

"And certain men came down from Judea and taught the brethren, 'Unless you are circumcised according to the custom of Moses, you cannot be saved'" (Acts 15:1).

Who was the main spokesmen at the Jerusalem council?

First, Paul put forth his reason why Gentiles should not be circumcised (Acts 15:12). Next, Peter rose up to tell how God had worked through him among the Gentiles (Acts 15:7–11). Finally, James, the half brother of Jesus, rose to the place of leadership in the church. He summarized the conclusion of the council (Acts 15:13–27).

How did the Lord lead Paul on the second missionary journey?

First, Paul decided not to take John Mark with him because the young man had abandoned them on the first missionary journey. So Paul used his reason to choose Silas to travel with him. Second, Paul began traveling through Syria and Asia Minor (Acts 15:41), using his natural inclination to go through his home regions. On the first journey he began in Cyprus, because Barnabas was from Cyprus and was going back home to minister. Third, the Holy Spirit used an "internal urge." As they went through Asia Minor, God would not let them go to the south or the north. "They were forbidden by the Holy Spirit to preach the word in Asia" (Acts 16:6) because "the Spirit did not permit them" (v. 7). Fourth, God used a supernatural vision to lead Paul: "And a vision appeared to Paul in the night. A man of Macedonia stood and pleaded with him, saying, 'Come over to Macedonia and help us'" (Acts 16:9).

Who was the man in the vision that invited Paul to Macedonia?

Some say the man was Luke, a Gentile, because immediately after Paul saw the vision, the "we" sections begin, implying that Luke joined Paul in ministry immediately after the Macedonian vision. However, a second interpretation is that the man in the vision was the Philippian jailor, the first man to be converted in Greece. In a third interpretation, some feel he is a "ubiquitous," or "universal," man who stood for all Greeks, inviting him to come and preach the gospel to them.

What ability did the young damsel have who constantly bothered Paul in Philippi?

The girl had the ability to tell fortunes (predict the future). The Bible said she had a "spirit of divination" (Acts 16:16), which means in the original "a spirit of a python." Since a serpent or a snake is the symbol of Satan, she was inspired and enabled by an evil demon.

Can a demon predict the future?

No, only God can predict the future, because only God knows the future. However, when a witch, psychic, or fortune-teller appears to predict the future, she (or he) does it in several ways. First, she has a natural inclination or insight into a person's personality. From that she determines what the person might do and make her prediction based on a "hunch." Second, demons have been observing and gathering knowledge about people since the beginning of time. They are able to make guesses based on what people might do.

Apparently this girl was able to tell the future with some accuracy, because she brought money to her masters.

Sometimes demons are able to control the future. For example, the demon in a medium tells what's going to happen, and another demon might arrange for the predicted situation to occur. One demon predicts you'll lose your business goods in an accident, while the other demon causes the accident to happen. Demons don't know the future, but they can have some accuracy in certain details that they can control.

How did Paul cast out the demon?

"And this she did for many days. But Paul, greatly annoyed, turned and said to the spirit, 'I command you in the name of Jesus Christ to come out of her.' And he came out that very hour" (Acts 16:18).

What was the reaction of Paul and Silas in prison?

"But at midnight Paul and Silas were praying and singing hymns to God, and the prisoners were listening to them" (Acts 16:25). The Greek word for *praying* is *proseuchomai*, which means "communion" or talking with God. The words *sang praises* come from the Greek word *hymomas*, which is the word from which we get *hymn*. They were "hymning," or singing praises to God. This is also the word from which the Hebrews get the *hillel*, which are the great songs of praise that the Jews would sing when they ascended up to Jerusalem, to the presence of God. In essence, Paul and Silas were not praying judgment on their captors, asking to get out of prison, or complaining about their mistreatment. Rather, they were fellowshipping with God and worshiping Him.

How did God release Paul and Silas from prison?

As Paul and Silas were fellowshipping with God and worshiping Him, "suddenly there was a great earthquake, so that the foundations of the prison were shaken; and immediately all the doors were opened and everyone's chains were loosed" (Acts 16:26). Though there is no proof for this, when I preach on this passage, I say that when God in Heaven heard two men in prison worshiping Him, He wanted to get closer to hear and receive their worship. Iron gates could not keep God out, but as God came to visit the prison and receive the worship of His servants, the gates "opened" to let God in. Notice, none of the prisoners fled when the gates opened and their shackles fell off. Technically, it was the jailor who freed Paul and Silas and took them to his home to wash their wounds, receive the Word of God, and be baptized.

What is one of the best gospel invitations found in Scripture?
"Believe on the Lord Jesus Christ, and you will be saved" (Acts 16:31).

Why does Paul apparently overlook some cities, and go to others?
"Now when they had passed through Amphipolis and Apollonia, they came to Thessalonica, where there was a synagogue of the Jews" (Acts 17:1). Notice in the above Scripture that Paul went to Thessalonica, while passing through Amphipolis and Apollonia. This is because Thessalonica had a synagogue, and Paul was still carrying the gospel to the Jews first (Rom. 1:16). The other two cities probably didn't have a synagogue or a Jewish presence.

What was required of Jason, Paul's host in Thessalonica?
"So when they had taken security from Jason and the rest, they let them go" (Acts 17:9). The security that was required of Jason was probably a peace bond. This was not unlike security that a church must post when renting a civic center or using other public facilities today. This security guaranteed that the church would not cause uproar in the city of Thessalonica, and if an uproar occurred, the bond was forfeited.

Did Paul compromise his stand in Athens?
When Paul got to Athens, many people feel that he compromised his message. First, they say he compromised his ministry on Mars Hill by preaching the gospel to philosophers (Acts 17:18) rather than emphasizing his ministry in the synagogue (Acts 17:7). Second, his message said very little about Scripture; rather, he quoted philosophers and used rational arguments with them. Third, there were very little results to his preaching. Fourth, when he finally mentioned the Resurrection, the crowd cut him off so he couldn't continue preaching (Acts 17:32).

On the other side of the argument, there are many who feel that Paul did not compromise his preaching. They say that he was in the center of God's will because, first, the nature of an audience determines the type of preaching. These were philosophers, who did not know the Scriptures nor would they take the Scriptures as verification of the truth; therefore, Paul tried to reach who they were, where they were. Also, Paul understood the nature of the city, and was attempting *cross-cultural evangelism*, reaching the Greeks at their capital city. (When Paul preached in synagogues, he was using *in-culture evangelism*.) And according to Acts 17:34, Paul did have some results, and his example has become a role model for others who preach the gospel among the educated or secular audiences.

Who were Priscilla and Aquila?

This was a godly couple used greatly of the Lord in the life of Paul. They were born in Pontus Asia Minor near the coast of the Black Sea, moved to Rome, and apparently were tent makers there. When Caesar Claudius commanded all Jews to leave Rome, they came to Corinth to set up their trade. It was there that Paul came to work for them, and they became leaders in the church of Corinth. When a traveling Jew named Apollos came to Corinth, everyone was impressed with his integrity, eloquent speech, and knowledge of Scripture. Yet Aquila and Priscilla thought he was not saved. They took him aside "and explained to him the way of God more accurately" (Acts 18:26). Later, the church of Corinth moved into their home, and when Paul wrote to Rome, they had moved to Rome, and established the church there.

Was Apollos saved?

Some people think he was not saved because Aquila and Priscilla had to explain "to him the way of God more accurately" (Acts 18:26). However, others believe that he was a Jew who had Old Testament salvation and who traveled preaching the Word of the Lord. The Bible describes him as "instructed in the way of the Lord; and being fervent in spirit, he spoke and taught accurately the things of the Lord, though he knew only the baptism of John" (Acts 18:25). Perhaps the issue is not whether he was saved or not. Apparently he had Old Testament salvation and repented under the preaching of John the Baptist. When Aquila and Priscilla taught him the way of God more perfectly, he came into full knowledge of Jesus Christ, the New Testament salvation.

When Eutychus fell three stories, did he die?

Eutychus was listening to the sermon Paul was preaching, when he apparently went to sleep and fell three stories to the ground. The Bible says he was "taken up dead. But Paul went down, fell on him, and embracing him said, 'Do not trouble yourselves, for his life is in him.' Now when he had come up, had broken bread and eaten, and talked a long while, even till daybreak, he departed. And they brought the young man in alive, and they were not a little comforted." (Acts 20:9–12). Some think that perhaps the boy was not dead, but only seriously injured. They point out that Paul did not think he was dead, because he said, "Do not trouble yourselves, for his life is in him" (v.10). Then Paul went and ate a meal with the disciples, and after he left, "they brought the young man in alive, and they were not a little comforted" (v. 12). However the author thinks the boy died because of the statement "was taken up dead" (v. 9). Paul prayed over the boy and said, "His life is in him" which was Paul's statement of faith in God's ability to do miracles (see James 5:16). Apparently the miracle had a delayed reaction, because the boy was presented alive after Paul left. Paul "talked" a long while, even till the break of day, so he departed. And "they brought the young man in alive" (Acts 20:11, 12).

How did the Holy Spirit forbid Paul to go to Jerusalem?

There were certain disciples who "told Paul through the Spirit not to go up to Jerusalem" (Acts 21:4). Later the Holy Spirit warned him through Agabus the prophet, who "took Paul's belt, bound his own hands and feet, and said, 'Thus says the Holy Spirit, "So shall the Jews at Jerusalem bind the man who owns this belt, and deliver him into the hands of the Gentiles"'" (Acts 21:11). Apparently the Holy Spirit through prophetic words spoke to Paul, telling him what would happen when he went to Jerusalem. In spite of the danger, Paul went to Jerusalem, where he was arrested as foretold by Agabus.

Did Paul sin by getting involved in Jewish vow and a Jewish sacrifice?

When Paul got to Jerusalem, the leaders of the church told Paul that the Jewish people were angry with him. So the church leaders asked Paul to demonstrate his loyalty to the Jewish people and the temple. They suggested, "Do what we tell you: We have four men who have taken a vow. Take them and be purified with them, and pay their expenses so that they may shave their heads, and that all may know that those things of which they were informed concerning you are nothing, but that you yourself also walk orderly and keep the law" (Acts 21:23–24). Paul obeyed the leaders of the church, apparently shaved his head, and went to the temple to offer a sacrifice. Acts tells us, "Then Paul took the men, and the next day, having been purified with them, entered the temple to announce the expiration of the days of purification, at which time an offering should be made for each one of them" (21:26). However, before Paul could carry out the sacrifice, the Jews created a riot and stopped him from offering a sacrifice.

Would Paul have sinned by submitting himself again to the Old Testament law?

Some Bible teachers think so. They point out that Paul's stinging rebuke of those going back under Old Testament law should have kept him from offering a sacrifice. Note the principle, "People fall at their strengths, not at their weaknesses." Paul's strength was his message of grace and his non-Jewish stance; however, he went against what he had known and preached; therefore he sinned.

Other people think he didn't sin. He was being respectful to the law. All he did was to pay the price of the sacrifice for four men and be present when the sacrifice was offered.

Did Paul violate Scripture by reviling the high priest?

When Paul was brought before the Sanhedrin, the high priest commanded that Paul be slapped in the mouth. Paul responded, "God will strike you, you whitewashed wall!" (Acts 23:3). Those who stood by told Paul he was reviling God's high priest and quoted to him the Law: "You shall not . . . curse a ruler of your people" (Ex. 22:28). When Paul heard this, he apparently apologized, for he said, "I did not know, brethren, that he was the high priest" (Acts 23:5). When Paul first entered the Sanhedrin, the Bible says, "Paul, looking earnestly at the council . . ." (Acts 23:1). The original Greek language indicates that Paul was straining to see who was there. He might have had poor eyesight, so he couldn't recognize who was in the Sanhedrin, also contributing to the fact that he didn't recognize the high priest.

Why did Paul appeal to Caesar?

Festus asked Paul in Caesarea if he was willing to go to Jerusalem and be tried of the Jews. It was then that the Jews planned to assassinate Paul. The Jews had requested that Paul be brought to Jerusalem because they wanted to kill him. Paul knew that Rome should protect him and that he should be tried under Roman law. So Paul, being a Roman citizen said, "For if I am an offender, or have committed anything deserving of death, I do not object to dying; but if there is nothing in these things of which these men accuse me, no one can deliver me to them. I appeal to Caesar" (Acts 25:11).

Why is the blinding of Jews mentioned at the end of Acts?

Jesus predicted that the Jews would be blinded because of their unbelief in refusing to believe Him and accept His ministry (Matt. 13:14–16). The final rejection of the Jews happened in Acts 28. The Jewish leaders in Rome came to see Paul, but they had not heard about the incident in Jerusalem, nor did they know why he was sent to Rome. Paul was able to present the gospel to them and press home the claims of Jesus Christ. "So when they had appointed him a day, many came to him at his lodging, to whom he explained and solemnly testified of the kingdom of God, persuading them concerning Jesus from both the Law of Moses and the Prophets, from morning till evening. And some were persuaded by the things which were spoken, and some disbelieved" (Acts 28:23–24). Because this was the final rejection of the message of Christ by the Jewish nation, Paul quoted Isaiah, saying, "Hearing you will hear, and shall not understand; and seeing you will see, and not perceive; for the hearts of this people have grown dull. Their ears are hard of hearing, and their eyes they have closed, lest they should see with their eyes and hear with their ears, lest they should understand with their hearts and turn, so that I should heal them" (Acts 28:26–27).

QUESTIONS ABOUT THE EPISTLE TO THE ROMANS

In what order did Paul probably write his epistles?

Paul probably wrote his epistles in the following order: Galatians, 1 Thessalonians, 2 Thessalonians, 1 Corinthians, 2 Corinthians, Romans, Ephesians, Philippians, Philemon, Colossians, 1 Timothy, Titus, 2 Timothy.

Who wrote the epistle to the Romans?

Paul wrote the book of Romans (Rom. 1:1) as his foundational book. Very few people have questioned Paul's authorship. The vocabulary, dramatic style,

logical development, and theological content are reflective of Paul's other letters. Apparently Paul dictated this to a secretary named Tertius (Rom. 16:22).

When did Paul write Romans?

Paul wrote Romans in A.D. 57 when he was in Greece (Acts 20:3–6), more
specifically in Corinth. Paul was living with Gaius (Rom. 16:23, 1 Cor.
1:14), and mentions Erastus, the treasurer of Corinth (Rom. 16:23).

How did the letter get to Rome?

After Paul finished writing the letter, there was a plot to kill Paul, so he went
by way of Philippi to return to Jerusalem. He gave the letter to Phoebe, who
was from a small church at Cenchrea near Corinth, and she forwarded the
letter to Rome (Rom. 16:1–2).

Why is the book of Romans placed first among Paul's writings?

Obviously Romans was not the first letter that Paul wrote, but it was considered his greatest work and is placed first among his letters because of its
doctrinal prominence.

What is the main thrust of the book of Romans?

The book of Romans has the most systematic presentation of doctrine of any
book in the Bible. But it is not just a theology book; it gives a logical examination of sin and an exposition of the death of Christ, His justification of
sinners, and man's response. The book also includes practical exhortations.
The message of Jesus Christ is more than theology or a set of facts one must
believe; it is the life of Jesus Christ, to be lived in godly holiness.

Who founded the church at Rome?

Paul did not plant the church at Rome. Tradition says that Peter was its
founder, but this is contrary to evidence. Some think that Jews who were
converted at Pentecost (Acts 2:10) returned to Rome and began the church.
Others think that the church began when Christians from other churches
moved to Rome, since by the time Paul wrote to the church of Rome, it was
predominately Gentile (see the Gentile names mentioned in Romans 16:11,
15–16). However, even though Gentile names were prominent, there were
some Jewish believers.

Why was Rome an important city?

Rome was the center of the Roman Empire. It had been founded in 553 B.C., and was considered the greatest city in the world. It was full of splendor with many buildings and had over one million inhabitants, though 90 percent of the people who lived there were slaves. The Roman citizens and government officials lived in splendor and opulence, while the slaves lived in squalor.

What is the key word in Romans?

The key word is *righteousness*, for God does more than save individuals. Those who accept Jesus Christ are declared righteous, "being justified freely by His grace through the redemption that is in Christ Jesus, whom God set forth as a propitiation by His blood, through faith, to demonstrate His righteousness, because in His forbearance God had passed over the sins that were previously committed" (Rom. 3:24–25).

What are the key verses in Romans?

"For I am not ashamed of the gospel of Christ, for it is the power of God to salvation for everyone who believes, for the Jew first and also for the Greek. For in it the righteousness of God is revealed from faith to faith; as it is written, 'The just shall live by faith'" (Rom. 1:16–17).

What does Paul mean by the word *salvation*? (Rom. 1:16)

Both the Greek and Hebrew words for salvation imply the ideas of deliverance and redemption, and are inclusive of the other great words that Paul uses to show the act of redemption: *justification, grace, imputation, forgiveness, sanctification,* and *preservation.*

In what sense is a person "saved"?

Salvation involves three verb tenses: (1) The believer *has been* saved from past sin and its penalty; (2) the believer *is being* saved from the domination of sin and its power; and (3) the believer *will be* saved in the future from the presence of sin.

What is the "righteousness of God"?

The righteousness of God is not an attribute of God, nor is it an attribute of a Christian. Righteousness, instead, is what Jesus Christ is Himself. Because

He fully did that which was right—He fulfilled the law; He fulfilled the act of redemption; He set aside the price of our penalty of sin when it was imputed to Him—He did the "right" thing to obtain salvation. Because of that, "Christ Jesus . . . became for us . . . righteousness" (1 Cor. 1:30).

What is "justification"? (Rom. 3:24)

Justification means "just-as-if-I've-never-sinned." I am not *made* perfect, but am *declared* perfect. When believers are declared righteous, they are as righteous as Jesus Christ, because they have His righteousness, which was transferred to Him (2 Cor. 5:21).

In what sense were we baptized into the death of Jesus? (Rom. 6:3)

Paul says that there is a spiritual baptism, and that when Jesus died, the believer died with Him; when Jesus was buried, the believer was buried with Him; and when Christ was raised from the dead, the believer was raised with Him. "Therefore we were buried with Him through baptism into death, that just as Christ was raised from the dead by the glory of the Father, even so we also should walk in newness of life. For if we have been united together in the likeness of His death, certainly we also shall be in the likeness of His resurrection" (Rom. 6:4–5).

What does Paul mean by the "old man"? (Rom. 6:6)

The "old man" means the old nature, or the sinful nature, that is in a person. The old man or old nature of a Christian was put to death with Jesus so that the believer may eventually live for Jesus Christ.

Whom is Paul discussing in Romans 7?

Some feel that Paul is discussing the Christian who is addicted or bound to sin, struggling to overcome his sin nature. Other people feel Paul is discussing an unsaved person who struggles with sin. Notice what Paul says about sin: "For the good that I will to do, I do not do; but the evil I will not to do, that I practice. Now if I do what I will not to do, it is no longer I who do it, but sin that dwells in me" (Rom. 7:19–20). Paul is saying that a person is dominated by sin when he lets the old sin nature rule his life.

What is the dominant theme of Romans 8?

The dominant theme is the Holy Spirit and what He will do for the believer who yields his or her life to Christ. "For the law of the Spirit of life in Christ Jesus has made me free from the law of sin and death" (Rom. 8:2). After Paul tells what the Spirit will do for the believer, he then tells the believer, "For as many as are led by the Spirit of God, these are sons of God" (Rom. 8:14). And then the Holy Spirit gives the believer confidence and assurance: "The Spirit Himself bears witness with our spirit that we are children of God, and if children, then heirs—heirs of God and joint heirs with Christ, if indeed we suffer with Him, that we may also be glorified together" (Rom. 8:16–17).

What does Paul teach about the Holy Spirit's intercession for the believer?

Paul says that the Holy Spirit will intercede to God the Father for believers, communicating with words that cannot be understood by humans. "Likewise the Spirit also helps in our weaknesses. For we do not know what we should pray for as we ought, but the Spirit Himself makes intercession for us with groanings which cannot be uttered" (Rom. 8:26).

What does Paul say about the Jews in Romans 9–11?

Paul writes to express his heart's passion that they might be saved: "For I could wish that I myself were accursed from Christ for my brethren, my countrymen according to the flesh" (Rom. 9:3).

How could God say, "Esau have I hated"? (Rom. 9:13 KJV)

It is obvious that the Lord loved Jacob, because Jacob used every means possible to choose God. Obviously Jacob wanted the birthright and the blessing. Even though Jacob used immoral means to get them, he still had a passion to get them, and God loved his choice, even if He did not approve of Jacob's scheming. When the Word says that God "hated" Esau, the word *hated* means "rejected." Because Esau rejected God by giving away his birthright and blessing, God says that He rejected Esau.

Does Paul teach that God is finished with the Jewish people and kingdom?

"I say then, has God cast away His people? Certainly not! For I also am an Israelite, of the seed of Abraham, of the tribe of Benjamin. God has not cast away His people whom He foreknew" (Rom. 11:1–2). This Scripture proves that God still has a future plan and purpose for the Jewish people.

What is "judicial blindness"?

God has blinded the Jews "judicially" because they have rejected Him. Paul talks about "eyes that they should not see and ears that they should not hear, to this very day" (Rom. 11:8). Later Paul says, "Let their eyes be darkened, so that they do not see" (Rom. 11:10). Paul describes this blinding in another place: "But their minds were blinded. For until this day the same veil remains unlifted in the reading of the Old Testament, because the veil is taken away in Christ. But even to this day, when Moses is read, a veil lies on their heart" (2 Cor. 3:14–15).

What is Paul teaching in the analogy of the wild olive branches?

In Romans 11:16–24, Paul is teaching that Israel is an olive branch that brought glory to God (the olive tree is an Old Testament symbol for Israel). But when Israel turned away from God, God took a wild olive branch (Gentiles) and grafted it into the olive tree. This is a picture of God's plan with Gentiles during the time of the Gentiles. However, the analogy also teaches that in the last days Israel shall turn to the Lord: "For if you were cut out of the olive tree which is wild by nature, and were grafted contrary to nature into a cultivated olive tree, how much more will these, who are natural branches, be grafted into their own olive tree?" (Rom. 11:24).

What does the phrase "all Israel shall be saved" mean? (Rom. 11:26 KJV)

Some feel that this will happen in the future, when every single Israelite will become converted and live in the kingdom. Others don't believe this refers to individual salvation, but to the nation of Israel (national salvation), who will live in the kingdom. It is understood that some Israelites will individually turn against God and not enter the kingdom. This is both individual and national salvation, so the nation of Israel shall be saved, as well as individual conversions.

What does the Bible teach about human government?

Paul teaches in Romans 13:1–7 that a Christian has several obligations to his government: (1) a Christian should be subject to government; (2) a Christian should not resist the government's power; (3) the government is to deal with lawlessness and the lawbreaker; (4) the government is the minister of God to do good for its citizens; (5) the government will bear the sword to protect from foreign invaders and from internal lawbreakers; (6) Christians should be subject to the government for conscience' sake; and (7) the Christian should pay taxes (vv. 6–7).

Is there a place for deaconesses in the church?

Phoebe delivered Paul's letter to Rome. Paul calls her a servant, that is, a *diakoness*. Since this one lady is called a deaconess, many people see this as the basis for the office of deaconesses in the church. Some feel that deaconesses are the wives of deacons, while others feel that deaconesses can be elected or appointed to an office based on their merit and/or service of Jesus Christ. Phoebe was a deaconess, and nothing is mentioned of her husband or that she is married to a deacon. Apparently she got her position based on her merit and service.

QUESTIONS ABOUT THE FIRST EPISTLE TO THE CORINTHIANS

Who wrote 1 Corinthians?

Paul is universally accepted as the author of 1 Corinthians: "Paul, called to be an apostle of Jesus Christ through the will of God, and Sosthenes our brother, to the church of God which is at Corinth" (1 Cor. 1:1–2).

Who planted the church at Corinth?

Paul planted the church in Corinth on his second missionary journey (Acts 18:1–7). He originally was a tent maker working for Aquila and Priscilla, and began his ministry reasoning with the Jews in the synagogue. Shortly thereafter, Titus and Timothy came from Philippi bringing a financial gift that enabled Paul to give full time to the church.

What was the condition of Corinth?

Corinth was a large cosmopolitan city of approximately seven hundred thousand people, of which two-thirds were slaves. The city was located on a small isthmus between the Aegean and Adriatic Seas. There was a port on each sea. Many ships were rolled across the narrow isthmus on wooden rails or dragged from one sea to the other; saving a two-hundred-mile trip around southern Greece. Nero and others attempted to dig a canal through the isthmus, but it was not done until 1893, and today the canal is a well-traveled sea-lane.

In Paul's day the city was filled with shrines and temples. The most prominent was the temple of Aphrodite, on top of the two-hundred-foot hill called Acrocorinthus. The temple contained over a thousand prostitutes whom people could visit as an expression of their worship of "the goddess of love." Because Corinth was a seaport, it contained business and government buildings, and because of its vice, many tourists came seeking sexual pleasure and corruption. The word *Corinth* was corrupted into *korinthiazomai*, which meant "debauchery and sexual freedom," from which came the phrase "to act like a Corinthian."

Why did Paul write the first epistle to the Corinthians?

Even though the city was filled with vice and corruption, the church grew, and many apparently believed in Jesus Christ. It was in Corinth that Paul moved his ministry from the local synagogue to the home of Titus Justus. Paul left the city in A.D. 52, and Apollos came to minister to the church (Acts 18:24–28).

On his third missionary journey, reports came to Paul from the household of Chloe (1 Cor. 1:11), and then the church sent a delegation of three men (1 Cor. 16:17) who told Paul about the quarrels, sin, relaxed standards, and other problems in the church. Apparently the three men who came bringing the letter to Paul wanted his opinion. In response to the problems of the church, Paul wrote about their divisions and bickering, their lawsuits, their immorality, their abuses at the Lord's Table, their abuses of spiritual gifts, and their questionable practices.

When was 1 Corinthians written?

Paul wrote the book in A.D. 56 from Ephesus (1 Cor. 16:5–8).

What is the key word in 1 Corinthians?

The key word is *carnal.* This was a carnal church filled with carnal people. The word *carnal* means "fleshly," and refers to those who were motivated by the flesh and lived to satisfy the flesh.

What are the key verses in 1 Corinthians?

"And I, brethren, could not speak to you as to spiritual people but as to carnal, as to babes in Christ. I fed you with milk and not with solid food; for until now you were not able to receive it, and even now you are still not able; for you are still carnal. For where there are envy, strife, and divisions among you, are you not carnal and behaving like mere men?" (1 Cor. 3:1–3).

QUESTIONS ABOUT THE SECOND EPISTLE TO THE CORINTHIANS

What is 2 Corinthians about?

In 1 Corinthians Paul wrote to rebuke the church of its sins expressed in divisions, lawsuits, immorality, questionable practices, and abuses at the Lord's Table, not to mention abuses of spiritual gifts. Since that time, the church had been racked by false teachers who said that Paul was not an apostle, and that he was arrogant, unimpressive in appearance and speech, dishonest, and lacking in love for the Corinthians. Paul had sent Titus to Corinth to deal with these difficulties, and when Titus returned, Paul wrote a letter expressing his thankfulness for the attitude of repentance of the majority, and to appeal to the rebellious minority to accept his apostleship. The book is an extended defense of Paul's character and calling as an apostle.

Who wrote the book of 2 Corinthians?

There is not doubt among the scholars of the Pauline authorship of this book. It begins, "Paul, an apostle of Jesus Christ by the will of God, and Timothy our brother, to the church of God which is at Corinth" (2 Cor. 1:1).

When did Paul write 2 Corinthians?

Paul probably wrote 2 Corinthians from Philippi in A.D. 56 (Acts 20:1–3).

What is the focus of 2 Corinthians?

One of the major themes of 2 Corinthians is Paul's defense of his apostolic office. This is especially evident in chapters 10–13. Many false apostles had risen in Corinth, and Paul had to discredit them, while establishing his own credibility.

What is the key word in 2 Corinthians?

The key word is *comfort*, which Paul extended to the people, and also to himself. In his letter, Paul showed his physical weakness, weariness, and pain. But it was more than just physical tribulation; there were spiritual and emotional pressures that pushed Paul to the breaking point. It was here that he needed the comfort that only God could give him.

What are the key verses in 2 Corinthians?

"Blessed be the God and Father of our Lord Jesus Christ, the Father of mercies and God of all comfort, who comforts us in all our tribulation, that we may be able to comfort those who are in any trouble, with the comfort with which we ourselves are comforted by God. For as the sufferings of Christ abound in us, so our consolation also abounds through Christ" (2 Cor. 1:3–5).

What was Paul's "thorn in the flesh"? (2 Cor. 12:7)

"And lest I should be exalted above measure by the abundance of the revelations, a thorn in the flesh was given to me, a messenger of Satan to buffet me, lest I be exalted above measure" (2 Cor. 12:7). Different Bible scholars have various views in attempting to identify this thorn.

Some believe that Paul's thorn in the flesh was his poor eyesight because of several passages that suggest this. Galatians 4:15 says, "For I bear you witness that, if possible, you would have plucked out your own eyes and given them to me." Then in Galatians 6:11 Paul says, "See with what large letters I have written to you with my own hand" (normally, a scribe wrote Paul's letters to the churches). In Acts 28:1–3, as Paul gathered firewood, he picked up what looked like a bit of firewood, but found when he laid it on the fire that it was a viper that was stiff from the cold. And as Paul stood before the council on another occasion, he was not able to recognize those at some distance from him. Apparently Paul did not even realize that he was speaking to the high priest. "I did not know, brethren, that he was the high priest" (Acts 23:2–5).

Others think Paul's thorn in the flesh was a physical incapacity from the various beatings Paul suffered, but there is no proof of that or any other opinion on what Paul's thorn was. God simply did not choose to reveal this truth. We may never know the answer until we get to heaven.

QUESTIONS ABOUT THE EPISTLE TO THE GALATIANS

Who wrote the epistle to the Galatians?

"Paul, an apostle (not from men nor through man, but through Jesus Christ and God the Father who raised Him from the dead), and all the brethren who are with me, to the churches of Galatia" (Gal. 1:1–2). Also, "Indeed I, Paul, say to you" (Gal. 5:2). At the end of the book, Paul actually says he wrote the book (Gal. 6:11), instead of dictating it to a secretary, as was his usual practice.

Where was the church of Galatia?

Actually, there was no one church to which this letter was written. This is the only letter that Paul wrote to a series of churches (Gal. 1:2).

Why did Paul write to the Galatians?

After he returned from evangelizing the churches in southern Galatia (the southern part of modern-day Turkey), Paul got news that the Christians had suddenly fallen to the false teaching of the Judaizers, who put them under the Law, including circumcision and keeping the temple rituals. These Judaizers professed to know Jesus, but required Christians to keep the Mosaic Law (Gal. 1:7; 4:17, 21; 5:2–12; 6:12–13).

Paul begins by setting forth his credentials as an apostle with a special message from God that salvation is by grace through faith. He declares that the Law makes people guilty and puts them in bondage, whereas Jesus Christ sets them free. Paul challenges the Galatians to enjoy their liberty in Christ.

When did Paul write the letter to the Galatians?

Paul and Barnabas evangelized the area on their first missionary trip (Acts 13:13–14:23). The Judaizers had come to Antioch in Syria where Paul and Barnabas had ministered. As Paul prepared to go the Jerusalem Council (Acts 15) to deal with the issue, he probably wrote Galatians from Antioch in A.D. 49, just before he went to the Jerusalem Council.

What is the key word in Galatians?

The key word is *law* because Paul deals with the law from several aspects. He constantly maintains, "I do not frustrate the grace of God: for if righteousness come by the law, then Christ is dead in vain" (Gal. 2:21 KJV).

What is the key verse in Galatians?

"Stand fast therefore in the liberty wherewith Christ hath made us free, and be not entangled again with the yoke of bondage" (Gal. 5:1 KJV).

QUESTIONS ABOUT THE EPISTLE TO THE EPHESIANS

Who wrote the epistle to the Ephesians?

The universal opinion is that Paul wrote it, and this opinion is supported by both internal and external evidence. "Paul, an apostle of Jesus Christ by the will of God, to the saints who are in Ephesus, and faithful in Christ Jesus" (Eph. 1:1).

Who planted the church at Ephesus?

At the end of Paul's second missionary journey, he visited Ephesus, where he left Priscilla and Aquila (Acts 18:18–21). The church was in existence when Paul arrived, so it is not known who planted the church.

What was the city of Ephesus?

Ephesus was one of the foremost Asian cities, located on the western coast of modern-day Turkey. It was a commercial center of Asia Minor and had a harbor for trade and travel. Ephesus was also a religious center where the famous temple of Diana (Roman name), or Artemis (Greek name), was built, considered one of seven wonders of the ancient world (Acts 19:35ff). Paul ministered in Ephesus for three years (Acts 18:23–19:41). When the word of God was spread throughout the province, many churches were planted. Because of Paul's ministry, the traffic of magic and images was seriously hurt, leading to an uproar in the huge Ephesian theater. It was then that Paul left the city.

When did Paul write Ephesians?

The book of Ephesians is considered one of the "Prison Epistles" written during Paul's first imprisonment (Eph. 3:1; 4:1; 6:20). The book was probably written in A.D. 60.

What is the thrust of the book of Ephesians?

Ephesians was a circulatory letter, that is, it was written to a number of churches and ended up in Ephesus where it stayed. Or it could have been written to Ephesus and from there circulated to a number of churches. Therefore, its reading tends to be impersonal to the people of Ephesus, rather than highly personal. Paul tells them in chapters 1–3 of their great wealth as Christians, which is their position in the heavenlies. In chapters 4–5 he reminds them of how they are to live as Christians. In chapter 6 Paul teaches them about the warfare as believers.

What is the key word in Ephesians?

The key word is *heavenlies*. Paul reminds the Christians that they are "in Christ," and because Christ is in heaven, they have a position or standing before God, and are perfect in Christ Jesus.

What is the key verse in Ephesians?

"Blessed be the God and Father of our Lord Jesus Christ, who has blessed us with every spiritual blessing in the heavenly places in Christ" (Eph. 1:3).

Years ago I heard a sermon describing the book of Ephesians as containing the wealth, walk, and warfare of the Christian. The sermon depicted the wealth as all of the benefits that a Christian has in Christ; the walk as how Christians are to live; and warfare as the spiritual combat we have with Satan. Of all of the books of the New Testament, there is perhaps more mentioned about spiritual warfare in Ephesians than in any other book.

QUESTIONS ABOUT THE EPISTLE TO THE PHILIPPIANS

Who wrote the epistle to the Philippians?
Both internal and external evidence indicates that Paul is the author of the book. "Paul and Timothy, bondservants of Jesus Christ, to all the saints in Christ Jesus who are in Philippi, with the bishops and deacons" (Phil. 1:1).

What is the key word in Philippians?
The key word is *joy*, indicating that Paul's joy was in the Lord Jesus Christ. He wanted his readers to participate in this joy: ". . . that your rejoicing for

me may be more abundant in Jesus Christ" (Phil. 1:26). Paul showed them that only in Christ is real joy possible, and as they modeled the humility and service of Jesus Christ (Phil. 2:5–6), they would have lives of peace and joy (Phil. 4:6–7).

What are the key verses in Philippians?
Paul exhorted the Philippians, "Rejoice in the Lord always. Again I will say, rejoice" (Phil. 4:4). He also said, "Fulfill my joy by being like-minded, having the same love, being of one accord, of one mind" (Phil. 2:2).

When was Philippians written?
Philippians is one of the Prison Epistles, written from a Roman jail. Paul wrote that everyone knew that he was in jail "so that it [would] become evident to the whole palace guard, and to all the rest, that [his] chains [were] in Christ" (Phil. 1:13). Paul first came to establish the church in Philippi in A.D. 51, and he wrote this epistle eleven years later, in A.D. 62.

What was the city of Philippi like?
King Philip of Macedonia, the father of Alexander the Great, took this small town and made it into a city, renaming it Philippi, after himself. The Romans captured it in 168 B.C., and the town was turned into a Roman colony and military outpost. The town did not have great commercial enterprises but was a military center. That's why there were not enough Jews to have a synagogue. Paul had to seek people praying by the river (Acts 16:13).

While in Asia Minor, Paul received the "Macedonian call" and crossed over the Aegean Sea to Greece and into Philippi. It was there that Lydia, a businesswoman who sold purple, was converted. It was also there that Paul and Silas were imprisoned. But after Paul and Silas had been beaten and put in prison, the jailer was converted. Because the city leaders had beaten Paul without a trial, they were embarrassed and released him (Acts 16:37–40). Perhaps because of this incident, the church enjoyed great freedom in the future. The city leaders respected the church.

What was the occasion for the writing of Philippians?
Paul wrote this letter to thank the Philippians for the financial gift that was sent to him in prison. Epaphroditus brought the money (Phil. 4:18), but this

was not the first time that they had sent money to Paul. They had done it on at least two other occasions (Phil 4:16). As a result, Paul said that the people in Philippi were his "fellow workers."

There was also a problem between two ladies (Phil. 4:2) in the church, and Paul wrote to tell them to solve their problems and work together.

What are the great and/or famous verses in the book of Philippians?

Many people have chosen as a life verse Philippians 1:21: "For to me, to live is Christ, and to die is gain." Others have chosen, "Let this mind be in you which was also in Christ Jesus" (Phil 2:5). Many people see a great benediction in Philippians 2:10–11: "That at the name of Jesus every knee should bow, of those in heaven, and of those on earth, and of those under the earth, and that every tongue should confess that Jesus Christ is Lord, to the glory of God the Father." Another verse that is often quoted is, "That I may know Him and the power of His resurrection, and the fellowship of His sufferings, being conformed to His death" (Phil. 3:10). Following this great commitment of Paul, many have quoted Philippians 3:14: "I press toward the goal for the prize of the upward call of God in Christ Jesus." In times of rejoicing and giving thanks, many people quote Philippians 4:6–7: "Be anxious for nothing, but in everything by prayer and supplication, with thanksgiving, let your requests be made known to God; and the peace of God, which surpasses all understanding, will guard your hearts and minds through Christ Jesus." Paul tells people how to meditate in Philippians 4:8, and this is another verse that people often memorize: "Finally, brethren, whatever things are true, whatever things are noble, whatever things are just, whatever things are pure, whatever things are lovely, whatever things are of good report, if there is any virtue and if there is anything praiseworthy—meditate on these things." Finally, one cannot mention the great verses of Philippians without repeating Philippians 4:13: "I can do all things through Christ who strengthens me."

QUESTIONS ABOUT THE EPISTLE TO THE COLOSSIANS

Who wrote the epistle to the Colossians?

Paul wrote the Epistle to the Colossians, along with three other Prison Epistles (Ephesians, Philippians, and Philemon), from prison in Rome. Paul identifies himself as the author in Colossions 1:1: "Paul, an apostle of Jesus Christ by the will of God, and Timothy our brother." He ends the letter by again indicating his authorship: "This salutation by my own hand—Paul. Remember my chains. Grace be with you. Amen" (Col 4:18).

What is known about the city of Colosse?

It was a very small city about a hundred miles east of Ephesus. The seven churches of Revelation were located nearby. The city of Colosse was located near a mountain pass on a road from Ephesus to the east. It is evident from the book that Paul never visited Colosse (1:8–10; 2:1).

What is the emphasis of Colossians?

Many have said that the books of Ephesians and Colossians were "sister letters." The book of Ephesians talks about the body of Christ, while Colossians talks about Christ, who is the Head of the body. While Ephesians focuses primarily on the believer, Colossians focuses primarily on the Head, Jesus Christ. Like the book of Ephesians, Colossians is divided into two sections. The first section is doctrinal (Col. 1–2), and the second section is practical (Col. 3–4).

What is the key word in Colossians?

The key word of Colossians is *preeminence*. Paul encouraged the Colossians to make Jesus Christ the preeminent One in their lives and church. Christ is the "head of all principality and power" (Col. 2:10), the Lord of Creation (Col. 1:16–17), the Reconciler (Col. 1:20, 22; 2:13–14), our Hope (Col. 1:5, 23, 27), full Deity (Col. 1:15, 19), the Creator and Sustainer of all things (Col. 1:16–17), the Head of the Church (Col. 1:18), and the All-Sufficient Savior (Col. 1:28, 2:3, 10, 3:1–4).

What is the key verse in Colossians?

"That in all things He may have the preeminence" (Col. 1:18).

When did Paul write Colossians?

This letter has all the evidences of the other Prison Epistles, so Paul wrote it A.D. 60 or 61 from Rome. He sent this letter with Tychicus and Onesimus to Colosse (Col 4:7–9; Eph. 6:21; Philem. 10–12). Onesimus was a slave whom Paul had led to Christ in Rome, and he sent Onesimus and Tychicus back to Colosse, each with a letter in his hand.

Why did Paul write Colossians?

Epaphras came to report the conditions of the church at Colosse to Paul. The church was threatened with heresy, so Paul wrote to "choke off" the heresy before it became a full-blown doctrinal problem for Colosse and all the other churches in the area.

What was the heresy in Colosse?

Part of the heresy was Gentile in nature (Col. 1:21, 27; 2:13), and part of it was Jewish in nature (Col. 2:11–17). We don't know all the details of the exact heresy; we can only surmise what it was from the way Paul refuted their arguments and attacked their false truth. We do know that they were involved in Greek philosophy (Col 2:4, 10:8), keeping the Jewish law (Col. 2:11–17), and Eastern mysticism (Col. 2:18–23). The people in Colosse also had a low view of the physical body and a wrong view of self-discipline. They thought that spirituality came by masochistic aestheticism (Col. 2:20, 23). The Colossian church was being tempted to legalistically obey circumcision, dietary laws, and the temple rituals. With it they were adding mystical experiences and the worship of angels. After answering all their problems, Paul reminded them, "If then you were raised with Christ, seek those things which are above, where Christ is, sitting at the right hand of God. Set your mind on things above, not on things on the earth. For you died, and your life is hidden with Christ in God. When Christ who is our life appears, then you also will appear with Him in glory" (Col. 3:1–4).

What is the unique thrust of Colossians?

Paul told the readers that "Christ is preeminent" in every part of life. Then he proceeded to give one of the loftiest views of Jesus Christ found anywhere in Scriptures (Col. 1:15–23). They were to be rooted in Christ, hidden in Christ, complete in Christ, and alive in Christ, and were to live in Jesus Christ, for without Christ their lives were nothing.

QUESTIONS ABOUT THE FIRST EPISTLE TO THE THESSALONIANS

Who wrote the first epistle to the Thessalonians?

Paul is the uncontested author of this book. Very few critics have claimed otherwise. "Paul, Silvanus, and Timothy, to the church of the Thessalonians in God the Father and the Lord Jesus Christ: Grace to you and peace from God our Father and the Lord Jesus Christ" (1 Thess. 1:1).

When did Paul write 1 Thessalonians?

Paul wrote the book shortly after he left the church in A.D. 51 in response to Timothy's report that the church was prospering, but that they had misunderstood the doctrine of the Second Coming of Jesus Christ, thinking that those who had died would not be taken in the rapture with living believers (1 Thess. 4:13–17).

What do we know about the city of Thessalonica?

Thessalonica was a prominent seaport and was the capital of the Roman province of Macedonia. Today, the city is known as Salonika. One of the reasons it was prosperous was that it was located on the main road from Rome to the East. Mount Olympus, the legendary mountain where the Greek Parthenon was located, could be seen from Thessalonica. Cassander, a Greek general, made this small town into a large city around 315 B.C. and renamed it after his wife, who was also the half sister of Alexander the Great. When the Romans conquered Thessalonica, it remained the capital city, but they made it a "free city," giving it freedom to govern itself. It became a commercial success, and during Paul's time, there were over two hundred thousand people in the city.

What is known about the church at Thessalonica?

When Paul went to the city, he began preaching in the synagogue of the Jews; however, a large number of Gentiles responded to the monotheistic teaching of Judaism and Christianity. They came to listen to what Paul had to say. Apparently, these Gentiles were turned off by paganism and the worship of many gods, and responded to the careful reasoning of Paul (Acts 17:10–12) and became saved. The Jews became very jealous of Paul's success, and a mob threatened to harm Paul and his company. When the mob didn't find Paul, they dragged Jason, Paul's host, before a secular judge and accused him of rebellion against Rome. "These that have turned the world upside down are come hither also (Acts 17:6 KJV). The political authorities took a *pledge*, a political bond from the Christians, guaranteeing no further uprising and that Paul would leave the city.

How long was Paul in the city?

Paul was probably there less than a month, that is "three Sabbaths" (Acts 17:2). During this short period of time, Paul had established a strong church and taught the people well. They understood prophecy and the return of Jesus Christ, and had reached out in evangelism to all the areas around them. "For from you the word of the Lord has sounded forth, not only in Macedonia and Achaia, but also in every place" (1 Thess. 1:8).

Most of the Thessalonian converts were Gentiles (1 Thess. 1:9; 2:14–16), and they continued to reach out to other Gentiles after Paul left the city.

What is the key word in 1 Thessalonians?

The key word is *example*. This church had become an example to all the other churches in the region in lifestyle, evangelism, learning, and growth in Christ.

What is the key verse in 1 Thessalonians?

"So that you became examples to all in Macedonia and Achaia who believe" (1 Thess. 1:7).

What is Paul's great passage on the return of the Lord?

"But I do not want you to be ignorant, brethren, concerning those who have fallen asleep, lest you sorrow as others who have no hope. For if we believe that Jesus died and rose again, even so God will bring with Him those who sleep in Jesus. For this we say to you by the word of the Lord, that we who are alive and remain until the coming of the Lord will by no means precede those who are asleep. For the Lord Himself will descend from heaven with a shout, with the voice of an archangel, and with the trumpet of God. And the dead in Christ will rise first. Then we who are alive and remain shall be caught up together with them in the clouds to meet the Lord in the air. And thus we shall always be with the Lord." (1 Thess. 4:13–17)

What was Paul's great prayer for the Thessalonians?

"And may the Lord make you increase and abound in love to one another and to all, just as we do to you, so that He may establish your hearts blameless in holiness before our God and Father at the coming of our Lord Jesus Christ with all His saints" (1 Thess. 3:12–13).

QUESTIONS ABOUT THE SECOND EPISTLE TO THE THESSALONIANS

Why did Paul write a second letter to the Christians in Thessalonica?

Apparently the person who delivered the first letter to the Thessalonians came back telling Paul that the people had developed another problem. Paul saw this problem as a seed that, if not nipped in the bud, would grow into full-grown heresy. The Thessalonians misunderstood the day of Christ, thinking that Christ had come and that they had been left behind. That produced another problem; some people were guilty of "laziness." They knew about the Lord's coming at any moment, so they had given up their jobs and were not working. Instead, they were waiting for Jesus to return and take them to heaven.

Who wrote the second epistle to the Thessalonians?

There is no question that Paul wrote 2 Thessalonians. "Paul, Silvanus, and Timothy, to the church of the Thessalonians in God our Father and the Lord Jesus Christ: grace to you and peace from God our Father and the Lord Jesus Christ. We are bound to thank God always for you, brethren" (2 Thess. 1:1–3). The word selection, style, and doctrine also support Paul's authorship.

When did Paul write 2 Thessalonians?

He probably wrote this letter a few months after he wrote the first letter to Thessalonica. Paul was still in Corinth with Silas and Timothy (Acts 18:5).

What are the key words in 2 Thessalonians?

The key words are *He shall come* (2 Thess. 1:10 KJV). The whole theme is that Jesus Christ shall come "to be glorified in his saints, and to be admired in all them that believe" (2 Thess. 1:10).

What is the key verse in 2 Thessalonians?

"When He comes, in that Day, to be glorified in His saints and to be admired among all those who believe, because our testimony among you was believed" (2 Thess. 1:10).

What is the theme of 2 Thessalonians?

The theme is the day of Christ. Notice the King James Version talks about the "day of the Lord" but the Greek word is *Christos,* meaning it should be "the day of Christ." This unfortunate translation has caused some to accept a post-Tribulation rapture position. The Christians of Thessalonica were upset because they thought that Christ had returned and missed them. So

Paul wrote, ". . . not to be soon shaken in mind or troubled, either by spirit or by word or by letter, as if from us, as though the day of Christ had come" (2 Thess. 2:2).

What guarantee did Paul give that the day of Christ had not come?
Paul said that if the "day of Christ" had come, (1) there would have been a falling away of saints from the gospel; (2) the man of sin, Antichrist, would have been revealed; and (3) the Antichrist would have exalted himself and would be sitting in the temple.

QUESTIONS ABOUT THE FIRST EPISTLE TO TIMOTHY

Who wrote the first epistle to Timothy?
"Paul, an apostle of Jesus Christ, by the commandment of God our Savior and the Lord Jesus Christ, our hope" (1 Timothy 1:1). The early church gave strong support for Paul in authorship of this letter, as did early-church fathers, such as Polycarp, Clement of Rome, Irenaeus, Tertullian, and the Muratorian Canon.

Where was Paul when he wrote 1 Timothy?
Paul was in a Roman prison cell, writing to Timothy, who was pastoring the church at Rome. Paul wrote, "To Timothy, a true son in the faith" (1 Tim. 1:2).

Paul called him, "my own son," because Paul was probably responsible for Timothy's salvation when Paul visited Lystra (Acts 16:1). Paul told Timothy, "Remain in Ephesus." This is because Timothy was then the pastor of the large and influential church at Ephesus.

Why did Paul write 1 Timothy?

Young Timothy was facing great odds and was unsure of himself. So Paul the "aged" (Philem. 9) wrote to encourage young Timothy to be strong, diligent, and to carry out the work of God. Because Timothy faced false doctrine, Paul told him to be faithful in leading the church, and to keep the church pure. Timothy was to avoid false teachers with wrong motivations. Timothy was to emphasize godliness, love, perseverance, and faith.

When was 1 Timothy written?

First Timothy was probably written in A.D. 62–63. Paul was at the end of his first imprisonment. He expected to be released, and in this book he writes that he expects to travel and preach again.

Was Paul released from prison?

In this first epistle to Timothy, Paul is upbeat and optimistic. Apparently, the Jews that had brought charges against him did not show up for his trial before Caesar (2 Tim. 1:8; 17; 2:9; 4:16–17). Some church traditions say that Paul went to Spain (Rom. 15:24–28). Others feel that he did not go to Spain, but went east, making a trip to the churches in Greece and Asia Minor. There he was joined by Timothy before being rearrested. Second Timothy tells of a second imprisonment where Paul had no hope of release and expected to die a martyr's death (2 Tim. 4:6–8, 18).

What are the key words in 1 Timothy?

The key words are *faithful sayings*. This phrase occurs throughout 1 and 2 Timothy. These were actual "sayings of faith," meaning that these were the oft-repeated slogans used by those in the church that reflected what they believed. "This is a faithful saying and worthy of all acceptance, that Christ Jesus came into the world to save sinners, of whom I am chief" (1 Tim. 1:15).

What is the key verse in 1 Timothy?

The key verse is introduced in 1 Timothy 3:15, where Paul says, "But if I am delayed, I write so that you may know how you ought to conduct yourself in the house of God, which is the church of the living God, the pillar and ground of the truth." Paul told Timothy to give heed to what he was saying so he would know how to lead the church of God. Then Paul broke into a "faithful saying." This is perhaps the earliest doctrinal statement that the early church used to express what it believed: "And without controversy great is the mystery of godliness: God was manifested in the flesh, justified in the Spirit, seen by angels, preached among the Gentiles, believed on in the world, received up in glory" (1 Tim. 3:16).

QUESTIONS ABOUT THE SECOND EPISTLE TO TIMOTHY

Who wrote the second epistle to Timothy?
Just as Paul wrote 1 Timothy, he also wrote 2 Timothy. The early church had two letters to Timothy from Paul. Apparently they added "B" to distinguish the second letter from the first. "Paul, an apostle of Jesus Christ by the will of God, according to the promise of life which is in Christ Jesus" (2 Tim. 1:1).

To whom was 2 Timothy written?
This letter was written to young Timothy. His name occurs more in Paul's writing than any other name. "To Timothy, a beloved son" (2 Tim. 1:2).

Who was Timothy?
Timothy had a Jewish mother, Eunice, and grandmother, Lois, who reared him in the Hebrew Scriptures (2 Tim. 1:5; 3:15). His father was a Greek (Acts 16:1), but Paul circumcised Timothy because of the Jews (Acts 16:1–3). Apparently, Timothy was converted the first time Paul visited Timothy's home in Lystra (Acts 16:1), and because of this, Paul calls him "son." When Paul traveled through Lystra on his second missionary journey, he took young Timothy with him for help in the ministry (young John Mark had left Paul on the first trip). Timothy was ordained to the ministry (1 Tim 4:14; 2 Tim. 1:6) and became a companion to Paul in the missionary tours (Acts 16–18). He was a preacher, and Paul left him in Ephesus, Macedonia, and Corinth to preach and lead those young churches. When Paul wrote the letter of 2 Timothy, young Timothy was leading the church at Ephesus (1 Tim. 1:3). Paul urged Timothy to come visit him in Rome before he died (2 Tim. 4:9).

Why was Paul imprisoned the second time?
Nero was Caesar (A.D. 54–68), but was both mentally and politically unstable. When half of Rome burned in July A.D. 64, Nero accused Christians of the fire, and inspired great persecution of Christians everywhere. Paul was arrested a second time and brought to Rome. No one stood with Paul in his defense in the Roman court (2 Tim. 4:16). He was abandoned by all of his followers (2 Tim. 4:10–11).

In Paul's first imprisonment in Rome, he was under house arrest. People could visit him freely, and he demonstrated a great spirit of hope that he would be released shortly. During Paul's second arrest, he was in a cold Roman cell (2 Tim. 4:13), people regarded him as an "evildoer" (2 Tim. 2:9), and he did not expect acquittal in spite of his first defense (2 Tim. 4:6–8, 17–18). Paul expected to die. So as winter approached, he wrote to Timothy, asking him to visit him (2 Tim. 4:21). He wanted his cloak and books.

When was 2 Timothy written?

It was probably written in the fall of A.D. 67, because winter was approaching.

How did Paul die?

Most believe that Paul was beheaded on the Apian Way outside of Rome.

What is the content of 2 Timothy?

While Paul had no hope or encouragement for his own life, he wrote Timothy a letter of encouragement to continue serving the Lord. Paul assured Timothy of his love, support, and prayers, and reminded Timothy of his spiritual heritage and responsibilities. Paul told Timothy to be strong when attacked, as Paul was during his trials.

What is the key word in 2 Timothy?

The key word is *doctrine*. Paul wanted Timothy to be strong in doctrine, because it is the foundation for all of life. The phrase "the faith" is used by Paul throughout 2 Timothy. Whereas faith usually refers to *saving* faith, in 2 Timothy the word *faith* is preceded by the article *the*. Timothy is told to defend *the faith*, as one defends a doctrinal statement, or statement of faith.

What is the key verse in 2 Timothy?

"Preach the word; be instant in season, out of season; reprove, rebuke, exhort with all longsuffering and doctrine" (2 Tim. 4:2 KJV).

QUESTIONS ABOUT THE EPISTLE TO TITUS

Who was Titus?

Titus was a young companion of Paul who was given the task of "setting in order" the church in Crete. While Titus is not mentioned in the book of Acts, there are thirteen references to him in Paul's epistles, revealing that he was one of Paul's closest companions. Paul led Titus to Christ and called him "a true son in our common faith" (Titus 1:4). Most say that Titus was born in Antioch of Syria, where Paul and Barnabas first started ministering together (Acts 11:19–26). When Paul went to the Jerusalem conference to confront the Judaizers over their legalism, he took Titus, an uncircumcised Greek believer, with him, where Titus became a testimony that Gentiles could be converted to Christ, yet have liberty from the law. Titus accompanied Paul on his third missionary journey (Acts 18:22), and was sent by Paul to Corinth on three different occasions (2 Cor. 2:12–13; 7:5–7, 13–15; 8:6, 16–24). Titus was not mentioned again until his name appeared with Paul during his second Roman imprisonment. Titus left to go to Dalmatia (2 Tim. 4:10), probably for missionary outreaches. Paul called Titus a "brother" (2 Cor. 2:13), a "partner and fellow worker" (2 Cor. 8:23), and his "son" (Titus 1:4).

This book to Titus is the third "pastoral epistle" (the others were 1 and 2 Timothy). Ironically, Titus had the same name as the Roman general who destroyed Jerusalem in A.D. 70.

Who wrote the epistle to Titus?

It is universally recognized that Paul wrote the book of Titus:

"Paul, a bondservant of God and an apostle of Jesus Christ, according to the faith of God's elect and the acknowledgment of the truth which accords with godliness, in hope of eternal life which God, who cannot lie, promised before time began, but has in due time manifested His word through preaching, which was committed to me according to the commandment of God our Savior; to Titus, a true son in our common faith." (Titus 1:1–4)

When did Paul write the epistle to Titus?

After Paul was released from his first Roman imprisonment, he went to Crete and spread the gospel throughout the island, leaving Titus there to finish organizing the churches (Titus 1:5). Therefore, Paul wrote this letter about A.D. 63. He was planning to spend the winter in Nicopolis, so he urged Titus to join him there (Titus 3:12).

What is the island of Crete?

Crete is a Mediterranean island that is approximately 150 miles long and 30 miles wide. The inhabitants were notorious for their immorality and lying (Titus 1:12–13). It is said that to live like a Cretan is "to play the liar."

When was the church at Crete established?

We know that Paul didn't plant this church, for there is no record of him visiting Crete before his trip to Rome (Acts 27:7–13). There were Jews from Crete at Jerusalem on the day of Pentecost who were probably converted and brought the gospel to their countrymen (Acts 2:11), but Paul spread the gospel upon his first release from Roman imprisonment (A.D. 63).

What is the focus of Titus?

Because of the immorality of the Cretans, Paul wanted Titus to stress the need for righteous Christian living. Some Judaizers—false teachers—were misleading the church about legal matters. Paul called these false teachers "those of the circumcision" (Titus 1:10).

In this letter Paul urged Titus to set the church in order by appointing elders, men of proven spiritual character who could oversee the ministry of the church. Paul was not just concerned with male leadership; he also mentioned how women both young and old should carry on ministry, and said that they had a vital function in the church. All were to be living examples of the doctrine they professed. Paul constantly stressed practical Christianity to Titus, emphasizing that the young minister should tell the people of their necessity to live out their salvation daily before the unsaved.

What is the key word in Titus?

The key word is *order*. Paul wanted the believers in the churches to live orderly lives.

What is the key verse in Titus?

"For this reason I left you in Crete, that you should set in order the things that are lacking, and appoint elders in every city as I commanded you" (Titus 1:5).

What are the "faithful sayings" found in Titus?

The "faithful sayings" are technically sayings of faith, or doctrinal statements. Paul told Titus, "This is a faithful saying, and these things I want you to affirm constantly, that those who have believed in God should be careful to maintain good works. These things are good and profitable to men" (Titus 3:8).

QUESTIONS ABOUT THE EPISTLE TO PHILEMON

Who was Philemon?

Philemon was a rich slave owner who lived in Colosse. He was a convert of Paul (v. 19), whom Paul called his "beloved friend and fellow laborer" (v. 1). Paul wrote to Philemon with much tact and tenderness asking him to take back his slave, Onesimus, who had probably robbed him and run away. Philemon's house was large enough for the church to meet there (v. 2), and he had been very helpful to other believers (vv. 5–7). His son, Archippus, was a leader in the church (Col. 4:17, Philem. 2). Philemon's house had guest quarters, and Paul asked Philemon to prepare a guest room for him because he was coming to visit.

Who was Onesimus?

Onesimus was a slave of Philemon who probably robbed his master or committed some other crime, then fled to Rome. Perhaps Onesimus thought that in Rome he could be lost among the large population of over a million people. Somehow, Paul came in contact with Onesimus and led him to Christ (v. 10). Maybe Onesimus heard about Paul while in Rome, and went to him for help. Onesimus became a servant or valet to Paul, helping him in many ways. But Paul knew that he had a responsibility to return Onesimus to his owner, so he sent Onesimus back to Colosse with Tychicus (the bearer of the letter to the Colossians). There were many people looking for runaway slaves, so Paul sent him with Tychicus for his safety.

What was the purpose of the epistle to Philemon?

Paul wrote a letter pleading Philemon to take Onesimus back and asking him to be as gentle with Onesimus as he would with himself. Paul suggested he would pay any debt that Onesimus owed. Paul realized that Philemon's love and forgiveness would overcome the problem.

Who wrote the letter?

No one doubts the authenticity of Paul, for he refers to himself in verses 1, 9, and 19. However, in the third century certain people said that the book of Philemon lacked doctrinal content, and they questioned whether it should be in the Canon. But church leaders like Jerome and Chrysostom endorsed the book, and the criticism evaporated.

When did Paul write Philemon?

The book of Philemon is one of the four Prison Epistles (see also Ephesians, Philippians, and Colossians), and was written about the same time that Colossians was written, A.D. 61 or 62. Paul was in his first Roman imprisonment and was not suffering or being persecuted. As a matter of fact, Paul expected to be released soon, so he told Philemon, "Prepare a guest room for me, for I trust that through your prayers I shall be granted to you" (v. 22).

What is the key word in Philemon?

The key word is *receive*. Paul was writing for Philemon to receive Onesimus back, with the same love and respect that Philemon would receive Paul. Paul said, "Receive him as you would me" (v. 17).

What are the key verses in Philemon?

"If then you count me as a partner, receive him as you would me. But if he has wronged you or owes anything, put that on my account. I, Paul, am writing with my own hand. I will repay—not to mention to you that you owe me even your own self besides" (vv. 17–19).

What was Philemon's son's role in the church at Colosse?

Philemon's son, Archippus, had a leadership role because Paul said, "And say to Archippus, 'Take heed to the ministry which you have received in the Lord, that you may fulfill it'" (Col. 4:17).

What is the popular nickname for the epistle to Philemon?

Philemon has been called a *postcard* that Paul wrote to Philemon because it is so short.

What Christian doctrine is presented in Philemon?

The core doctrine of forgiveness is seen in this book. Just as Jesus Christ took our sins upon Himself and forgave us all of our offenses, so Paul asked Philemon to forgive the crimes that Onesimus had done against him. Previously, Onesimus was a worthless slave to him, but now Onesimus was a brother in Christ. Paul was motivated by his love for both Onesimus and Philemon in asking that the slave be taken back, not just as a slave, but as a brother. Paul pledged to pay for the debt of Onesimus. We see here a picture of Onesimus as a sinner who has run away from God the Father. Paul is a picture of the intercessory work of Jesus Christ before the Father, pleading for the slave to be forgiven and accepted back by the Father. Philemon is a picture of the Father, the One who owns us, against whom we have sinned.

QUESTIONS
ABOUT
THE EPISTLE
TO THE HEBREWS

What is the focus of the epistle to the Hebrews?

The readers were exhorted to "go on to perfection" (Heb. 6:1) and not go back into Judaism, but to continue serving Jesus Christ, even if it involved persecution.

What is the key word in Hebrews?

The key word is *better*. Christ is better than the angels, better than Moses, better than the Aaronic priesthood, and better than the Old Testament Law. The book centers on the superiority of Christ to Old Testament rituals.

What are the key verses in Hebrews?

The word *better* is used thirteen times in Hebrews, showing that Christ is better than the old. "Having become so much better than the angels, as He [Christ] has by inheritance obtained a more excellent name than they" (Heb. 1:4). The author writes, "Seeing then that we have a great High Priest who has passed through the heavens, Jesus the Son of God, let us hold fast our confession. For we do not have a High Priest who cannot sympathize with our weaknesses, but was in all points tempted as we are, yet without sin. Let us therefore come boldly to the throne of grace, that we may obtain mercy and find grace to help in time of need" (Heb. 4:14–16).

The author wrote chapter 11, "The Christian Hall of Faith," to demonstrate the faith of great men and women in the Old Testament, and to show that Jesus is better, because He was the focus of their faith. "Therefore we also, since we are surrounded by so great a cloud of witnesses, let us lay aside every weight, and the sin which so easily ensnares us, and let us run with endurance the race that is set before us, looking unto Jesus, the author and finisher of our faith, who for the joy that was set before Him endured the cross, despising the shame, and has sat down at the right hand of the throne of God" (Heb. 12:1–2).

Who wrote the book of Hebrews?

There is great debate over the authorship of Hebrews. After much study, we can only agree with the early church father, Origen, who said, "Who it was that really wrote the Epistle, God only knows." Many are sure that this is Paul's "fourteenth" epistle, because the logic and development is Pauline. The Eastern Orthodox Church (the Greek Orthodox Church and other orthodox churches) have steadfastly maintained that Paul was the author. However, the Western Church, that is, the Roman Church, does not support that conclusion.

When I was a student in seminary, my Greek professor required that we read the entire book in the Greek text and come to class prepared to discuss who wrote the book. After reading the Greek text, all students agreed that Paul did not write the book of Hebrews: (1) the Greek style of writing is far more polished than anything that Paul wrote; (2) Paul consistently claims to be an apostle, but the language of 2:3 is not Pauline, "which at the first began to be spoken by the Lord, and was confirmed to us by those who heard Him"; (3) every one of Paul's letters has his customary greeting, which includes his name—a salutation not found in Hebrews; (4) while Paul quoted the Old Testament from both the Hebrew and Septuagint, the writer of Hebrews did not know the Hebrew language and quoted only from the Septuagint; (5) Paul used all of the compound titles of Jesus, Lord, and Christ, but the writer of Hebrews does not use them; (6) Paul concentrates heavily on the ministry of Christ on the cross, while Hebrews concentrates heavily on His present intercessory work in heaven; and (7) Paul writes with the legal style of a lawyer, while Hebrews is written with medical terminology found in Luke and Acts, and the author followed Greek syntax in developing his thoughts.

I think the book of Hebrews is a sermon or a series of sermons that Paul preached in the churches when he traveled on his missionary journeys. Luke, the companion of Paul, heard these sermons so many times that he could repeat them. Therefore, the book of Hebrews is a sermon or sermon series of Paul's, but it is written in the language and style of Luke. Neither Paul nor Luke takes credit for the book—Paul because he didn't pen the words, and Luke because they were not his ideas.

When was the book of Hebrews written?

Clement of Rome quoted from the book of Hebrews in A.D. 95, so we know that it was written earlier than that date. The book of Hebrews does not mention the destruction of the temple or that the sacrificial system was terminated. Since the Roman general Titus destroyed the temple in A.D. 70, the book of Hebrews must have been written prior to that. Also, Timothy was still alive (13:23). The writer says that the Jewish system was about to be removed (12:26–27). All of this suggests that Hebrews was written between A.D. 64 and 68. Paul's name is not mentioned because he would have been recently martyred.

To whom was the book of Hebrews written?

The people who got the book of Hebrews were believers (3:1) who had come to faith through the testimony of eyewitnesses of Christ (2:3). They had been saved for a long time, for they were not novices (5:12), and they had successfully endured hardships in their stand for Jesus Christ (10:32–34). This book is a description of Christians who lived in Jerusalem. They had gone through several phases of persecution, had seen James beheaded, and had been persecuted both by the Jews and Rome. The writer of Hebrews said that more persecution was coming (12:4–12). Since some leaders were on the verge of going back into Judaism to avoid persecution from Rome and the Jews, it seems obvious that the writer was urging them not to give up or go back. They needed to know that Christ was better than Judaism, and for readers who went back into Judaism, "there no longer remains a sacrifice for sins" (Heb. 10:26), meaning the Jewish sacrificial system could not forgive their sins. The readers were reminded that if they sacrificed a lamb, "they crucify again for themselves the Son of God, and put Him to an open shame" (Heb. 6:6).

Why is Paul not mentioned in the salutation or throughout the book?

The Christians in Jerusalem would have rejected anything to do with Paul, because Paul's ministry was to the Gentiles, and the people of Jerusalem characterized Paul as one who rejected the Law of Moses, or at least was "soft" on Old Testament Law.

What is chapter 11 called?

Chapter 11 has been called the "Honor Roll" or the "Hall of Faith" because it lists the great Old Testament heroes who faithfully endured persecution and served Jesus Christ, "looking for better things."

What is God's ultimate means of self-revelation? (Heb. 1:1–2)

The book of Hebrews tells us that God has already spoken to us in these last days "by his Son" (1:2). Throughout the Old Testament God has spoken in a number of ways—visions, dreams, poetry, biography, sermons, miracles, angels, and eyewitnesses who wrote down what God was doing. But the ultimate means of God's self-revelation is in Jesus Christ.

What can we know about angels?

The first chapter tells us that Christ is superior to angels (1:4). Angels are servants of God who are His messengers (1:14). They are spirit beings who cannot be seen but can become visible in human form, and possess intellect, emotion, and will. Angels have great power, but are not omnipotent. Angels have great wisdom, but are not omniscient. There are a great number of angels (Heb. 12:22), but they are not limitless.

Why does the book of Hebrews contain warnings?

The book of Hebrews contains five warning passages (2:1–4; 3:7–4:13; 5:11–6:20; 10:19–39; 12:18–29). Each of the warnings says that Christ is better and warns these Jewish Christians (or anyone else) not to go back to the Jewish law or the temple sacrifices.

Are sign gifts available today?

The writer of Hebrews describes sign gifts: "God also bearing witness both with signs and wonders, with various miracles, and gifts of the Holy Spirit" (Heb. 2:4). These sign gifts were given to confirm apostolic revelation (2 Cor. 12:12, Heb. 2:2–4), and most Christians do not expect them today. Just as it is necessary to erect a scaffolding to aid in the construction of a building, so sign gifts were the spiritual scaffolding used by God to give credibility to His revelation, the Word of God. Since the Bible is the foundation of the church, when the written Word of God was complete, God removed the temporary scaffolding, that is, the sign gifts. Sign gifts were given primarily to Jews (1 Cor. 1:22), but the church ministers primarily to Gentiles who seek wisdom (1 Cor. 1:22), so sign gifts are not necessary. The apostles were given the revelation of God and repeated it in oral tradition; therefore they needed signs to authenticate their message (2 Thess. 2:15). Remember, the sign gifts, such as the gift of apostles, were foundational gifts needed in the first century for preaching and for writing. However, since there are no apostles today, there are no sign gifts today. Paul implied that these gifts may cease (1 Cor. 13:8), and he referred to these gifts seemingly in the past tense, which he would not do if they were still active and prevalent at the time of the writing (2:3).

There are a group of people today who feel the gift of apostles has been given to the church, and they validate it by the miracles and/or healings that are done by the modern-day apostles. These modern-day apostles speak "words of prophecy" or "words of revelation." However, modern-day apostles do not elevate these "words" to the level of Scripture. Rather, they seem to communicate on the level of what most Christians call "illumination."

In what sense was Christ "without sin"? (Heb. 4:15)

The words *temptability* and *impeccability* describe Christ in His temptation. Christ was tempted in all parts of His being, but that does not mean He was tempted with all parts of sin and evil (James 1:13). The word *impeccability* means Christ, as God, could not have sinned. The word *temptability* means that Christ was tempted but not tempted to sin. He was tempted to do what only God could do, like turning stones into bread.

What is the intercessory work of Christ?

In His present work in heaven, Christ is interceding for Christians (Heb. 7:25), "Therefore He is also able to save to the uttermost those who come to God through Him, since He always lives to make intercession for them." This is like preventive medicine that a mother gives to keep her child from getting sick. Likewise, Christ prays in heaven for the believers during times of weakness and temptation to keep them from sin.

In what sense did Christ "purify heaven"? (Heb. 9:12)

In the Old Testament the blood was used primarily for atonement (*kaphar*) for individuals. But in a secondary sense, the blood of bulls and goats cleansed the Holy of Holies in the Temple of God. So the blood of Jesus Christ is primarily to satisfy the wrath of God and pay the price of redemption for believers. But also, when Jesus the eternal High Priest entered heaven, He purified it "by his own blood" (Heb. 9:12).

Are angels ranked in order? (Heb. 12:22)

The writer of Hebrews suggests, "an innumerable company of angels" (Heb. 12:22). This suggests that angels exist in orderly arrangements, perhaps with specialized responsibilities. As an illustration, Michael the archangel (Jude 1:9) was the highest in the order of angels. Gabriel appears to be the messenger angel of God, usually delivering a message for God. Cherubim are portrayed as serving God, usually attached to His throne, while seraphim were angels assigned to the altar and were concerned about the holiness of God.

QUESTIONS ABOUT THE EPISTLE OF JAMES

Who wrote the epistle of James?

Obviously the book was written by a person called James: "James, a bond-servant of God and of the Lord Jesus Christ, to the twelve tribes which are scattered abroad: greetings" (James 1:1). There were four Jameses mentioned in the New Testament: James the father of Judas, not Iscariot (Luke 6:16); the apostle who was called James, the son of Alphaeus (Matt. 10:3); James the son of Zebedee (Matt. 10:2) (but we know this James was not the author of this book because he was beheaded; see Acts 12:2); and James, the half brother of Jesus, who was one of the pillars of the church (Gal. 1:19).

Who was James, the author of Hebrews?

Tradition tells us the author was the half brother of Jesus, because he used the same word for "greeting" (*chairein*) found in the letter he wrote after the Jerusalem council (Acts. 15:23). James did not believe that Jesus was Messiah during His life (John 7:5). Jesus appeared to him after the Resurrection (1 Cor. 15:7), and he was among the believers praying in the Upper Room for the coming of the Holy Spirit on the day of Pentecost (Acts. 1:13–14). Shortly after he became the acknowledged leader of the church in Jerusalem (Acts 12:17; Gal. 2:9, 12), he became the spokesman for the Jerusalem council in Acts 15. He continued to observe the Old Testament Law, even though he was the leader of the church in Jerusalem (Acts 21:18–25). Tradition tells us he was extremely godly, and was nicknamed "camel knees" because of his constant kneeling in prayer. He died a violent martyr's death right before Titus destroyed Jerusalem in A.D. 70.

To whom is the book of James written?

James writes to "the twelve tribes which are scattered abroad" (James 1:1), which means the Hebrew Christians living outside of Palestine. The entire book reflects "Jewish thought." The recipients of this book were being tested for their faith, persecuted by unsaved Jews and/or the Roman government.

James probably wrote the book early in the life of the church, before or around A.D. 45. If so, this would be one of the first books written in the New Testament since it does not mention Gentile Christians or their relationship to Jewish Christians that would have come after the ministry of Paul. It has no distinctive theology, which would have been true of early Christianity. The book of James has little verbal similarity to the Gospels, which probably had not been written by then. James uses the word *synagogue,* whereas Gentile Christians were assembling in churches, and does not emphasize the office of *elders, bishops,* or *pastors.* James emphasizes the Jewish aspect of ministry, i.e., teachers or elders (3:1, 5:14). He does not mention the issues involved in the council of Jerusalem (A.D. 49) because it probably hadn't happened yet. Therefore the book of James was written early in the life of the church.

What is the key word in James?

The key word of James is *trials* or *temptations.* The recipients of the letter were going through various trials of their faith, and James was writing to help them endure trials for the glory of God.

What are the key verses in James?

The key verse is "Blessed is the man who endures temptation; for when he has been approved, he will receive the crown of life which the Lord has promised to those who love Him" (1:12). Because these Christians were undergoing trials and temptations, James wrote, "My brethren, count it all joy when you fall into various trials, knowing that the testing of your faith produces patience" (1:2–3).

What is the thrust of James?

While James told them to overcome trials and temptations, the basis of their faith was the Word of God. James is a book of active faith, saying that faith without works is dead. Those who had verbal faith did not have enough; they had to put faith into action. Faith endured trials, overcame temptations, obeyed the Word of God, harbored no prejudice against the poor, demonstrated itself by good works, and controlled the tongue, that small part of the flesh that directed the entire body. Faith produced separation from worldly activities, and those with faith waited patiently for the coming of the Lord (5:7).

QUESTIONS ABOUT THE FIRST EPISTLE OF PETER

Who wrote the first epistle of Peter?
The church has universally accepted the authorship of Peter the apostle. The internal evidence indicates, "Peter, an apostle of Jesus Christ, to the pilgrims of the Dispersion in Pontus, Galatia, Cappadocia, Asia, and Bithynia" (1 Peter 1:1).

To whom was 1 Peter addressed?
Peter wrote to Christians who lived in Asia Minor. Peter reminded them that they had been scattered there, but we are not sure when. Some say

549

these were Christians who were saved at Pentecost who went home to serve Christ. Others feel they were scattered at a later time (Acts 11:19). Some believe they were Jews converted during the first or second missionary journeys of Paul, so they were exhorted to keep their "conduct honorable among the Gentiles" (1 Peter 2:12). However, others feel the recipients were not saved Jews, but Gentiles. This is because they were saved "out of darkness" (1 Peter 2:9). They once "were not a people but are now the people of God" (1 Peter 2:10), and they no longer engaged in debauchery and idolatry (1 Peter 4:3–4). This description does not fit Jewish Christians but describes Gentiles. However, Peter was the apostle "to the circumcised" (Gal. 2:9), not to the Gentiles, so this letter's scope would be to Jewish believers.

When was 1 Peter written?

We know little that Peter did after the Jerusalem council (Acts 15). We do know that he spent part of his life in Rome, and tradition tells us he was crucified upside down prior to Nero's death in A.D. 68. This letter was written from Babylon (1 Peter 5:13), but we are not sure what "Babylon" means. Some feel Babylon is Rome, because it would have been a "spiritual Babylon" because of its ungodly environment. Others feel that Peter traveled to the actual city of Babylon on the banks of the Euphrates River because there was a great number of Jews in that city and an extremely large synagogue. However, Peter mentions Mark (5:13), who was with Paul in Rome (Col. 4:10), another argument that "Babylon" is a reference to Rome. The book was probably written shortly before Nero began persecuting the church in A.D. 64.

What is the focus of 1 Peter?

The focus is on persecution that the readers are suffering because of their stand for Jesus Christ. These were Jewish believers, who conducted themselves in the way of the New Testament and witnessed to their neighbors. They were undergoing persecution for their faith, so Peter wrote, "Think it not strange concerning the fiery trial which is to try you, as though some strange thing happened to you" (1 Peter 4:12 KJV). Peter reminded them that they were partakers of the sufferings of Christ by their trials and sufferings.

What is the key word in 1 Peter?

The key word is *suffering*, the dominant theme throughout the book.

What is the key verse in 1 Peter?

The key verse is "But rejoice to the extent that you partake of Christ's sufferings, that when His glory is revealed, you may also be glad with exceeding joy" (1 Peter 4:13).

In what sense is every believer a "royal priesthood"? (1 Peter 2:9)

Every believer has the privilege and responsibility of praying directly to God. In the Old Testament, a priest from the tribe of Levi was designated as an intercessor for each Jew. In the New Testament, every Christian is a priest and can pray directly to God.

QUESTIONS ABOUT THE SECOND EPISTLE OF PETER

Why did Peter write a second letter?

In the first letter, Peter deals with the problems of trials and temptations that were coming from the outside. In this second letter, Peter was dealing with internal problems in the church, warning believers about false teachers who were spreading false doctrines among them.

Who wrote the second epistle of Peter?

Obviously the writer of 1 Peter is also the writer of 2 Peter. The author says, "Simon Peter, a bondservant and apostle of Jesus Christ, to those who have obtained like precious faith with us by the righteousness of our God and Savior Jesus Christ" (2 Peter 1:1).

How do we know that the apostle Peter wrote this letter?

The writer says, "Beloved, I now write to you this second epistle" (2 Peter 3:1), so that Peter who wrote the first epistle also wrote the second. Also, he refers to the Lord's prediction about his death (2 Peter 1:14). Jesus had told Peter that he would die a violent martyr's death (John 21:18–19). Finally, Peter was on the Mount of Transfiguration with the Lord, and he makes reference to his eyewitness of that event in this book (2 Peter 1:16, 18).

When was 2 Peter written?

Obviously it had to be written after the first epistle in A.D. 64. Paul was probably still living (2 Peter 3:15), so it must have been written around A.D. 65 or 66. Paul was martyred in A.D. 66 or 67, and Peter was martyred in A.D. 67 or 68 by Nero.

What is the key word in 2 Peter?

There are two answers to this question. First, Peter is greatly concerned about false teaching (2 Peter 2:1), so he emphasizes the word *knowledge* that the readers of his letter must have about the Lord Jesus Christ (2 Peter 1:2–3, 5–6, 12, 14, 16, 20; 2:9, 20–21; 3:3, 17–18). Also, when looking for a key word, note the word *ignorance*. The readers were not to be ignorant but to understand doctrine.

What are the key verses in 2 Peter?

Peter focused on false doctrine that was threatening believers and reminded them of Jesus Christ. "But there were also false prophets among the people, even as there will be false teachers among you, who will secretly bring in destructive heresies, even denying the Lord who bought them, and bring on themselves swift destruction" (2 Peter 2:1). Another key verse is 2:9: "The Lord knows how to deliver the godly out of temptations and to reserve the unjust under punishment for the Day of Judgment."

What does Peter say about the inspiration of Scripture?

Peter says, "For prophecy never came by the will of man, but holy men of God spoke as they were moved by the Holy Spirit" (2 Peter 1:21). These writers were "moved," which means that they were "borne along" or "picked up and carried" as they were delivering God's message. When the writers were penning the words of Scripture, the Holy Spirit guided their words so that what they wrote accurately expressed the mind of the Holy Spirit, without error.

How will judgment come in the future?

Peter suggests that the ancient world was flooded (2 Peter 3:6), but in the future God will send fire to destroy the world "until the day of judgment and perdition of ungodly men" (2 Peter 3:7).

What is the will of God concerning unsaved people?

God is "not willing that any should perish" (2 Peter 3:9). This expresses God's desire that every person be saved. Obviously, all are not saved, so the will of God is not carried out in every place. This "will of God" is not His plan, but this "will of God" is His passion for all people to become a Christian.

QUESTIONS ABOUT THE FIRST EPISTLE OF JOHN

Who wrote the first epistle of John?

Although John's name is not found in the book, the church universally has said John the apostle wrote the book. The church father Polycarp, who knew John in his youth, said that John wrote this book.

Why is John's name not in the book?

Because John was so well known and his style of writing was so significant, it was not necessary to include his name. Everyone would have recognized John's authorship. The style is similar to the gospel of John, and the author follows the same emphasis on light and darkness, love, and life. John says that "God is light" (1 John 1:5) and "God is love" (4:8).

When did John write this first letter?

The First Epistle of John was probably written after the gospel of John was finished. However, it is difficult to determine an exact date. It was probably written somewhere between A.D. 90 and 95. The persecution of Diacletian began in A.D. 96.

What is the focus of 1 John?

This is a fatherly letter written to his children to remind them to be steadfast in truth, even when false teaching was beginning to creep into the church. Also, John was reminding them not to sin and to be true to God.

How does John characterize God?

First of all, John said that "God is light" (1 John 1:5), so He wants His children to walk in light, not darkness, and when they walk in the light, the blood of Jesus Christ will continually cleanse them of sin (1:7). But if they do sin, they are to confess their sins (1:9). If they continually walk in light, that is a demonstration that they are children of God.

John also said, "God is love" (4:8), and if His children do not love, they do not know God. To John, love was more than words; love was action. John said that those who do not love do not know God.

A third key to John's writing is eternal life ("God is life"). Those who walk with God possess His eternal life. And how does one get eternal life? "He who has the Son has life; he who does not have the Son of God does not have life" (5:12).

What is the key word in 1 John?

The key word is *know*, which is mentioned thirty-two times in the book. There is a hymn, "Blessed Assurance," which is really the theme of 1 John. When you know you are saved, you have assurance that your life is blessed by God.

What is the key verse in 1 John?

The key verse in 1 John is, "These things I have written to you who believe in the name of the Son of God, that you may know that you have eternal life, and that you may continue to believe in the name of the Son of God" (1 John 5:13).

What can a believer know?

When believers love one another, they can know they are saved (1 John 5:2). When they get their prayers answered, they can know they are saved (5:12, 13). When the Word of God gives them confidence (5:11) and when believers keep themselves from sin, they can know that they are saved (5:18). When they realize the whole world is lost, they can know that they are saved (5:19). And when the Son of God comes into their lives, they can know that they are saved (5:20).

Why is 1 John such a simplistic book?

John writes with a limited vocabulary, telling people that knowing God is a very simple thing, not complex or compound. Why? Because just as you know what light is by seeing it, you can walk in light. You can know what love is by experiencing it, so you can know that God wants you to simply know Him.

In what sense is Christ our advocate? (1 John 2:1)

An *advocate* is a lawyer who represents his client before a court of law. So Jesus is the Advocate for Christians. When Christians sin, Christ pleads their cases before the Father to restore them to fellowship with God.

How does John classify temptation?

John classifies temptation in a threefold manner: "Do not love the world or the things in the world. If anyone loves the world, the love of the Father is not in him. For all that is in the world—the lust of the flesh, the lust of the eyes, and the pride of life—is not of the Father but is of the world" (1 John 2:15–16).

According to John, who is Antichrist? (1 John 2:22)

The term *antichrist* refers to anyone who takes the place of Christ or opposes Christ. There is a specific person named "Antichrist" during the Tribulation who will carry out Satan's strategy on earth. That Antichrist has many other names such as "that wicked one" (2 Thess. 2:8 KJV), "the son of perdition" (2 Thess. 2:3), and "the willful king" (Dan. 11:36). He is an immensely powerful political leader who through his statesmanship will bring the entire world together to fight the cause of God upon the earth. However, he will not be revealed until after the rapture (2 Thess. 2:3). John called anyone who followed the rulership of Satan on this earth "antichrist," because they were under the leadership of Satan. John wanted Christians to know that the "spirit of antichrist" was already at work in the world (1 John 4:1). Anyone who denies the deity of Jesus Christ is antichrist.

How can a Christian have assurance?

The Bible clearly teaches that Christians can have an inner assurance that they are saved (not the same as eternal security, which is a doctrinal fact). Their assurance is an internal confidence (1) because the believer has Christ in his heart (1 John 5:12), (2) because of the witness of the Word of God (1 John 5:10), (3) because his prayers are answered (1 John 5:14–15), (4) because he understands Scripture (1 John 5:20) and keeps God's commandments (1 John 5:18), (5) because he loves the brethren (1 John 3:14), and (6) because he has the inner witness of the Holy Spirit (Rom. 8:16).

QUESTIONS ABOUT THE SECOND EPISTLE OF JOHN

Who wrote the second epistle of John?
John the apostle wrote the book, as he did the First Epistle of John. Conservative scholars have attributed these two books to the apostle John because of their similarity of style, vocabulary, and structure. Also, the moods of 2 John and 1 John are similar, indicating that they have the same author.

Why is John's name not mentioned?
Those who received this letter knew the author's identity well. So John did not need to use his name. Rather, he designates himself as "the Elder": "The

Elder, to the elect lady and her children, whom I love in truth, and not only I, but also all those who have known the truth" (2 John 1).

Who received this letter?

This letter was written to the "elect lady and her children" (2 John 1). Some feel this "elect lady" is a specific woman who was a leader in one of the churches. However, the phrase "elect lady" is probably a descriptive term for a local church. The "children" are the members of that church. Since the church was the bride of Christ, John would have used this wording to describe a church as a lady.

Why is this book so short?

In writing to this church (probably in Asia Minor near Ephesus), John commended them for their stand in truth and love against false teachers. This book has only 303 words and is the shortest book in the Bible. After John made his point, he concluded this letter.

What are the key words in 2 John?

The key words are *in truth and love*. The people in this church held the truth of God, yet they loved one another. John wrote to remind them "whom I love in the truth" (v. 1).

What is the key verse in 2 John?

The key verse is, "Grace, mercy, and peace will be with you from God the Father and from the Lord Jesus Christ, the Son of the Father, in truth and love" (2 John 3).

When was 2 John written?

Obviously it would have been written after 1 John, probably around A.D. 90. All three of John's epistles were written from Ephesus.

QUESTIONS ABOUT THE THIRD EPISTLE OF JOHN

Who wrote the third epistle of John?

Again, the apostle John wrote this book, although he does not give his name. He calls himself "the Elder," a term that seems to be his designation in his final years of ministry. He is probably the only apostle alive at this time. We know that he wrote it because it has the same style and content as the gospel of John and 1 and 2 John.

When was 3 John written?

This is the only letter that he wrote to an individual, and it was probably written after 1 and 2 John were delivered. Therefore, it was probably written around A.D. 95.

Where did John write this letter?

Since the letter is similar to 1 and 2 John, he probably wrote it from Ephesus, where he wrote the other two letters.

Who was Diotrephes? (3 John 1:9)

Diotrephes was involved in an Asian church (near Ephesus), and made himself the ruling authority in the church. He criticized John's authority, rejected teachers and letters (perhaps 2 John) sent out by the apostle John, and would not receive the truth. Those in the church who received John's messages were kicked out of the church by Diotrephes. The name *Diotrephes* has come to stand for those who are self-willed and arrogant church leaders.

Who was Gaius?

Gaius was a Christian in this church, who received the letters and messages sent by John. He was obviously a distinguished leader in this local church.

There are three other people in the New Testament named Gaius—a common Roman name. These men are: Gaius who traveled with Paul (Acts 19:29), Gaius of Derbe (Acts 20:4), and Gaius in Corinth (1 Cor. 1:14). But these three are probably not the recipient of this letter.

Who was Demetrius?

He was the one who came to John telling him about the hospitality of Gaius and the hostility of Diotrephes. "Demetrius has a good testimony from all, and from the truth itself. And we also bear witness, and you know that our testimony is true" (3 John 12).

What are the key words in 3 John?

The key words in 3 John are *love and truth*. In 2 John the two words were reversed, "truth and love," because truth comes first, and out of it grows love. In 3 John the standard has been reversed, and it is "love" first, then "truth."

What is the key verse in 3 John?

The key verse is "The Elder, to the beloved Gaius, whom I love in truth" (3 John 1).

QUESTIONS ABOUT THE EPISTLE OF JUDE

Who wrote the epistle of Jude?

The author gives his name and identifies himself as James's brother: "Jude, a bondservant of Jesus Christ, and brother of James, to those who are called, sanctified by God the Father, and preserved in Jesus Christ" (Jude 1).

There are two major views as to which Jude wrote this book. Some feel Jude is the physical half brother of Jesus, because the author identifies himself as the brother of James (another physical half brother of Jesus). He refers to apostles as "they" (Jude 1:17–18), and has strong Jewish content. However, other people feel this is the Jude who was the apostle, that is, "Judas . . . not Iscariot" (John 14:22). This Judas remained faithful when Judas Iscariot denied the Lord and sinned. Because of Judas's faithfulness and his name, this Judas was very aware of false teaching and treachery. As he traveled throughout the early church, people rejected this Judas because of his name, which reminded them of Judas Iscariot. So he changed his name to Lebbaeus Thaddaeus (Matt. 10:3). A change of name removed barriers from his preaching the gospel. Therefore, this Judas would have understood the barriers of false teaching against which he wrote. However, later in life, Lebbaeus Thaddaeus changed his name back to Judas, or Jude. (Remember Judah is the Hebrew name, Judas is the Greek name, and Jude is the Latin name, the same name with different pronunciations and spellings.) He changed his name back because he was ministering to Latins. The early church called this man Trionomous, "the man with three names."

When was Jude written?

The New Testament is silent concerning the later years of Judas, so we do not know when it was written, but because of its similarity to 2 Peter, many believe that this book was written around the same time, shortly after A.D. 66.

To whom was Jude written?

The readers of this letter were not identified in a particular circle, church, or ethnic group. There are no geographical clues where it was written. So Jude was writing to all believers everywhere.

What is the message of Jude?

Jude was warning of dangerous libertines who were living ungodly lives, and their lives were destroying their doctrine. But he also warned of false doctrine and laid the foundation with negative examples of moral obedience, like Sodom and Gomorrah and the disobedient angels who sinned in the beginning.

What are the key words in Jude?

The key words are *contend for the faith*. Throughout this book the author wants people to fight against heresy, go to war against sin, and engage false teachers who are attacking their faith.

What is the key verse in Jude?

"Beloved, while I was very diligent to write to you concerning our common salvation, I found it necessary to write to you exhorting you to contend earnestly for the faith which was once for all delivered to the saints" (Jude 1:3).

QUESTIONS
ABOUT
THE REVELATION

What is the focus of the Revelation?

The Revelation is not primarily a focus on prophetic events, but on Jesus Christ. The first verse indicates it is "The Revelation of Jesus Christ" (Rev. 1:1). The word *revelation* means "unveiling or disclosure," and thus, it is the final disclosure of who Jesus Christ is. This book is a self-revelation, because Jesus Christ is giving these revelations to John the Revelator to write down.

What is the title of the book?

The book is called "The Revelation of Jesus Christ," also known as *Apocalypse,* a transliteration of the word "unveiling" or "disclosure."

Who wrote the book of Revelation?

The book is written by the apostle John, who identifies himself four times in the book (Rev. 1:1, 4, 9, 22:8). The church has almost universally accepted John as the author, and when you look at the internal material, it emphasizes John's distinctive words, such as *lamb, true,* and *word,* and his themes of light versus darkness, love versus hatred, and good versus evil.

When was Revelation written?

Revelation was written when John was on the isle of Patmos, a small, desolate, volcanic rock island in the Aegean Sea, where Romans banished criminals and political offenders. It was probably written during the persecution of Diocletian, about A.D. 95 or 96.

To whom was the book written?

The book was written to seven churches, beginning with the church in Ephesus, and then proceeding clockwise in a large circle (Rev. 2–3). This book was probably taken in clockwise sequence and read to all of the seven churches. It was probably quickly copied and passed throughout the Mediterranean world; hence, the early and wide acceptance of this book.

Where is Patmos?

It is a small island about sixty miles from Ephesus in the Aegean Sea. John was kept there as a political prisoner but was released. Tradition says he died peacefully in his sleep in Ephesus.

What is the focus of Revelation?

Just as Genesis is the book of beginning, Revelation is the book of the end. It is God's final statement about the return of Jesus Christ to the earth. John writes, "Behold, He is coming with clouds, and every eye will see Him, even they who pierced Him. And all the tribes of the earth will mourn because of Him. Even so, Amen" (Rev. 1:7).

What is the key word in Revelation?

The key word is *prophecy;* the predictions that have been prophesied in the Old Testament and by Jesus are fulfilled in this book. Many books have prophetic messages, but the book of Revelation deals primarily with prophetic events and their fulfillment.

What is the key verse in Revelation?

"Blessed is he who reads and those who hear the words of this prophecy, and keep those things which are written in it; for the time is near" (Rev. 1:3).

How is Jesus Christ seen in chapter 1?

He is identified by His name, Jesus Christ (Rev. 1:1), and is called "Him who is and who was and who is to come" (v. 4). Jesus is called the "faithful witness, the firstborn from the dead, and the ruler over the kings of the earth" (v. 5). He is identified as the one "who loved us and washed us from our sins in His own blood" (v. 5), who "cometh with clouds," and who is "pierced" (v. 7 KJV). Jesus identifies Himself as "Alpha and Omega, the beginning and the end" (v. 8). He calls Himself "Lord" and "the Almighty" (v. 8). Jesus is described as having "a great voice" (v. 10 KJV), which is a reference to His being the Word of God (John 1:1). Jesus is also called "the Son of man" (v. 13), a reference to His humanity. Yet "His countenance was as the sun" (v. 16 KJV). When Jesus speaks to John, He identifies Himself, "I am He that lives, and was dead, and behold, I am alive forevermore." Jesus said that He has "the keys of hell and of death" (v. 18). Jesus is the one who is walking in the middle of the seven churches (v. 20) and who has the churches and their pastors in His hand (v. 20).

What promises were made to the seven churches?

To each church "that overcometh," He promised a reward. Jesus told the churches, "He that has an ear, let him hear what the Spirit says to the churches."

What is "the book" that is mentioned in Revelation 5:6–7?
Some believe it is the "Book of Life," which contains the names of all believers in Jesus Christ. Only Christ Himself could open this because He alone is the "Lamb that has been slain." Others believe the book is the "title deed to heaven and earth," and only the Lamb can open this title deed. The "god of this world" has been confined to hell, and God finally rules without Satan or any alternate demonic voice.

What is the "new song" that is sung in heaven?
The new song is a worship hymn to God Himself singing, "Worthy is the Lamb."

INDEX

ABOUT THE AUTHOR

Dr. Elmer Towns co-founded Liberty University with Jerry Falwell and now serves as Dean of The B. R. Lakin School of Religion there. He is also co-founder of Church Growth Institute, author of popular and scholarly works, seminar lecturer, and dedicated worker in Sunday school. He has since written more than eighty books, including several bestsellers. In 1995 he received the Gold Medallion Book Award for *The Names of the Holy Spirit*. Dr. Towns served as President of Winnipeg Bible College for five years and taught at Trinity Evangelical Divinity School in Chicago. He and his wife reside in Forest, Virginia.

APPRECIATION

I could not have produced this volume without the help of Linda Elliott, typist, editor, and proofreader. Appreciation also goes to Renee Grooms, my administrative assistant, for typing, as well as to Jill Walker, a graduate assistant from Liberty University.

Thanks to Victor Oliver for suggesting this project for Thomas Nelson Publishing.

Appreciation to President John Borek at Liberty University for giving me a platform to teach and write this book as dean, School of Religion. My associate dean, Jim Stevens, looks after administrative details so I can give attention to projects like this. Many thanks to him as well.

Appreciation to Harold Willmington, Dean, Liberty Bible Institute, for his fellowship on our weekly TV program on the Liberty Broadcast Network, *The Bible Hot Seat,* where we answer many of these questions. Also, my gratitude to Jerry Falwell, who has allowed me to answer some of the questions mailed to him over the past thirty-two years. Rather than answering the same questions over and over, I direct people to the answers posted on my home Web page. That way, as many as possible can get answers to their questions (visit www.elmertowns.com and click on "Theological Q & A"). I have over seven hundred questions entered on this database.

Appreciation to all my students over the years, who have asked me questions (many included here), and appreciation for their patience with my answers.